UNIVERSITY OF MAINE

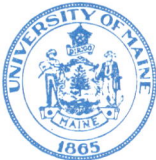

Raymond H. Fogler Library

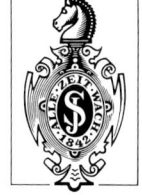

Pavol Ivanyi (Ed.)

Realm of Tolerance

With a Foreword by M. Boiron

With 72 Figures and 60 Tables

Springer-Verlag Berlin Heidelberg New York
London Paris Tokyo Hong Kong

Pavol Ivanyi, MD PhD
Central Laboratory of the Netherlands Red Cross
Blood Transfusion Service
and Laboratory for Experimental
and Clinical Immunology
Plesmanlaan 125
NL-1066 CX Amsterdam
The Netherlands

Proceedings of a meeting in memory of Professor Milan Hašek
October 5-8, 1988 in Ommen/Amsterdam

Supported by FONDATION DE FRANCE

Cover: Letter from Milan Hašek dated October 10, 1984;
by curtesy of M. Malkovský

ISBN 3-540-51056-7 Springer-Verlag Berlin Heidelberg New York
ISBN 0-387-51056-7 Springer-Verlag New York Berlin Heidelberg

Library of Congress Cataloging-in-Publication Data
Realm of tolerance / Pavol Ivanyi (ed.). p. cm. "Proceedings of a meeting in memory of
Professor Milan Hašek, October 5-8, 1988, in Ommen/Amsterdam"-T.p. verso.
Bibliography: p. Includes index.
ISBN 0-387-51056-7 (U.S.: alk. paper)
1. Immunological tolerance-Congresses. 2. Hašek, Milan. I.Ivanyi, P. (Pavol), 1930-.
II. Hašek, Milan. QR188.4.R43 1989 616.07'9-dc20 89-33873 CIP

This work is subject to copyright. All rights are reserved, whether the whole or part of
the material is concerned, specifically the rights of translation, reprinting, re-use of
illustrations, recitation, broadcasting, reproduction on microfilms or in other ways, and
storage in data banks. Duplication of this publication or parts thereof is only permitted
under the provisions of the German Copyright Law of September 9, 1965, in its version of
June 24, 1985, and a copyright fee must always be paid. Violations fall under the
prosecution act of the German Copyright Law.

© Springer-Verlag Berlin Heidelberg 1989
Printed in Germany

The use of general descriptive names, registered names, trademarks, etc. in this publication
does not imply, even in the absence of a specific statement, that such names are exempt
from the relevant protective laws and regulations and therefore free for general use.

Product Liability: The publisher can give no guarantee for information about drug dosage
and application thereof contained in this book. In every individual case the respective user
must check its accuracy by consulting other pharmaceutical literature.

Typesetting, printing and binding: Appl, Wemding
2123/3145-543210 - Printed on acid-free paper

Foreword

I have been very interested in this project from the first moment for a number of reasons. First, I was of course aware of the significance of Milan Hašek's discovery of immunological tolerance: his work represents a milestone in our understanding of the immune system. Moreover, this discovery found important applications in the broad field of transplantation, including bone marrow transplantation, which is a major concern in leukemia therapy.

A second reason for my interest was the knowledge that Milan Hašek had established what is called the Prague school of immunology, from which a great number of scientists have originated. I have known several of them personally, for instance, Marika Pla at the Hospital Saint-Louis and Radslav Kinsky who has been working with Guy Voisin in Paris for 20 years. In addition, there have been many contacts between French scientists and members of Hašek's group, e.g., the cooperation of the Iványis with Jean Dausset at the Hospital Saint-Louis.

A third aspect was the personality of Hašek himself. Although I never met him personally, I know he had multiple and friendly contacts with many French scientists such as Jean Dausset, François Jacob, Jean Bernard, Georges Mathé, Guy Voisin, and François Kourilsky. Two of them have contributed to the Proceedings with personal recollections of Milan Hašek. It is revealing of Milan Hašek's personality that, 20 years after the dispersal of his group, the very idea of holding a meeting in his memory could arise.

I therefore found highly appealing the original proposal to bring together 27 former coworkers of Hašek for a workshop where they could present their current research and also recount their personal memories and experiences of working and living abroad. This appeared to be a very creative project, and we gave credit to the organizers, Marika Pla and Pavol Iványi.

The result is the present book, which, I think, does show that we made a very good decision in supporting the proposal. This volume will stand as a permanent reminder of a small piece of history, maybe not so much important as exciting due to the involvement of the human personalities who have all contributed in their specific manner to the further development of science. The reference section itself illustrates how various and important these contributions have been. This volume is certainly the best acknowledgement of the interest and confidence that Fondation de France, in the great French tradition of favoring international scientific contacts, showed in the organization of the meeting "Realm of Tolerance."

May 1989

Michel Boiron
Director of the Institute
of Haematology
Centre Hayem
Hôpital St. Louis
Paris

FONDATION DE FRANCE

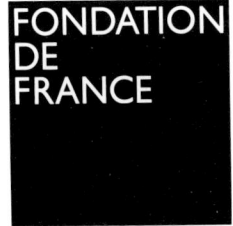

The FONDATION DE FRANCE is a private, state-approved, non-profit institution established in 1969 thanks to the efforts of Général de Gaulle and André Malraux.

The FONDATION DE FRANCE provides an essential link between the French people's generosity and the needs and aspirations of contemporary society. It acts as catalyzer, fulfilling a double mission: collecting funds from individuals and private enterprise in order to further social, cultural and scientific development, and providing persons or businesses who wish to pursue their own projects for the benefit of the general public, the means to do so under its aegis.

The FONDATION DE FRANCE works via priority programs, defined through observation of the numerous grant proposals which are submitted each year. Particular effort has been made to foster scientific and medical research, especially in the field of leukemia.

In 1982, the FONDATION DE FRANCE and a group of specialists in hematology, directed by Professor Jean Bernard, decided by common assent to create the Foundation Against Leukemia. The new foundation had as its goals the support of new directions in research, better conditions for patients in care, the development of new methods of treatment for leukemia, and the encouragement and promotion of international exchange.

With this in mind, the Foundation Against Leukemia funded the symposium „Realm of Tolerance" held in Ommen/Amsterdam in October, 1988. Dedicated to the memory of Professor Milan Hašek, this international meeting provided an opportunity for researchers trained in his school to present and compare their current work in the fields of immunology, genetics and oncology.

The FONDATION DE FRANCE is pleased to participate in this concerted scientific action, which is invaluable for the development of research.

Preface

In this book, former members of the Institute of Experimental Biology and Genetics of the Czechoslovak Academy of Sciences in Prague dedicate their research accomplishments to the memory of their late director, Milan Hašek.

Professor Milan Hašek discovered immunological tolerance in 1953 in experiments on embryonal parabiosis of chicken. He exposed the chorioallantoic membranes of a pair of eggs, joined the membranes together, and thus forced the two developing embryos to exchange blood after their vessels had fused together. Hašek also built up a group of coworkers interested in various, interrelated aspects of genetics, immunology, virology, and tumor research. He became the head of the department and later director of the Institute. Prof. M. Hašek was removed from his post as director in 1970 but continued to work at the Institute as a member. Milan Hašek died in 1984 at the young age of 59 years.

Approximately twenty-seven academics, all of whom were previously associated with Hašek's Institute, are now working throughout North America or western Europe. Many were close collaborators of Hašek, and all of them knew him personally. Most of them had left the Institute – and the country – around the year 1968.

In these Proceedings the participants of the meeting at Ommen/Amsterdam, in September, 1988, summarize and discuss the experimental work they have carried out *after* leaving the Prague Institute. Some manuscripts are embellished with introductory and/or concluding remarks (or drawings) about personal memories of Milan Hašek and life at the Institute, as well as the author's first experiences abroad. Finally, a complete bibliography of work published *after* leaving the Prague Institute is listed. This is a list of more than 1000 papers and books written or edited.

How was this meeting organized? During my scientific travels over the last few years, whenever I met colleagues from the Institute in Prague, the possibility of an "Institute meeting" was frequently raised. On Thanksgiving Day in 1987, I was staying with Tamara Rakusan and Jan Cerny in Galveston, Texas, and it was decided that I should try to organize one. However, I was unable to raise funds. While talking about the project – with my irresistible enthusiasm – to Marika Pla, she replied eagerly: "I shall try ... in Paris." And she succeeded. We obtained support from the FONDATION DE FRANCE. Professor Boiron explains in his Foreword the reasons for their decision to fund our meeting. There are not enough words to express our gratitude for their generosity.

I am also thankful to Professors J. Dausset, F. Jacob, A. Mitchinson, and M. Simonsen, with whom Hašek had various personal contacts, for their willingness to contribute their personal memories to this book. We also found a publisher, personified for me by Dietrich Goetze and Barbara Montenbruck, whom I thank for their skills and enthusiasm for realizing this book so quickly.

And so, we organized the meeting together with Marika. This was quite an experience! Twenty-five former coworkers of Hašek's Institute participated in a 3-day meeting in Ommen, a small place near Amsterdam. (Three colleagues could not come, but they have contributed to the Proceedings.) Some of us had been enthusiastic about this meeting from the very beginning, others remained sceptical about its value for a long time. But soon after arriving and the first discussions, it definitely became clear that this would be a great event. Someone commented: "These have been the most wonderful days since my departure from Prague. It is a dream fulfilled." This only goes to illustrate that we were quite an unusual team of scientists and friends in Prague ... thanks to Hašek.

Two problems were raised by most participants before the meeting. First, which language should we use? Could we talk about immunology in Czech? The problem was solved by Jan Cerny as he gave the first talk on theoretical immunology in Czech; it was possible! The second question was whether we would listen to each other at all, because our topics of interest had become quite diverse. However, the lectures were followed avidly until 10.00 p.m. and discussed with interest. Even the last speaker of the day wanted to use his or her 60 min, and at the end of the meeting the number of participants was identical to that at the beginning. Discussions of specialized topics by individuals with diverse scientific backgrounds were actually quite stimulating.

However, the haunting question remains: why did we actually organize this meeting? What could be the broader significance of such an effort, if any? We hope that this book provides an answer to those who are really seeking one: *Realm of Tolerance*.

Moreover, it is a story of the rise and gradual transformation of a scientific school that was created by an inspired leader. Milan Hašek had to cope with a complex world. And his personality was also complex. Both points come across clearly from the many ways in which Hašek is perceived and remembered by the authors of this volume. Diverse views have been expressed even by Hašek's old friends from outside the Institute who have written the introductory memorials. We, the participants at the meeting, are also very diverse people. Yet there must have been very strong feelings rooted in Prague which finally allowed us to experience so much enjoyment after so many years. For this we thank Milan Hašek, our director and friend.

Amsterdam, May 1989   Pavol Ivanyi

Table of Contents

Milan Hašek: In Memoriam

Once upon a time ...
J. Dausset 3

An imposing stature ...
F. Jacob 6

It took a few years ...
N. A. Mitchison 7

My old friend ...
M. Simonsen 9

Tolerance, Transplantation and Immune Network

From Horses to Mice: Graft Rejection and Tolerance
R. Kinsky 13

Tolerance and the Immune Network. T Cells Reactive
to the Variable Domains of Immunoglobulins
J. Cerny 17

Milan Hašek, Lymphokines and Retroviruses
M. Malkovský 29

Genetic Requirements for Interactions Between Cells
for Murine Islet Allograft Rejection.
Class I and Class II Antigens in Mouse Islet Rejection
V. Hauptfeld-Dolejsek 36

Chicken Major Histocompatibility Complex
and Its Role in Disease
K. Hala 43

Tolerance, the Thymus, and H-Y
L. Jerabek 50

Autologous Mixed Lymphocyte Culture:
Immunoregulatory Aspects
F. Pazderka 60

Immunogenetics (MHC)

Mickey, Hugo, and Eve: A Study in the Evolution
of the Major Histocompatibility Complex
J. Klein 73

From Histocompatibility to Cancer
P. Demant 80

HLA Antigens and Matching for Kidney Transplantation
P. T. Klouda 90

HLA Subtypes
H. Mervart 94

Zeroing in on the *H-2* Complex
D. Klein 109

Of Men and Mice
M. Pla 117

Individual Differences Among Syngeneic Mice
in Immune Response to Alloantigens and Modified
Self-MHC-Antigens
P. Ivanyi 122

Immunology and Cytology in Bacterial, Viral and Tumor Diseases

Immunological Analysis of Mycobacterial Disease
J. Ivanyi 137

Genetic Control of Susceptibility to Mycobacterial Infections
E. Skamene 145

From Serology of the Chicken MHC to Polymorphism
of Malaria Antigen Genes
J. S. McBride 154

Virus-Induced Neutropenia
T. A. Rakusan 160

Tumor Immunotherapy
P. Koldovsky 168

Radiation-Enhanced Oncogene Expression
V. Klement 180

Oncogenes: A Pathologist's View
L. R. Donner 189

Natural Killer Cells:
Odyssey from Laboratory Artifact to Clinical Reality
E. Lotzová 195

Allergy to Drugs and Other Chemicals
Diagnosed by the Presence of Specific Memory Cells
in Human Blood
D. M. V. Stejskal 213

Contribution of Cytogenetics to Cancer Research:
Endometrial Adenocarcinoma
D. Simon 226

Bibliography 239

Appendix A: FONDATION DE FRANCE 301

Appendix B: Memoranda 303

Name and Subject Index 307

List of Contributors and Participants

Balcarová-Ständer, Jitka
Rahmengasse 3/1, 6900 Heidelberg, Federal Republic of Germany

Cerny, Jan
Department of Microbiology and Immunology, University of Maryland Medical School, Baltimore, MD 21201, USA

Demant, Peter
The Netherlands Cancer Institute, Dept. of Molecular Genetics, Plesmanlaan 121, 1066 CX Amsterdam, The Netherlands

Donner, Ludvik R.
Dept. of Surgical Pathology, Scott and White Clinic, 2401 South, 31st Street, Temple, TX 76508, USA

Engelberth, Jana
Dr. H. Colijnlaan 230, 2283 XV Rijswijk (ZH), The Netherlands

Hála, Karel
Institut für allgemeine experimentelle Pathologie, Fritz-Pregl-Straße 3, 6020 Innsbruck, Austria

Hauptfeld-Dolejsek, Vera
Department of Genetics, Washington University School of Medicine, St. Louis, MO 63110, USA

Ivanyi, Juraj
MRC, Tuberculosis & Related Infections Unit, Royal Postgraduate Medical School, Hammersmith Hospital, Du Cane Road, London W12 0HS, United Kingdom

Ivanyi, Pavol
Central Laboratory of Blood Transfusion Service, Plesmanlaan 125, 1066 CX Amsterdam, The Netherlands

Jerabek, Libuse
Stanford University School of Medicine, Department of Pathology,
Stanford, CA 94305, USA

Kinsky, Radslav
U 262 INSERM, Clinique Baudelocque, 123 Bld de Pont-Royal,
75674 Paris, France

Klein, Dagmar
MPI für Biologie, Abteilung Immunogenetik, Corrensstraße 42,
7400 Tübingen, Federal Republic of Germany

Klein, Jan
MPI für Biologie, Abteilung Immunogenetik, Corrensstraße 42,
7400 Tübingen, Federal Republic of Germany

Klement, Vasek
Dept. of Radiation Oncology, Division Radiation Medicine,
2025 Zonal Av., Los Angeles, CA 90033, USA

Klouda, Peter T.
U.K. Transplant Service, Southmead Hospital, Southmead Road,
Bristol BS10 5ND, United Kingdom

Koldovska-Libicka, Eva
2345 E. Edison Street, Tucson, AZ 85719, USA

Koldovsky, Pavel
HNO Klinik der Universität Düsseldorf, Forschungslabor,
Moorenstraße 5, 4000 Düsseldorf 1, Federal Republic of Germany

Lotzová, Eva
Section of Natural Immunity, Department of General Surgery,
MD Anderson Cancer Center, 1515 Holcombe Blvd., Box 18,
Houston, TX 77030, USA

Malkovský, Miroslav
University of Wisconsin-Madison Medical School, Dept. of
Medical Microbiology, 436 Services Memorial Institute,
1300 University Avenue, Madison, WI 53706, USA

McBride, Jana S.
Department of Zoology, University of Edinburgh,
West Mains Road, Edinburgh EH9 3JT, United Kingdom

Mervart, Helena
Canadian Red Cross Society, National Reference Laboratory,
1800 Alta Vista Drive, Ottawa, Ontario K1G 5J5, Canada

Pazderka, Feldzgeritta
Departments of Medicine and Laboratory Medicine, University of Alberta, Room 226, CRC Building, 8249 - 114 Street, Edmonton, Alberta, Canada T6G 2R8

Pla, Marika
Mouse Immunogenetics, U93 INSERM, Hôpital Saint Louis,
2 Place du Dr. A. Fournier, 75010 Paris, France

Rakusan, Tamara A.
Dept. of Pediatrics, C-71, University of Texas, Medical Branch, Galveston, TX 77550, USA

Simon, Daniela
The Wistar Institute of Anatomy and Biology,
36th Street at Spruce, Philadelphia, PA 19104, USA

Skamene, Emil
Montreal General Hospital, McGill University,
1650 Cedar Avenue, Room 7113, Montreal, Quebec H3G 1A4, Canada

Stejskal, Vera
Safety Assessment, AB Astra, 151 85 Sodertalje, Sweden

Milan Hašek: In Memoriam

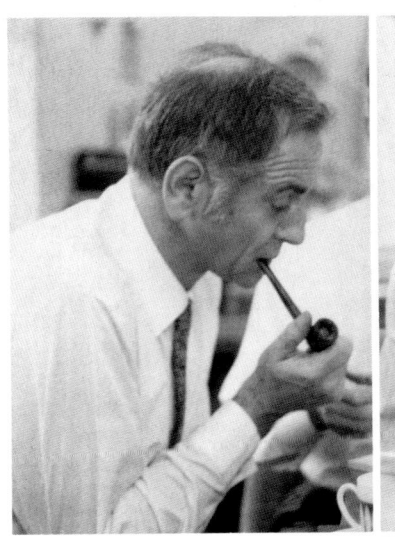
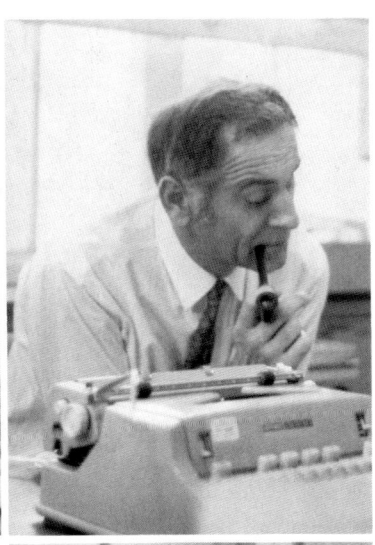
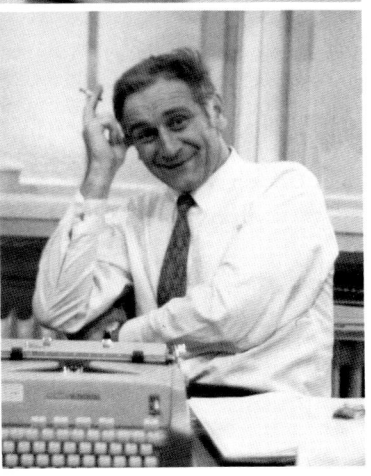

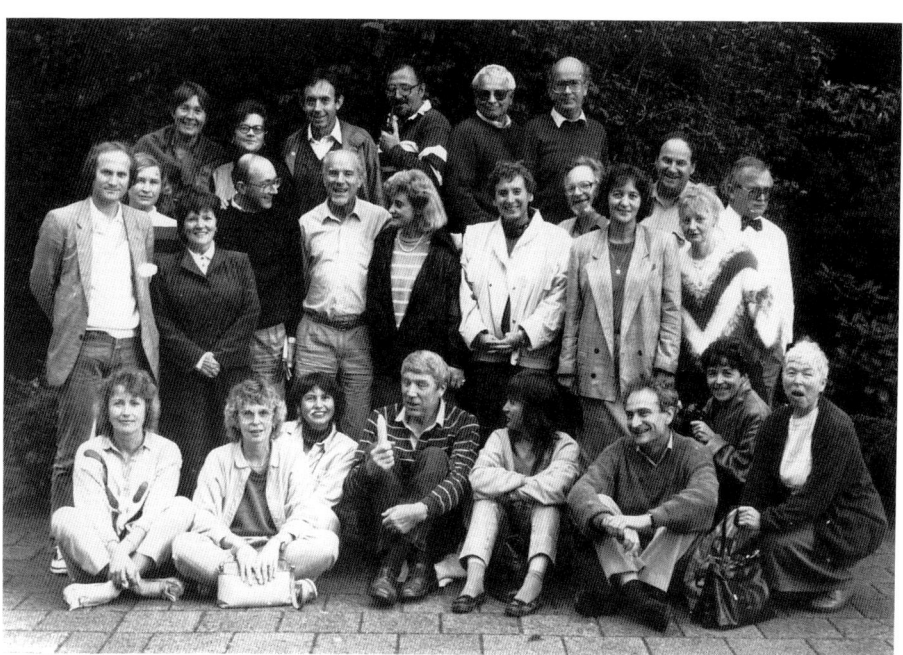

Participants of the meeting.
From left to right:
back: D. Ivanyi, F. Pazderka, E. Skamene, J. Cerny, K. Hala, P. Koldovsky
middle: M. Malkovský, J. Engelberth, H. Mervart, P. Demant, P. Ivanyi, L. Jerabek, V. Stejskal, P. Klouda, T. Rakusan, V. Klement, M. Pla, L. Donner
front: D. Klein, V. Hauptfeld, D. Simon, J. Klein, J. Balcarova, J. Ivanyi, A. Skamene, E. Koldovska-Libicka

Once upon a time there was a giant, a giant in every respect: with an impressive stature, a force of character, infinite generosity of heart, and a noble spirit. He was broad-minded and a courageous humanist. His dynamism and zest were irresistible. He was highly talented, even a genius. Such was the person we knew and loved: Milan Hašek. Oaks are normally not felled, but, alas, he was.

We owe to him the extraordinary Czech school of biology which was created out of nothing but himself in a city devastated by war but with an indestructible soul: a city where the flame of the ancient, deeply rooted Czech culture was still burning.

I enjoyed the distinguished privilege of meeting Milan Hašek when he was already at the height of his fame, at the time when he ought to have at least shared the Nobel Prize with F. Macfarlane Burnet and Peter Medawar, awarded for the great discovery of immunologic tolerance. The material then at his disposal now seems totally rudimentary: some animals, a great deal of imagination, experimental skill, and above all intelligent interpretation.

But that is not all.

He was a great school director, as proved, 30 years after this memorable discovery, by the respects his numerous pupils still insist on paying him. Although they are scattered throughout the world, they are united in spirit and language and met to extol his memory with the Amsterdam/Ommen colloquium and the publication of this volume. Milan Hašek had indeed known how to gather brilliant pupils around him and had been able to enthuse them with his optimism and to convey to them his intellectual values: he had thus formed a nursery of first-rate immunogeneticists. It was completely natural for this group to tackle the study of the major histocompatibility complex of various species: chicken, mouse, and of course man.

In 1965, at the very beginning of the great adventure posed by human histocompatibility, I had the chance to welcome Pavol and Dagmar Iványi to my laboratory. Taking advantage of the patient and systematic techniques they had learnt in Prague, we described together the Hu-1 system, which later became HL-A and then HLA.

This ist how the "Paris connection" with Prague came into being. It is certainly not out of place at this point to tell the story of the small flat in the avenue Rapp. In a building doomed soon to be demolished, we had found very inexpensive but very precarious living quarters for our friends the Iványis. Demolition was delayed for years, during the course of which many Czech scientists came to stay in this flat, either in turn or sometimes crammed together. Despite the sparseness and lack of comfort, this flat became a real phalanstery, a home of Czech freedom.

I was thus given the completely unexpected opportunity of getting to know and value the spirit of friendship which united all these young people in happiness and enthusiasm. It must be stressed that they had no contacts on an international level but they were, however, all moved by a burning ambition which proved to be, as we may see today, entirely justified.

These ties won me several memorable visits to Prague and its surroundings. I was able to visit the Institute of Experimental Genetics, then under the direction of Milan Hašek, and to see for myself that the laboratories, although sparsely equipped, were crammed with ideas.

As for the town itself, despite the dreariness of the buildings and the oppressing weight of all the blackened stone, there was a sense of humor, a dynamism, and a matchless vitality bursting forth from those badly lit alleys and crying out the refusal of a proud people with intellectual roots a thousand years old, moulded by hundreds of years of oppression.

After the humor of the poor soldier Švejk, after the 6/4 graffiti scrawled on every wall on the evening of the soccer match against the Russian team which was beaten 6 to 4, after the artistic talents such as, for example, the originality of the shadow theater, after the more or less clandestine surrealistic paintings and the music of Dvořák or other composers - work was obviously now the best answer.

The greatest effort went into the study of the major histocompatibility complex and, alongside Bar Harbor, Prague became the second scientific center in the world specializing in the H-2 system.

Here we should recall again the memorable meeting in the castle of Liblice close to Prague, where George Snell presented the huge table of the numerous loci and alleles which were supposed to exist in the mouse complex. The table was several meters high and wide.

It is to Peter Démant that we owe our thanks for establishing the link between man and mouse. When he went on a sabbatical year to Bar Harbor a few months later, he took with him the concept of a human complex composed of, at that time, only two loci (HL-A and -B) with several alleles. Thanks to the application of this concept to the mouse, Snell's huge table became less complex and could be arranged into two allelic series, K and D. This was probably the most important contribution made by the HLA complex to the H-2 complex as a token of its gratitude and indebtedness.

In the meantime, Pavol Iványi and his team had brought new insights into the various, especially endocrinous, functions the H-2 complex could carry out, thus foreshadowing the discovery of the class III and IV "squatter" genes.

It was in the midst of this studious and highly productive atmosphere that the invasion of Prague struck like a thunderbolt. Milan Hašek, Pavol Iványi, Jan Klein, and myself were in Japan on that very day, and I remember their feelings and, above all, how they painfully argued with their conscience. Each of them took his decision according to his own personal criteria, and each decision deserves our respect.

Everyone is aware of the consequences: the immunogenetic school splintered and was gradually sapped of its vitality. Milan Hašek lost his working place, and most of his pupils scattered throughout the world.

A considerable number of them, more than 20, left and founded immunogenetic centers outside Czechoslovakia, studying mainly the mouse but also the chicken, primates, etc. In this connection, the contribution of Jan Klein deserves special mention. Here is another giant who is at the root of the discovery of the other genes of the H-2 complex: the class II genes which are known to be of the utmost importance in immunology. In his turn, he has founded a fine school which stands comparison with Milan Hašek's in terms of brilliance and originality.

If all the cities where Hašek's pupils have settled were pinpointed with little flags on a map of the world, it would be astonishing to see how scattered they are: Amsterdam, Paris, Miami, etc.

But this geographic dispersal has not prevented the continuance of the close ties between these laboratories, despite the distances separating them – anyway, in science there is no such thing as distance any more. The Hašek "family" has remained a united family. The Amsterdam/Ommen meeting and this book are proof.

His pupils remain united not only by memories, but also by the Czech culture, the language, and the scientific education, all of which were formed in the same mold.

I have had the privilege of witnessing this venture which some would justifiably call a drama, but which, under difficult conditions and even outright misery, finally proved beneficial for science in general, if not for Czech science.

I was able to admire the self-sacrifice, the stoicism of many, the lack of dispondency, and the will to overcome difficulties. At the end of the day, the success of this immunogenetic diaspora will have possibly served science better than would have been the case had it not happened.

In my opinion, this book pays homage not only to the great scientist and the great school director that Milan Hašek was, but also to the extraordinary catalytic role played by all his pupils throughout the world.

The last image I have of Milan Hašek, at the Gare de l'Est a few months before his death, is of the happy face of a man who exhibited a sense of satisfaction upon having come to the Collège de France to give a series of lectures.

Jean Dausset
Collège de France
Rue d'Ulm, Paris

An imposing stature; his face broad and open under an opulent head of hair; a direct look, full of enthusiasm; a very deep voice; in short, the "presence" of an actor or an orator. Anyone who met Milan Hašek but once could never forget him. I met him in August 1965 in Brno, on the occasion of the symposium organized by the Academy of Sciences of Czechoslovakia to commemorate the centenary of Mendel's first dissertation. It was the time of the Prague "spring". The garden where Mendel had cultivated his peas had been restored and his statue had been reerected. In the church adjoining the monastery where Mendel had lived, two hundred American biologists and two hundred Soviet biologists had attended, side by side, a mass celebrated by a bishop who looked like Max Delbrück.

The night before, the Czech Academy had given a grand reception. The world's geneticists debated, ate, and drank heartily to the memory of the founder. Suddenly, I noticed that Lise, my wife, had disappeared. I searched for her among all the groups. Lise was not there. I felt alarmed and ran back to the hotel. Lise was not there. I came back to the reception to look for her in all the rooms. Lise was nowhere. Finally I found her. She was calmly seated in a small room reserved for the members of the Academy and the organizers of the symposium. There, instead of pâté and beer, they were sampling caviar and vodka. Lise was engaged in a long philosophical discussion with Milan Hašek!

I did not meet Milan Hašek again until 20 years later, a few months before he died. He had come to Paris to give lectures at the invitation of Jean Dausset. He had changed. But his bearing was still imposing and his voice very deep. He still had the same presence.

Milan Hašek had numerous disciples. Many of them have become eminent researchers and teachers in a variety of countries. We are obliged to them for having organized a colloquium and published this book to the memory of one of the greatest biologists of this century.

François Jacob
Professeur au Collège de France
et à l'Institut Pasteur

It took a few years to recover from the war, but by the 1950s young scientists were beginning to rush round the world again. In 1955 I was 27 years old, had come back from the United States to Edinburgh and wanted to be off on my travels again. My university was full of wonderful biologists; in the basement Peter Mitchell was earning his future Nobel Prize for work on transport into mitochondria; but not enough of them could help me to study immunology. Politically I had found the United States just after McCarthy pretty unattractive and felt proud of Britain's move to the left under the post-war Labour government, of which my father was an active supporter in Parliament. So it seemed logical to go and look at socialism in action in the Eastern block, and when John Humphrey told me that Šterzl had discovered how to transfer antibody production by injecting rabbits with one another's RNA, off I went. My professor in Edinburgh, Michael Swann, did not seem to mind how long I took, and in those days the train cost practically nothing. At Šterzl's request, the Czechoslovakian Academy of Science looked after me, and they did so with great generosity for which I still feel very grateful.

Jaroslav Šterzl must have found me a thoroughly awkward visitor, although he certainly never said so. I could not speak a word of Czech, could not get those RNA experiments to work, and would not join in the highly organised team-work of his section of the Academy at Dejvice. Most of the laboratory work was done by enchanting female assistants, and, as well as an inability to speak foreign languages, my fine British education had left me completely unable to speak to girls. I began to feel out of sorts.

Jaroslav Šterzl, Mirka Hrubešová and Zdeněk Trnka went on looking after me in the most hospitable way, but I was slipping away. Out at the other end of the building it felt much more like home. Somehow they worked different hours there, and the dragon who locked up everywhere else did not seem to penetrate that far, so one could mess about in the evening and at the weekends. That took the pressure off and left everyone free to spend as much of the rest of the day as they liked in chatting. That suited me fine, as I had a lot to learn. So I started to work there in Milan's biology section, instead of with Jaroslav in microbiology. Most of Milan's research work was with eggs, and somehow peering at softly illuminated embryos was much more fun than rabbits: it is hard to warm to rabbits, they are so ridiculously large for such a stupid animal. At that time Milan had a bizarre collection of birds: guinea fowl, turkeys and geese; the birds themselves were pretty stupid too, but that did not seem to matter so long as they went on providing their wonderful eggs. The truth, I suppose, was that I had found someone to admire, and that was what mattered to a forlorn but enthusiastic young man.

What I admired most in Milan was his intellectual generosity and enthusiasm for science. He seemed totally willing to listen, and always seemed to have time to spare to sit down and talk a topic through. In those talks his aim was to fish out of the pool of ideas whatever could be assimilated into his own thinking. He was determined to build a decent research programme for his group, so everything had to be sifted through for nuggets that would come in useful. He had a shrewd grasp of what could be managed with the resources available to him, and very wisely concentrated on whole-animal-based immunology rather than launching out into elaborate in vitro technology. But the main thing was birds and their eggs, for they were his secret weapon to keep up with the riches of the West!

The project that I undertook in his laboratory ended in catastrophe. We were going to identify turkey cells grafted into chicken eggs by means of antibodies. To our surprise many of the erythrocytes in the chimeras had both chicken and turkey markers. Milan was delighted, for that smelled of Michurinism at the cellular level. But alas, Morton Simonsen came out with the graft-versus-host reaction, and we became suspicious: sure enough, the "turkey markers" were simply turkey antibodies, made against their host cells and masquerading as part of the erythrocytes to which they had bound.

Perhaps I nerver understood where all that Michurinism sprang from. Was Milan simply following the party line? Surely not, for one became hypersensitive to cynicism in scientific circles in Prague that year, and he came across as a true believer at that time. I suppose that those ideas had indeed led Milan to his great egg-chimera experiment, and that success blinded his critical faculties. And of course he was a tremendously positive person who would far rather welcome an idea than discard one.

After that year we remained friends. Věra Hašková came and worked with me for a while in Edinburgh. We are very fond of one another, and she became a friend of my whole family. I kept going back to Prague until 1968. The last time that Milan and I sat down together properly was in that year, at my house in Mill Hill. My wife Lorna and I tried passionately to argue him into staying in Prague, which of course he did although no doubt for other reasons. Maybe that was a sad mistake.

N. A. Mitchison
Department of Zoology and Cell Biology
University College London
Gower Street, London WC1E 6BT, UK

My old friend Milan Hašek died suddenly and unexpectedly, according to everybody I have talked to, in November 1984. The feeling that he tragically died long before his time was really up comes naturally to me because he was 4 years younger than I and he had seemed as strong and vigorous as ever when I met him, for the last time, about 6 months before he died. I first met Milan in Prague in 1954. Because of common interests and common ways of thinking in many respects, we developed and maintained a life-long friendship.

As a matter of fact, my first contact with Czechoslovak immunology did not begin with Milan Hašek but with Jaroslav Sterzl. Jaroslav and I met in Rome in September 1953 at the International Congress of Microbiology. As I remember, we really found each other through shared political and humanitarian convictions. If anybody should ask what politics had to do with international microbiology in 1954, the answer is: quite a lot. Some major countries were known to be preparing for biological warfare, and others were suspected of it. Some of us, being young and idealistic strongly felt that this was utterly wrong and we wanted the Congress to adopt a resolution calling on all microbiologists in the world to refuse their services in preparation for biological warfare. In the end, we succeeded in passing a resolution to that effect. Among the very active conspirators in that anti-biological warfare plot was a strong British contingent, including among others John Humphrey, and a young, newly married couple Donald Michie and Anne McLaren, to whom I shall soon come back in connection with Milan.

One thing Milan and I had in common is the fact that we were young together when cellular immunology was also young and mostly took its leads from a very few and scattered laboratories which were devoted to problems of transplantation immunology. I am now thinking back to the time of 1953-1954. At the beginning of 1953 I had published, and defended, my doctoral thesis at the University of Copenhagen, in which I had demonstrated that kidney transplantation from dog to dog was an immunological problem. The motions I went through before I came to that conclusion were largely similar to what Medawar et al. had already been doing in the 1940s in England by skin grafting in rabbits. This, of course, was well before the era of chemical immunosuppression which was later to put clinical organ transplantation on the map, and tissue typing was still very primitive and essentially confined to the mouse. The hopes of ever overcoming the boundaries of biological incompatibility in organ transplantation were frankly dim in those days. Such was the setting in which the discovery of immunological tolerance was made, lighting a flame of hope that eventually proved to be warranted.

Immunological tolerance, as you will recall, was discovered first as a naturally occurring event when Ray Owen, in the United States, found blood group chimerism in dizygotic calf twins, resulting from spontaneous vascular anastomoses in their plancentae. In the experimental exploration of Owen's findings there are two great names in my book: Medawar and Hašek.

These two men and their respective co-workers opened up the field of induced antigen-specific suppression of the immune response which still remains a major challenge to immunological theory and practice alike. Medawar coined the term "immunological tolerance" and eventually received the Nobel Prize together with Burnet. Milan had no Nobel Prize although his own original experimental demonstration of immunological tolerance in chicken embryos was performed independently and simultaneously with Medawar's. Milan also published his first findings simultaneously with Medawar (1953), but he published in Russian and in a journal practically unknown in the West, rather than publishing in *Nature* and in English. It is to Medawar's credit that, when he somehow learned of Hašek's work, he also gave full credit to its experimental substance although not, of course, to the Mitchurinist ideology and terminology in which Milan's early writings on immunological tolerance were dressed for reasons which were poorly understood in the West and certainly not appreciated.

I first learned about the experimentally induced immunological tolerance in the New York Academy of Sciences from Medawar's first presentation of his findings in February 1954. I spent most of 1954 in England working on that interesting new discovery and wanted to investigate to what extent tolerance could be extended across species barriers. While living in England in 1954, I spent a lot of time with my old friends from Rome, Donald and Anne. They went to Prague for their summer holidays and came back full of enthusiasm for a marvelous Czech they had met, Milan Hašek, who seemed now to be doing work very similar to mine. Later in the year, I received an invitation from the Academy of Sciences in Prague to attend a meeting in Liblice. There I finally met Milan himself, saw his laboratories, compared notes with him, and suggested that we should publish our findings on tolerance in chickens to other avian species simultaneously, as in fact we did in *Nature*.

In the following years, I went back to Prague many times. Eventually, Prague became quite fashionable with Western immunologists, thanks first and foremost to the schools of experimental immunology created there on Danish standards, by Milan Hašek and Jaroslav Sterzl, both very young men, when they were given the opportunity to form their own laboratories.

Milan Hašek naturally became, and remained, the chief of his own institute until he was replaced after 1968, but even then he retained his scientific interests and remained an active force in immunology until his death.

Milan was not only a natural chief of the institute, he was also a chieftain. He was loyal to his friends and fair to everybody. His work belongs forever to the history of immunology. We will treasure the memory of Milan in our hearts!

Acknowledgement. This paper was a Memorial Talk delivered at Marianske Lazne, April 22nd, 1985.

Morten Simonsen
Professor of Immunology
University of Copenhagen

Tolerance, Transplantation and Immune Network

From Horses to Mice: Graft Rejection and Tolerance

R. Kinsky

I first met Milan Hašek in Dejvice (Prague) in 1956 while trying to find a research team prepared to accept me. My previous practical experience was limited to horse breeding and to a fair linguistic knowledge due to my family background. Milan immediately received me as a friend – which was unfortunately unusual in the 1950s since our small population was somewhat artificially divided into many "classes" depending on one's parents' social origin. Our family estates had been nationalized since 1948, and, worst of all, my close relatives had all left the country since then. Nevertheless, Milan seemed to approach these regulations with great courage and magnanimity. The attitude of his co-workers, mainly Marta Vojtišková and others, only reflected Milan's own example of kind interest and tolerance. I soon became actively involved in his main topic dealing with immunological tolerance, having exchanged horses for mice, and my first experiments were performed with Pavel Koldovsky.

In 1957 I accompanied Milan to Paris as an interpreter and became engaged to Thamar Amilakvari, a distant French cousin of Georgian origin, whom I married in Paris in 1958. Milan seemed to approve my choice and after that, whenever he came over, he visited us in Paris where I started to work in Prof. Raoul Kourilsky's department of immunopathology at the St. Antoine Hospital. With Guy A. Voisin we designed several research projects largely inspired by Milan's original ideas. We focused our attention on the active components of tolerance in the mouse system and on the various applications of passive and active enhancement, mainly in the prevention of the graft-versus-host (GVH) disease. My French PhD thesis was dedicated to Milan Hašek who became an honorary member of the French Immunology Society.

I remember Milan's lectures in Paris, at the Collège de France and elsewhere, where he displayed an extraordinary effortless aptitude to make himself understood in French with a disarmingly restricted vocabulary. He made ingenious use of his deep bass voice added to persuasive slow gestures in order to attract attention to the key problems which had to be understood. There were few words but many excellent ideas expressed in an economic and clear fashion. He was also the center of all social events which often ended in singing or displaying his unusual physical strength, lifting furniture with one hand while emptying noggins and joking with everybody.

Soon his co-workers started to come to Paris, and I always enjoyed having them in our house or helping them to survive whenever some practical arrangements were needed. It was therefore an immense pleasure for me to attend the meeting in Brno in 1980 held in Milan Hašek's honor although his ailing health was beginning to cause us concern. I saw him for the last time a few months before his death when he stayed in Paris at the invitation of Prof. Jean Dausset. My wife and sons will always remember Milan as one of our closest friends. It is rare to have known a man to whom so many owed so much.

After having joined, in 1958, the Center of Immunopathology at the St. Antoine Hospital, founded and directed by Prof. Raoul Kourilsky, I developed several research topics with Guy A. Voisin dealing with transplantation immunology. Emphasis was placed on the role of antibodies in transplantation reactions, and it was shown that both passive and active enhancements known only in some restricted tumor systems were a general phenomenon implicated even in specific acquired tolerance. These results were further extended into a concept of specific immunoregulation. The Ig isotypes involved in enhancement and specific acquired tolerance were thoroughly studied and new methods designed for their revelation. On several, although too rare occasions I could discuss our results with Milan Hašek who usually gave me some valuable suggestions and criticisms which helped me in future scientific approaches.

In 1960 I joined Avrion Mitchison in Edinburgh (Scotland) where we started to induce tolerance to allogeneic skin grafts in chickens using erythrocyte suspensions as tolerizing agents. Chicken erythrocytes, unlike mice erythrocytes, proved to be efficient in tolerance induction. Avrion Mitchison always belonged to Milan Hašek's friends, and we of course exchanged our impressions and positive feelings concerning his group.

Back in Paris I designed certain active enhancing protocols which significantly prolonged allogeneic skin grafts in two distinct rabbit breeds. The role of the spleen in active enhancement was clearly established. In collaboration with the Cancer Research Institute in Villejuif, I studied the consequences of a systemic GVH reaction in mice on blood leukocyte counts and on selective drops of serum immunoglobulin levels.

The GVH model was extensively used for the application of antibody-mediated specific modulation of this transplantation reaction. The active counterpart of this model consisted in donor preimmunization using lyophilized allogeneic spleen cells. Here again an efficient, although dose-dependent effect on immune protection against the GVH disease was achieved. In my PhD thesis (1967) I thanked Milan Hašek for all his initial support and encouragement.

Specific acquired tolerance was studied in mice. The blood of animals injected i.v. with allogeneic spleen cells at birth was sampled at various periods of life while the animal tolerated permanent skin grafts. The presence of specific antibodies and enhancing factors was found in a large proportion of mice. Spleen cells from tolerized donors were also able to transfer some degree of tolerance. These results led to the concept of "active tolerance," further developed by Ivan Hilgert in Prague with whom I have collaborated ever since. In 1968 I returned to Edinburgh where James Howard was involved in the study of immune paralysis to the polysaccharide S III. We first showed that tolerant mice displayed a positive rosette formation with S III-coated RBCs in spite of a total absence of circulating antibodies. Another topic I studied in Edinburgh concerned the origin of Kupffer's cells in mice. This consisted in placing mice in parabiosis, one partner carrying the T6T6 chromosome marker. The presence of this marker in some Kupffer's cells located in the liver of the normal CBA parabiotic partner proved the passage of blood-borne precursors from the $T6^+$ parabiont into the other. In Edinburgh I again met my old friends Marta Vojtiškova and Alena Lengerová from Prague, and the unfortunate August 1968 events in our home country caused us much concern.

Back in Paris in 1969 I started to work on transplantation anaphylaxis. Indeed, anaphylactic antibodies, thermolabile IgE, and thermostable IgGl were found in mouse sera obtained after repeated allogeneic immunizations. The method designed to reveal these antibodies made use of soluble *H-2* antigenic material presenting a total absence of toxicity. These substances were prepared by Ivan Hilgert from Milan Hašek's group. Hundreds of mice were injected and skinned for passive cutaneous anaphylaxis (PCA) until the proper conditions for antigen concentrations and ways of antigen preparation were established. Beside PCA, an in vitro method consisting in direct allogeneic anaphylactic mast cell degranulation (DAAD) was designed for further studies. Isolated anaphylactic antibodies were also found to be capable of inducing lethal shocks in newborn as well as adult mice. In Paris we further aimed to find an answer for discrepant results cited in the literature concerning the involvement of Ig isotypes in passive enhancement of allogeneic tumor grafts. This study involved preliminary work concerning the efficiency of immune complexes prepared with purified Ig isotypes and soluble *H-2* antigens. Since, in our hands, larger doses of IgG2a antibodies usually inhibited Sa I tumor growth, this effect could be converted in enhancement of the same target graft by previous complexing of cytotoxic IgG2a antibodies with the specific $H\text{-}2^a$ soluble antigen. The contribution of H. T. Duc in this and other studies was most valuable.

The target antigens in passive enhancement of Sa I grafts was further shown to be linked to class I epitopes of the *H-2* system using various congenic strain combinations for antibody preparation as well as absorption procedures.

Anti-idiotypic antibodies were studied for enhancing properties in the mouse. While no tumor enhancement was obtained, these anti-recognition structure (RS) antibodies reacting with parental cells could efficiently inhibit a local GVH reaction in the popliteal lymph node assay. Anti-idiotypic antibodies were disclosed in allogeneic pregnant mice using a radioimmune assay. This and other works in the field of reproductive immunology were initiated in close collaboration with Gérard Chaouat.

Immune responses, both at humoral and cellular levels, were studied with Ivan Hilgert in males and females of several mouse strains and hamsters. A clear difference in antibody production kinetics and cellular responses was noticed between both sexes as well as differences in allogeneic tumor rejections.

With George Douvas (USA) we showed the involvement of suppressor cells in mice treated for passive enhancement. Again with Ivan Hilgert we studied another way of transplantation tolerance induction in mice using a continuous treatment with lentil lectin (LcA). Here again suppressor cells were disclosed, presenting specific effects for the test skin graft antigens. Murine T and B lymphocytes were studied morphologically using classical staining procedures and electron microscopy with Nikola Vujanović (Yugoslavia) and Philippe Lebouteiller. Some characteristic distinctions concerning size, surface, and nuclear-cycloplasmic ratios were described.

Our work in reproductive immunology was predominantly centered on the immunomodulating effects of placental glycoproteins. The methods used involved the modulation of anti-sheep RBC (SRBC) plaque-forming cells (PFC) responses and various in vivo and in vitro transplantation models. This fascinating study was carried out with Gérard Chaouat in collaboration with Gopal Gupta (India), Thamar Mekori (Israel), Miljenko Dorić (Yugoslavia) and Pierre Bobe.

The role of histamine in the modulation of local GVH reactions was studied with Claude Ramazeilles. Histamine and serotonin were efficient in preventing GVH responses, as was also the supernatant of degranulated mast cells. Histamine H_2 receptor-bearing cells were isolated by panning and proved to have suppressor properties. The transplantation of fertilized eggs was carried out in the murine species with Koljo Vlachov (Bulgaria) and later Ricardo Cibotti (Argentina). Surrogate mothers were examined for their reactivity to fully allogeneic transplanted embryos and presented positive in vivo and in vitro responses of various types.

More recently we have turned our attention toward the immuno-modulatory properties of sperm lactate dehydrogenase (LDH)-C4 in a series of experiments performed with Gopal Gupta (India). An effect of this sperm-specific isozyme was noticed on the suppressor versus helper cell ratio in mice treated either i.p. or intrarectally. LDH-C4 therefore seemed to favor suppressor mechanisms while preferentially hampering helper cellular components. This work was based on fluorescence-activated cell sorter (FACS) and enzyme-linked immuno-adsorbent assay (ELISA) studies, mixed lymphocyte reaction, cytotoxic T cell lympholysis, and GVH.

Since I left Milan Hašek's group with his approval in 1958, I have visited various countries, working in the United States at Duke University in Durham (North Carolina), several times in Edinburgh (Scotland), the last time with Spedding Micklem (1984), in the Federal Republic of Germany (with Günther Hermann and Pavel Koldovsky) and in Israel (with Isaac Witz). I have tought immunology in Paris and other French cities, as well as in Tunisia, Morocco, and Algeria and have made friends in all these countries. In 1980 I was invited to Brno (Czechoslovakia) to honor Milan Hašek at a symposium organized by his local co-workers. When Milan came to our house the year before his death, my wife and I still enjoyed his always pleasant company. I am certain the same feelings will be always shared by all his numerous co-workers and pupils both in our old home country and all around the world.

Tolerance and the Immune Network.
T Cells Reactive to the Variable Domains
of Immunoglobulins

J. Cerny

Introduction

Personal Note

Professor Milan Hašek is famous for his discovery of immunological tolerance. However, I believe that Hašek's greatest scientific achievement was the creation of the Institute for Experimental Biology and Genetics (IEBG) in Prague, Czechoslovakia, an unparalleled research center of its time. In the atmosphere of enthusiasm, free thinking, and individual freedom at the IEBG, Milan Hašek launched the careers of dozens of young scientists whom he fished out of the muddy waters of Czechoslovak society of the 1950s and 1960s, with admirable intuition and personal courage. Many of those scientists left the institute after 1968 to live and work abroad. Their contributions to scientific development in various countries represent the continuing influence of Milan Hašek on international science.

It is difficult to describe to the Western scientist the process by which Hašek selected his associates in the social system borne of the Marx Brothers' movies (no pun intended). My own situation was colorless compared to the stories of my colleagues as narrated in other chapters of this book. Having graduated from the preventive branch of the Charles University Medical School, my future was predetermined by the so-called distribution scheme according to which graduates were sent, by the Secretary of Health, to particular locations of the country for specific jobs. These assignments were dictated by the perceived needs of the society, but the political profile of the individual as well as the whimsy of bureaucrats played a major role in the process. Escape from the "distribution" was nearly impossible. Fortunately, I had worked as a student in various laboratories, including the IEBG, in my later years of medical school, and Milan Hašek had heard of my interest in research. One telephone call from Hašek – himself an influential member of the political establishment – to the Secretary of Health had performed the miracle, and I became a graduate student at the IEBG.

My personal remembrance of Milan Hašek is blurred. If one is allowed an exalted parallel, looking up to him was like staring straight into the sun. His vitality and confidence were exhilarating and intimidating at once. Suffice to say that my odyssey through American universities and cities – from Philadelphia to Boston, to Galveston, and to Baltimore – has been a continuous, fruitless search for another place like the IEBG and another leader like Milan Hašek. I know now that I shall never find them, not the least because one cannot find one's lost youth. The meeting of former members of IEBG in Ommen in 1988 was as close to the realization of the dream as we will ever get.

From Immunological Tolerance to the Idiotype Network

The concept of immunological tolerance was, not surprisingly, one of the main research topics at the IEBG. It still remains a key issue of immunology, the science of self/non-self discrimination. The mechanisms by which the potentially self-reactive lymphocytes are excluded from immune response, or regulated, are not yet fully understood. In the last decade, the notion has arisen that some types of self-reactions may be "allowed" to take place and may perform physiological, hitherto unknown functions. One such function was formulated by Jerne (1974) in the so-called idiotype network hypothesis. The concept is based on the fact that the variable regions of each immunoglobulin molecule have unique shapes, called idiotopes. The network hypothesis holds that the idiotopes are recognized by complementary, anti-idiotopic lymphocytes. Moreover, the anti-idiotopic (self-reactive) lymphocytes are not silent; rather, they actively regulate the function of the idiotope-bearing lymphocytes. The original network hypothesis was based solely on the interaction of complementary immunoglobulins, the idiotope-bearing (Id^+), and the anti-idiotopic (anti-Id) molecules. Even in its "simple" form, the network is extremely complex and poses difficult conceptual problems. The complexity has increased further by the introduction of T cells and T cell idiotopes, i.e., the variable domains of the antigen receptors expressed by the T lymphocytes. An experimenter who sets out to explore the validity of the network hypothesis must reduce his or her experimental system to a particular type of interaction. I shall limit the subsequent discussion to the special case of T cells that recognize the self-idiotopes on immunoglobulin molecules. In other words, I shall describe the evidence, from my own experimentation, for the existence of anti-Id T cells that react against the Id^+ B cells and that regulate the production of the Id^+ antibody in response to the antigen stimulation.

Autologous anti-Id T Cells: Concept and Working Hypothesis

The stimulation of anti-Id T cells by syngeneic Id^+ immunoglobulins was first described by Janeway et al. (1975). In their experiments, as well as in much of the subsequent work from a number of laboratories, the Id-specific T cells were activated by repeated injections of animals with syngeneic or autologous immunoglobulins. However, by the year 1980, we and others had accumulated enough data to support the notion that the anti-Id T cells were being activated by a physiological process in the course of antigen-driven immune response (Cerny 1984; Eichmann 1978; Baker 1975; Abbas 1982; Rajewski and Takemon 1983). In other words, we postulated that administration of an antigen triggers the specific Id^+ B cells which, in turn, activate the anti-Id T cells that regulate the antibody response (Fig. 1).

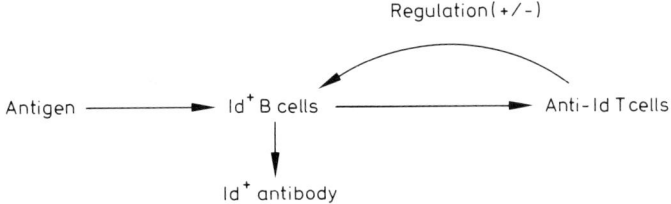

Fig. 1. Schema of reactions following immunization: antigen triggers the specific, idiotype-positive (Id$^+$) B cells which, in turn, activate the anti-Id T cells that help (+) or suppress (−) the production of Id$^+$ antibody

We have studied this scenario using a reductionist model of antibody response to *Streptococcus pneumoniae* R36a (Pn) in mice. This antibody response is dominated by molecules expressing the well-characterized T15 idiotopes (T15$^+$ antibody). Moreover, the anti-Pn response is T independent, in the sense that the triggering of B cells by Pn does not require the presence of the antigen-specific T helper cells. This has allowed us to study the regulatory effects of the putative anti-T15 T cells without the concomitant regulation by anti-Pn T cells.

We observed that immunization of mice with Pn leads to activation of T cells in the spleen that were able to bind the T15$^+$ immunoglobulin. Moreover, these T cells were able to actively regulate the T15$^+$ antibody response, either in an adoptive transfer experiment or in a read-out culture. Both helper cells (T$_H$) and suppressor cells (T$_S$) were identified depending on the manner of antigen administration and time after immunization (Cerny and Caulfield 1981; Cerny et al. 1986).

The key question raised by these studies was: what is the physiological stimulus for the activation of anti-Id T cells in the course of immune response? If we find that signal, can we employ it as a tool to clone the anti-Id T cells in vitro and to formally establish their identity?

The T15-binding T cells appear in the spleen very early (day 2–day 3) after immunization (Kelsoe and Cerny 1979). Therefore we hypothesized that the most likely events leading to the activation of anti-T15 T cells were:

1. Increasing numbers of antigen-driven T15$^+$ B cells that trigger the activity and the expansion of anti-T15 T cells by a cognate, cell-to-cell interaction.
2. Complexes of antigen (Pn) with the antibody molecules (T15) that are produced in the early stages of the B cell response.

Both hypotheses have been tested experimentally, as discussed in the next two sections. The reader will notice that we did not consider the soluble serum antibody as a likely candidate for stimulation of anti-Id T cells. This notion has been borne out in every instance by control experiments.

Activation of Anti-Id T Cells by an Antigen-Antibody Complex

The experimental design for testing the hypothesis that anti-Id cells are activated by an antigen-antibody complex is shown in Fig. 2. Normal T cells were incubated with complexes prepared from the Pn polysaccharide and the purified antibody

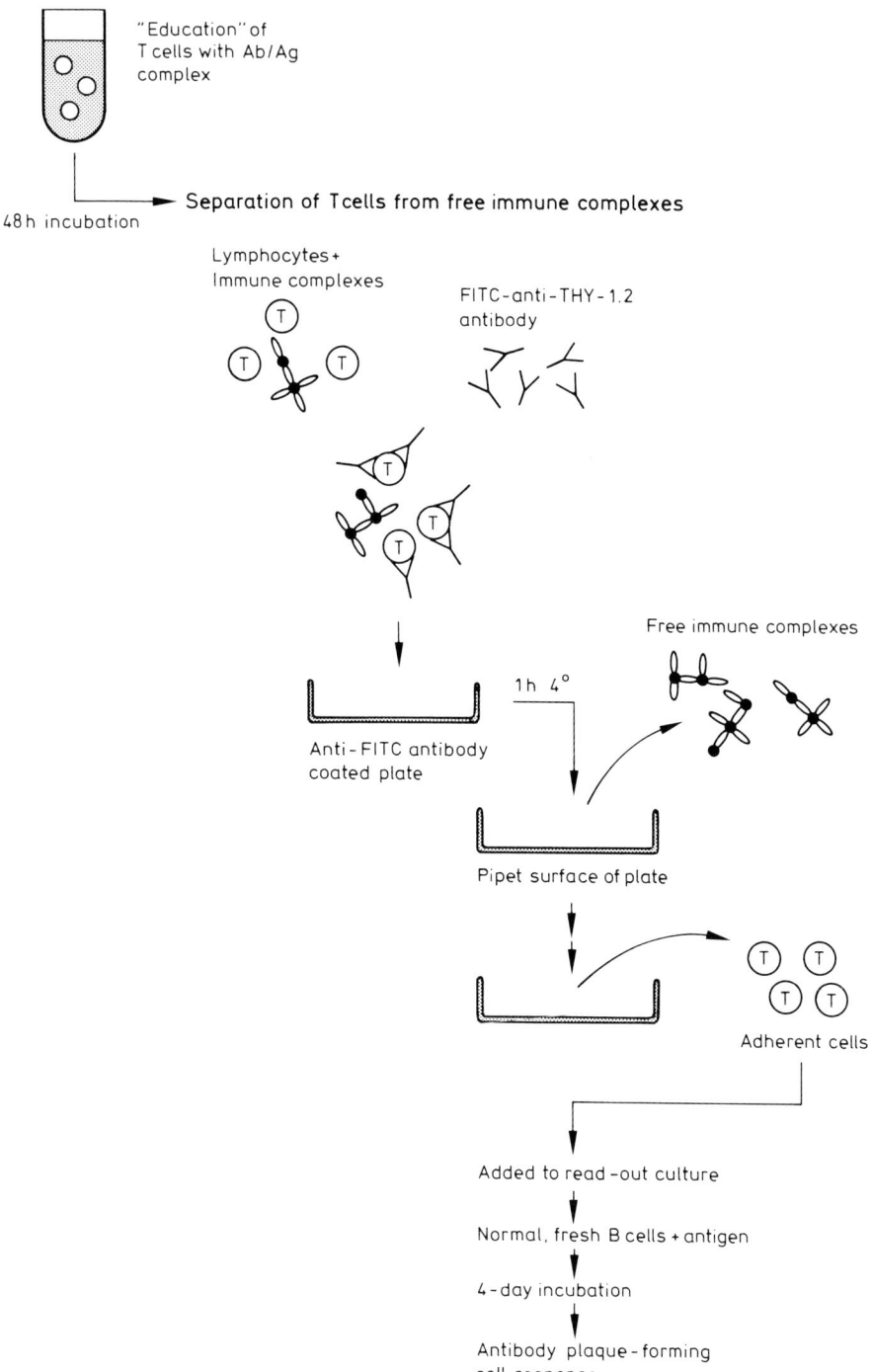

Fig. 2. Activation of T cells with Ag/Ab(Id) complex in vitro. The crucial step in the procedure is the removal of residual immune complex before the addition of educated T cells into the read-out culture

Table 1. Immunoregulatory activity of T cells that have been exposed to the antigen/T15 idiotype complex

T cells educated with:	Effect on antibody response in vitro to:		Effect on anti-Pn response by:	
	Pn	TNP-BA	T15$^+$ B cells	T15$^-$ B cells
Pn	None	None		
T15$^+$ antibody	None	None		
Pn/T15$^+$ complex	Suppression	None	Suppression	None
Control immune complexes	None	None		

(T15+ anti-Pn). After 2 days in culture, the T cells were purified free of any immune complex, and their activity was measured in a second, read-out culture consisting of normal, syngeneic B cells stimulated with Pn. Would the "educated" T cells regulate the antibody response of B cells, as measured by the number of antibody plaque-forming cells (PFC) generated in the read-out culture? The results of detailed experiments (Caulfield et al. 1983) are summarized in Table 1. The T cells that were educated with the Pn/T15$^+$ antibody complex specifically inhibited the anti-Pn response in vitro. Neither the antigen nor the idiotope alone produced such an effect. The antibody responses to control antigens, such as trinitrophenyl (TNP) coupled to *Brucella abortus* (BA) (TNP-BA), were not suppressed. Most important is the result at the right-hand side of Table 1, where the T cells were tested for their ability to suppress the T15$^+$ and T15$^-$ B cells. The T15$^+$ B cells were splenocytes (T-depleted) from normal BALB/c mice. T15$^-$ B cells were from mice that had been neonatally injected with anti-T15 antibody. The injection eliminates all T15$^+$ lymphocytes, and, when the mouse reaches adult age, it reacts to Pn immunization by producing antibody that lacks in T15 idiotopes. As seen from Table 1, the educated T cells were unable to inhibit the activity of T15$^-$ B cells, suggesting strongly that the suppression involved the recognition of the T15 Id by the T cells.

These experiments indicate clearly that immune complexes may alter the course of antibody response by activation of idiotope-specific T_S cells. Since the soluble idiotope alone seems unable to activate the T cells, a whole set of new questions must be raised about the molecular recognition of immunoglobulin-variable domains by T cells. Also, we were not able to activate any helper/amplifier T cells by the immune complex. Repeated attempts to establish anti-Id T cell lines with the immune complexes failed (M. Caulfield, personal communication).

Production of Anti-T15 T Cell Lines with T15$^+$ B Cells

In order to test the hypothesis that anti-Id T cells are activated by contact with autologous Id$^+$ B cells, we needed a source of large numbers of T15$^+$ lymphocytes. This was accomplished by transfection of a B cell lymphoma line, BCL$_1$, B$_1$ (BALB/c) with the T15 immunoglobulin transgene. The resulting stable transfec-

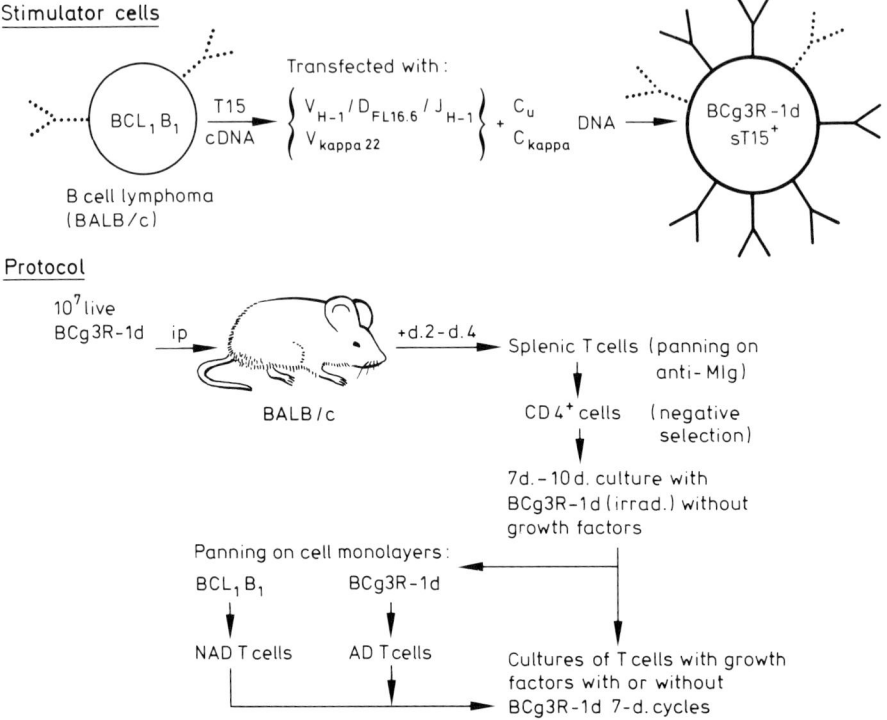

Fig. 3. Protocol for establishment of T cell lines by stimulation with syngeneic T15⁺ transfectant B cells

Table 2. Cell surface markers on the T cell lines

Antibody[a], incubation		Membrane fluorescence-positive[b] lymphocytes, live (%)
First	Second	
Thy-1.2/FITC	None	>90
L3T4	Goat a-mouse IgG/FITC	70->90
None	Goat a-mouse IgG/FITC	<0.5
TEPC15	Goat a-mouse IgA/FITC	10->30[c]
M511	Goat a-mouse IgA/FITC	<2
None	Goat a-mouse IgA/FITC	<0.5

[a] Two-step membrane staining.
[b] Range of positively stained cells found in various passages from three independently derived T cell lines. At least 300 cells were scored each time.
[c] Expressed as the proportion of the Thy-1.2⁺ cells counted in the parallel preparation from the same cell suspension.

tant BCg3R-1d cell was used as a "stimulator cell" for the syngeneic T lymphocytes. After repeated rounds of co-culture, outlined in Fig. 3, stable T cell lines were obtained. The surface phenotype of the T cells is shown in Table 2. The stable CD4$^+$ lines were studied in detail (Cerny et al. 1988), and their properties can be summarized as follows:

1. The T cells grow only in the presence of the T15$^+$ stimulator cells (BCg3R-1d), but not with T cell growth factors alone. Moreover, the cell lines do not grow in the presence of syngeneic splenocytes plus soluble T15$^+$ molecules (data not shown).
2. The established T cells bind the soluble T15$^+$ immunoglobulin in a competitive radioimmunoassay. Figure 4 shows an example of such an assay. The T cell line binds the T15$^+$ molecule TEPC15 very well, while the binding of immunoglobulins M603 and M511 is lower or nil, respectively. The proteins M603 and M511 have idiotopes which are different from TEPC15, even though their isotype is the same (IgA) and they react with Pn. Therefore the binding of TEPC15 by the T cells is truly Id specific. Moreover, it requires the intact immunoglobulin molecule because the isolated chains (H and L) are not bound (Fig. 4).
3. The T cells discriminate between somatic idiotopic variants of T15 (Table 3). These variant immunoglobulins, all of which react with Pn, differ from each other by changes in the expression of the conformational T15 determinants. The changes come about as somatic mutations of the germline-encoded T15. The fine differences in the idiotopy of these variant molecules have been mapped

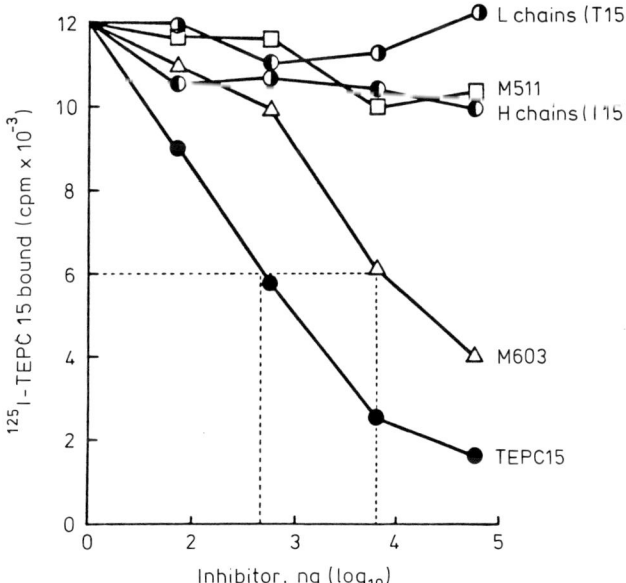

Fig. 4. Binding of ^{125}I-TEPC15 by the T3-F24 cell line (10^5 cells/tube, in duplicate) in the presence of increasing amounts of unlabeled inhibitors: ●, TEPC15; △, M603; □, M511, and isolated heavy (◐) and light (◑) chains of TEPC15. The *dotted lines* indicate the ID$_{50}$ concentrations for TEPC15 (600 ng) and for M603 (6000 ng)

Table 3. Idiotype binding studies on long-term T cell lines

Cell line	Assay date	T15 Id+ Ig								T15 Id− Ig	
		TEPC15 (α)			HPCM-6	HPCG-11	HPCG-14	7-22	293	M603	M511
		Intact	L chain	H chain	(μ)	(γ3)	(γ1)	(μ)	(μ)	(α)	(α)
T3-F24	08/20/87	200								1500	>60000
	10/02/87	600	>60000	>60000						6000	>60000
T4-EF	08/20/87	750	>60000	>60000							
	10/22/87	1500	>60000	>60000	500	6000				20000	>60000
	12/01/87	600			400		24000	4000	>60000		
T5-2	07/06/87	500								3000	>60000
T5-3	08/20/87	200								2000	>60000
T5-4	08/20/87	400								4500	>60000
	09/24/87	400	>60000	>60000	600	5000		>60000	>60000	5000	>60000
	10/23/87	650	>60000	>60000	200	2200		11000	12000		
T9	09/30/87	900			200	150		1200	900	6000	>60000
	10/20/87	200	>60000	>60000	100	150		2000	200	600	40000
	02/25/88	600				200	15000				

Inhibition potential of various immunoglobulins (ID_{50}, ng) in competition with ^{125}I-TEPC15 (600 ng)

Table 4. Binding of T15 idiotype-bearing immunoglobulins by monoclonal antibodies and by T cell lines

Reactivity pattern	Monoclonal antibody[a]	T cell line[b]	Relative binding (ID$_{50}$, µg/l) of T15 immunoglobulin variant					
			TEPC15	HPCM-6	7-22	293	HPCG-11	HPCG-14
I	AB1-2		0.3	20.0	10.0	1.0	50.0 [c]	20.0
	B24-44		0.5	8.0	1.0	3.0	10.0	10.0
II	MaId5-4	T-9	0.2	0.3	0.2	0.05	1.0 [c]	10.0
			0.6	0.6	2.0	0.6	0.1	15.0
III	B36-75		1.5	1.5	>500.0	>500.0 [c]	>500.0	>500.0
	B39-38		0.8	10.0	>500.0	>500.0	80.0	200.0
		T5-4	0.6	0.4	20.0	40.0	5.0	
		T4-EF	0.6	0.5	4.0	>60.0	6.0	25.0

[a] Monoclonal anti-Id raised against the S107/V$_K$ 22 germline-encoded immunoglobulins (TEPC15/HOPC8) have been described in Strickland et al. (1988). These anti-Id have been tested for binding of the T15 variant molecules in a competitive radioimmunoassay with ^{125}I-TEPC15.
[b] Binding of T15 variants by T cell lines (from Table 3).
[c] Boxed values indicate a weak binding (high ID$_{50}$) of the same T15 Id variant by both the monoclonal anti-Id and the T cells that is distinctive from the other reactivity patterns.

with monoclonal anti-idiotypes (Strickland et al. 1988). For example, the cell line T4-EF (Table 3) binds the immunoglobulin HPCM-6 very well, whereas HPCG-14 is bound poorly, and the 293 is not bound at all. HPCM-6 shares all idiotopes with TEPC15, HPCG-14 differs in five idiotopes and 293 differs in three, as shown by the analysis of these molecules with a panel of monoclonal anti-Id (Strickland et al. 1988). Indeed, it appears that the repertoire of certain T15-binding T cell lines is comparable to the particular monoclonal anti-T15 antibodies. In Table 4, the cell line T-9 binds the T15-variant immunoglobulins similarly, as does the monoclonal anti-T15 probe MaId 5-4. On the other hand, the cell lines T5-4 and T4-EF have binding profiles comparable to the anti-idiotopes B36-75 and B39-38. Collectively, these results suggest that the T cells bind the same V region epitopes as do monoclonal antibodies.

4. The proliferative responses of the T15-binding T cells to the T15$^+$ B cell, BCg3R-1d are shown in Fig. 5 and 6. The response is enhanced by addition of anti-CD3 antibody, and it is inhibitable equally well either with antibody to class II MHC molecules or with antibody to the T15 conformational idiotopes. However, the soluble T15 is unable to trigger the T cell proliferation (data not shown), even though it binds to the T cell receptor.

Based on the data summarized above, we speculate that the anti-Id T cells generated by stimulation with Id$^+$ B cells represent a unique phenotype that differs from the classical antigen-specific T cells. The majority of antigen-specific T cells recognize the foreign protein antigens as small peptide fragments generated from intracellular enzymatic breakdown ("processing"). The peptides are recognized by the T cells in complex with MHC-encoded glycoprotein on the surface of the presenting cells. In contrast, the anti-Id T cells generated with autologous B lymphocytes appear to recognize the intact immunoglobulins. Indeed, minor structural

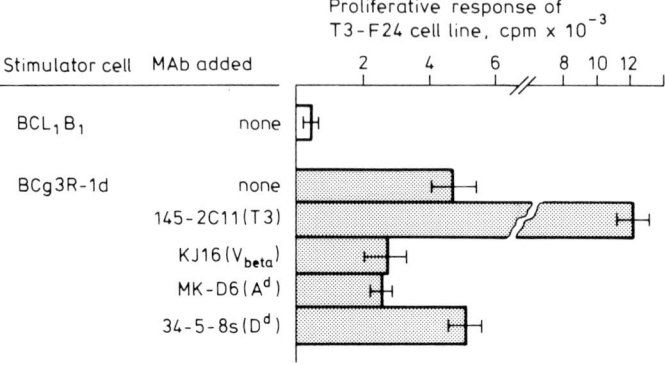

Fig. 5. Proliferative responses of T cell lines (10^4 cells/well) against irradiated, fixed stimulator cells (10^4/well) in a 3-day culture, measured by the uptake of ^{3}H-thymidine. The T cell responses were inhibited by addition of various monoclonal antibodies *(MAG)* into the culture media as shown

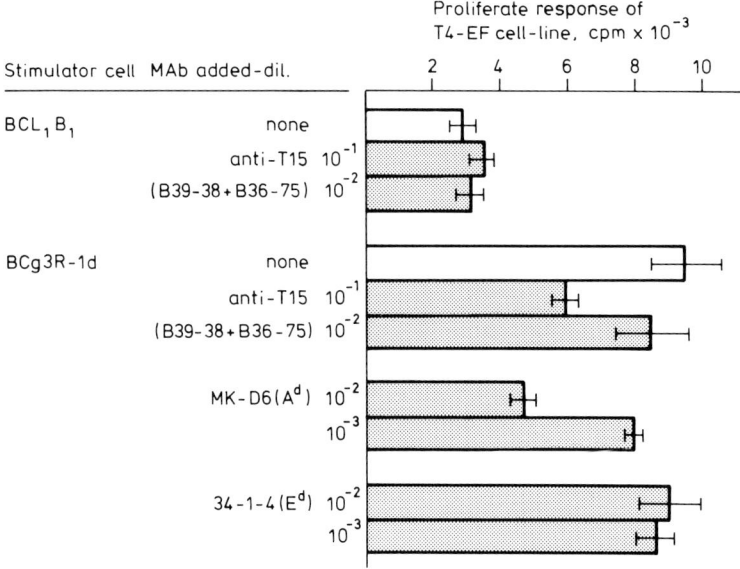

Fig. 6. Effect of different dilutions of monoclonal antibodies. See also Fig. 5

changes in the V domains of these immunoglobulins alter the recognition very dramatically. The full activation of these T cells does nonetheless require the recognition of class II molecules on the Id$^+$ B cell. This leads us to propose a working model of a T cell receptor that recognizes a complex of intact immunoglobulin with class II molecules on the B cell surface. Our preliminary data indicate that the presentation of the T15 idiotope with an inappropriate (allogeneic) class II molecule is not sufficient for the anti-Id T cell activation, but it inhibits specifically the response of these T cells to the self class II/T15 complex. The formal resolution of our working hypothesis will depend on our ability to clone the T cells.

The knowledgeable reader will point out that Id-reactive T cells previously isolated in two laboratories (Hannestad et al. 1986; Bogen et al. 1986) have been shown to recognize small peptide sequences from the V_L region in an MHC-restricted manner. However, these T cells were generated by immunization of mice with soluble Id^+ molecules. Under these circumstances, the immunoglobulins are apparently processed by the immune system in a manner similar to other proteins, and the resulting T cells fall under the paradigm of peptide recognition. Our T cell lines have been generated in a different manner. It seems reasonable to propose that the repertoire of Id-specific T cells depends on the manner of their activation.

Conclusion

The concept of immunological tolerance to self had undergone much alteration from its original form proposed in the 1940s and 1950s. Here I have discussed evidence suggesting that T cells may remain responsive to at least some of the self epitopes that are presented to them on the variable domains of immunoglobulins, and that such T cells may participate in the regulation of antibody response. Are these phenomena biologically important? One cannot be sure at this point, since the methodology of these experiments is highly artefactual. The field of tolerance is waiting for another genius who would bring us to a higher level of understanding with a solution as simple and elegant as was Hašek's original experiment with chicken embryos. How I wish it were possible to discuss my data with Milan Hašek again, to rely on his intuitive powers, and to draw encouragement from his ironic but kind comments. Alas, I am grown up now and on my own. And I must go on with my work hoping that at the end, Milan would not regret his telephone call to the Secretary of Health that started my life in immunology.

References

Abbas AK (1982) Immunologic regulation of lymphoid tumor cells: model system for lymphocyte functions. Adv Immunol 32: 301
Baker PJ (1975) Homeostatic control of antibody responses: a model based on the recognition of cell-associated antibody by regulatory T cells. Transplant Rev 26: 3
Bogen B, Malissen B, Haas W (1986) Idiotope-specific T cell clones that recognize syngeneic immunoglobulin fragments in the context of class II molecules. Eur J Immunol 16: 1373
Caulfield MJ, Luce KJ, Proffitt MR, Cerny J (1983) Induction of idiotype-specific suppressor T cells with antigen-antibody complex. J Exp Med 157: 1713
Cerny J (1984) Autologous idiotope-specific T cells in regulation of antibody response. In: Greene MI, Nisonoff A (eds) Biology of idiotypes. Plenum, New York, p 381
Cerny J, Caulfield MJ (1981) Stimulation of specific antibody-forming cells in antigen-primed nude mice by the adoptive transfer of syngeneic anti-idiotypic T cells. J Immunol 126: 2262
Cerny J, Cronkhite R, Stout JT (1986) Rapid changes in the regulatory potential of autologous anti-idiotopic T cells during an antigen-driven primary response. J Immunol 136: 3597
Cerny J, Smith JS, Webb C, Tucker PW (1988) Properties of anti-idiotypic T cell lines propagated with syngeneic B lymphocytes. I. T cells bind intact idiotypes and discriminate between somatic idiotypic variants in a manner similar to the anti-idiotopic antibodies. J Immunol 141: 3718

Eichmann K (1978) Expression of idiotypes on lymphocytes. Adv Immunol 26: 195

Hannestad K, Kristoffersen G, Briand JP (1986) The T lymphocyte response to syngeneic light chain idiotopes. Significance of individual amino acids revealed by variant chains and idiotope-mimicking chemically synthesized peptides. Eur J Immunol 16: 889

Janeway CA Jr, Sakato N, Eisen HN (1975) Recognition of immunoglobulin idiotypes by thymus-derived lymphocytes. Proc Natl Acad Sci USA 72: 2357

Jerne NK (1974) Toward a network theory of the immune system. Ann Immunol (Paris) 124C: 373

Kelsoe G, Cerny J (1979) Reciprocal expansion of idiotypic and anti-idiotypic clones following antigen stimulation. Nature 279: 333

Rajewsky K, Takemori T (1983) Genetics, expression and function of idiotypes. Ann Rev Immunol 1: 569

Strickland FM, Gleason JT, Cerny J (1988) Serologic and molecular characterization of the T15 idiotype. Mol Immunol 24: 637

Milan Hašek, Lymphokines and Retroviruses

M. Malkovský

In the Beginning

I will never forget, for many reasons, the moment I first met Milan Hašek. It was in 1972 when I attended (as an undergraduate student) a scientific meeting held at the "Dejvice" branch of the Institute of Experimental Biology and Genetics of the Czechoslovak Academy of Sciences in Prague (now the Institute of Molecular Genetics), the institute Milan Hašek founded. In one of the men's rooms of the Institute I met a tall man whom I thought I had never seen before. Nevertheless, he started to tell me a joke - talking to me as if to someone he had known for years: "There were two university students, one from Oxford and the second one from Cambridge, having done what we are doing now. The Oxford student says: 'We are taught in Oxford that after p***ing we should wash our hands.' The second student replies, 'Most interesting, but we are taught in Cambridge how not to p*** on our hands!'" At that time I did not have the slightest idea who the man was and how decisive my encounters with him would be.

I joined Milan's Institute as an undergraduate student in 1973, and in the years that followed we started to meet more frequently and became friends. After obtaining my MD and PhD degrees, I continued to work there as an "external employee" (paid by the Charles University) until 1981 when I moved to London. Two weeks after my arrival in London, I received my first message from Czechoslovakia. It was a postcard with a picture of Prague's old town with eight hand-written words. "*Alea iacta est* (the dice is cast). Good luck! Ever yours Milan."

Immunoregulation and Human Retroviruses

Mitogenic Signalling and Immunological Tolerance

In many experimental systems, mitogenic signals interfere with the establishment of immunological tolerance. For instance, interleukin-2 (IL-2), which participates in potent DNA synthesis-inducing signals in lymphocytes, impairs the induction and maintenance of acquired immunological unresponsiveness to alloantigens (Malkovský et al. 1984, 1985; Loveland et al. 1986; Irschick et al. 1986; Holáň 1987, 1988). Interestingly, the reactivity of tolerant cells against the tolerogen is re-established when they are exposed to IL-2 (Lehtonen et al. 1986; Essery et al. 1988).

It is noteworthy that IL-2 reverses unresponsiveness to mycobacterial antigens (Colizzi 1984), converts a stimulus causing unresponsiveness into an immunogenic stimulus (Colizzi et al. 1985) and overcomes *Ir* gene hyporesponsiveness (Kawamura et al. 1985). Blocking proliferation during T cell recognition of alloantigens by an inhibitor of IL-2 production (Malkovský et al. 1982) results in functional inactivation of antigen-specific T cells (Asherson et al. 1985), and antibodies against the IL-2 receptor (IL-2R) induce unresponsiveness (Kirkman et al. 1985; Kupiec-Weglinski et al. 1986; Diamantstein and Osawa 1986). Since the induction of T cell un-

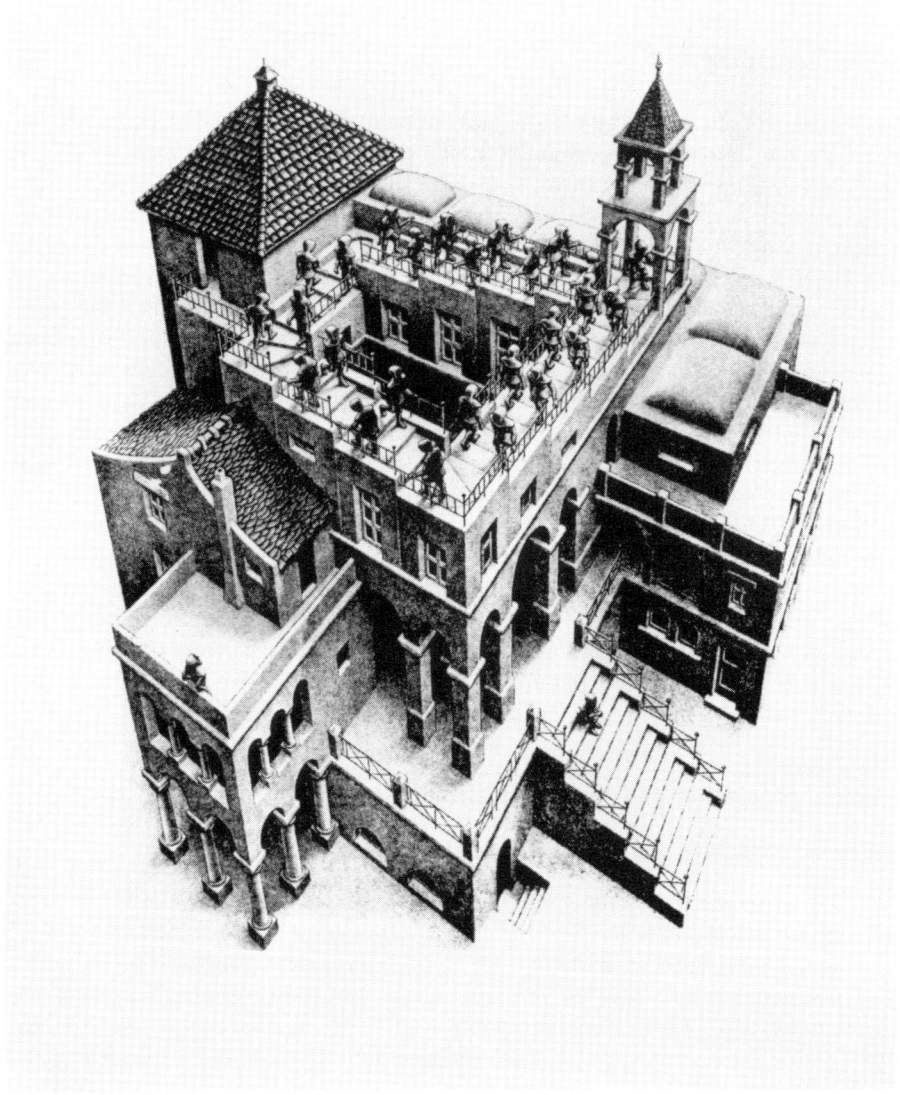

Fig. 1. Ascending and Descending by M.C. Escher (lithograph, 1960)

responsiveness has the same specificity as T cell activation (Jenkins and Schwartz 1987), it has been proposed that antigenic stimuli associated with insufficient IL-2 (nonmitogenic conditions) are tolerogenic, whereas the same stimuli are immunogenic if a sufficient amount of IL-2 (mitogenic conditions) is present (Malkovský and Medawar 1984; Malkovský 1987; de Boer and Hogeweg 1987).

However, it appears that IL-2 stimuli may not be potent enough to interfere with unresponsiveness in systems of "weak" antigens (Malkovský et al. 1986; Holáň 1989) and that some mitogenic antibodies can induce unresponsiveness (Tomonari 1988). Also, it is conceivable that additional signalling through CD2, CD3, CD4, CD8, CD11a, CD18, interleukin receptors, antigen receptors, etc. may be involved in keeping the balance between immunity and unresponsiveness. Indeed, preliminary results of J. Lamb and his colleagues (personal communication) indicate that the induction of unresponsiveness in some T cell clones can be abolished by IL-4. Moreover, various signals are capable of influencing each other, for example, signals through CD18 down-regulate signalling through CD3 (van Noesel et al. 1988), T cell receptors, and IL-2R (Malkovský 1988). A detailed analysis of various signalling pathways is now a major research priority, as the level of our understanding of the biological reasons for the seemingly "infinite" number of molecular activation signals and their interactions co-ordinating the "ascendent and descendent" phase of the immune response is not dissimilar to that of the reason for the illusively infinite walk of ascending and descending monks in Fig. 1.

Immunological and Antiviral Effects of Interferons

Interferons (IFNs) are involved in the regulation of various functional activities in many cell types (Pestka et al. 1987). We have studied their effects on induction of lymphokine (IL-2)-activated killer (LAK) activity, proliferation of lymphocytes, and virus yield. After incubation for 2-4 days with IL-2, purified lymphocytes show maximal LAK activity against various target cells as assessed by a 5-h ^{51}Cr release assay (Malkovský and Sondel 1987). Addition of exogenous IFN-α to cultures of lymphocytes plus IL-2 results in significant inhibition of LAK activity, but addition of IFN-γ has no effect (Fig. 2). Similarly, human immunodeficiency virus (HIV) replication in T cells was not impaired by the addition of IFN-γ, whereas it was blocked by addition of IFN-α (Fig. 3). Furthermore, IFN-γ potentiated, but IFN-α diminished, the proliferative response of lymphocytes to IL-2 (Table 1). We conclude that, in T cell systems, IFN-γ should not be regarded as an antiviral agent, but rather as a co-stimulator of T cell growth. It is pertinent to mention in this context that similar observations were made by Landolfo et al. (1988) in the mouse.

HIV, Its Receptor, and Anti-HIV Activity of Nonspecific Killer Cells

The CD4 molecule is an important constituent of the HIV receptor, and as yet no other relevant component has been demonstrated (Dalgleish and Malkovský 1988). However, the nature of the viral receptor merits further study, since the CD4 glycoprotein has not been detected on some HIV-infectable cells. This may

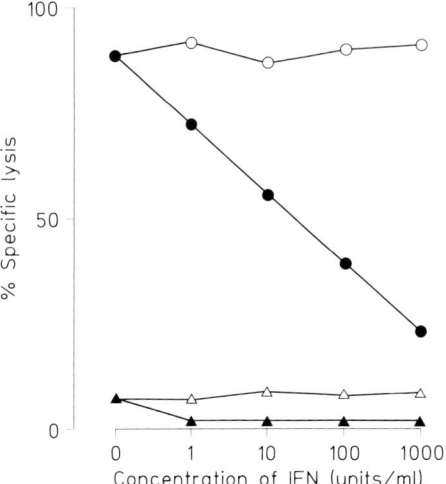

Fig. 2. Human peripheral blood mononuclear effector cells were depleted of monocytes and incubated (10^6 cells/ml) for 64 h in the absence *(triangles)* or presence *(circles)* of IL-2 (Biogen; 500 units/ml) and various concentrations of IFN [*open symbols*, IFN-γ (Biogen); *solid symbols*, IFN-α (Wellcome)] under standard conditions (Malkovský et al. 1987). The specific lysis of target cells was measured using a standard ^{51}Cr-release assay (Malkovský et al. 1983). Very similar data were obtained with different target cells. The figure illustrates a representative experiment using radiolabeled T24 target cells

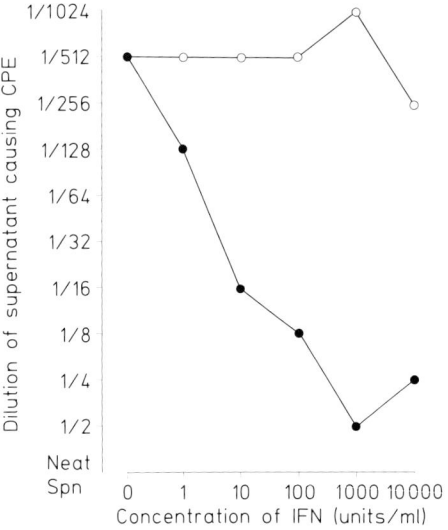

Fig. 3. Human peripheral blood lymphocytes were infected with the Ma isolate of HIV-1 (10^4 infectious units/ml), washed and incubated for 7 days (10^6 cells/ml) in the presence of IL-2 (50 units/ml) and in the absence or presence of various concentrations of IFN. The highest dilution of the resulting supernatants capable of inducing the cytopathic effect *(CPE)* on JM cells (2×10^5 cells/ml) was recorded. *Open circles*, IFN-γ; *solid circles*, IFN-α

Table 1. IL-2-induced DNA sythesis in lymphocytes: effects of IFNs

DNA synthetic response (cpm)[a]

Units/ml	IFN-α	IFN-γ
0	1200	1200
1	1000	1100
10	850	1250
100	600	1400
1000	300	2850
10000	250	900

[a] Human peripheral blood lymphocytes were stimulated with IL-2 (500 units/ml) in the absence or presence of various concentrations of IFN. A total of 10^5 cells were incubated in 96-well tissue culture plates in 0.2 ml RPMI 1640 medium supplemented as previously described (Malkovský et al. 1987). After 48 h, the cells were pulsed with ^{3}H-thymidine (0.5 µCi per well; 6 h) and the incorporation of tritiated thymidine was measured by liquid scintillation counting (Malkovský et al. 1982). The incorporation in the absence of IL-2 ranged between 100 and 200 cpm (with or without IFN-α) and between 200 and 450 cpm (with IFN-γ).

have important implications for HIV receptor-targeted prevention and therapy (Dalgleish et al. 1988).

Recently we have shown that HIV-infectable cells, which do not display surface CD4 detectable by conventional techniques, express low levels of CD4 mRNA (undetectable by Northern blotting but demonstrable using S1 nuclease analysis). Thus infection with HIV may be one of the most sensitive methods of revealing the CD4 positivity of human cells (Malkovský et al. 1988).

We have also found that, after infection with HIV in vitro, some natural killer (NK)-resistant cells become NK sensitive and their susceptibility to LAK cells increases (Malkovský et al. 1988). It is possible that HIV-infected cells which are accessible and susceptible to these nonspecific cytotoxic cells may be effectively eliminated in vivo. This could explain, at least in part, the presence of low numbers of virus-positive cells in the peripheral blood and other tissues of HIV-infected individuals and may be important for the pathogenesis of HIV-associated disorders.

Concluding Remarks

Since Milan's first message in 1981, our correspondence increased continuously, despite the fact that some of our letters never arrived and some were received after more than 2 months' delay. This was probably supposed to curtail the amount of information we exchanged, but it had quite the opposite effect. We wrote to each other more frequently (to check whether or not the previous letter had arrived) than we would otherwise have done and we also discovered "alternative pathways" (not strictly associated with complement activation) of how to get the message through the Iron Curtain. The last of Milan's letters, dated October 10, 1984, arrived on November 12, 1984. The letter was full of enthusiasm and plans for the future, but Milan probably never had a chance to read my reply which I wrote the same day. Two days later, on November 14, 1984, Milan Hašek passed away. When I finally accepted the idea that Milan was no longer among us, I realized more acutely than ever how vitally important to me were the times when my path crossed Milan's. What and where would many of us be without Milan's "injections" of enthusiasm, generosity, and wisdom? I wonder ...

References

Asherson GL, Colizzi V, Malkovský M, Colonna-Romano G, Zembala M (1985) The role of interleukin-2 as one of the determinants of the balance between immunity and unresponsiveness. Folia Biol (Praha) 31: 387-395

Colizzi V (1984) In vivo and in vitro administration of interleukin 2 containing preparation reverses T-cell unresponsiveness in *Mycobacterium bovis* BCG-infected mice. Infect Immun 45: 25-28

Colizzi V, Malkovský M, Lang G, Asherson GL (1985) In vivo activity of interleukin-2: conversion of a stimulus causing unresponsiveness to a stimulus causing contact hypersensitivity by the injection of interleukin-2. Immunology 56: 653-658

Dalgleish AG, Malkovský M (1988) Advances in human retroviruses. Adv Cancer Res 51: 307-360

Dalgleish AG, Kennedy RC, Sattentau Q, Chanh T, Beverley P, Maddon P, Axel R, Malkovský M (1988) The T4 molecule: its possible use in therapeutic strategies against AIDS. In: Bolognesi D (ed) Human retroviruses, cancer and AIDS: approaches to prevention and therapy. UCLA Symposia on molecular and cellular biology. Liss, New York, pp 283-288

de Boer RJ, Hogeweg P (1987) Immunological discrimination between self and non-self by precursor depletion and memory accumulation. J Theor Biol 124: 343-369

Diamantstein T, Osawa H (1986) The interleukin-2 receptor, its physiology and a new approach to a selective immunosuppressive therapy by anti-interleukin-2 receptor monoclonal antibodies. Immunol Rev 92: 5-27

Essery G, Feldmann M, Lamb JR (1988) Interleukin-2 can prevent and reverse antigen-induced unresponsiveness in cloned human T lymphocytes. Immunology 64: 413-417

Holáň V (1987) Successful induction of specific hyporeactivity to rat skin xenografts in newborn mice. Effect of immunoregulatory molecules. Transplantation 44: 809-812

Holáň V (1989) Modulation of allotransplantation tolerance induction by interleukin-1 and interleukin-2. J Immunogenet 15: 331-338

Irschick E, Niederwieser D, Spielberger M, Schönitzer D, Lochs A, Margreiter R, Huber C (1986) Acquired donor-specific CML unresponsiveness under cyclosporine treatment is reversible by exogenous IL-2. Transplant Proc 18: 1316-1318

Jenkins MK, Schwartz RH (1987) Antigen presentation by chemically modified splenocytes induces antigen-specific T cell unresponsiveness in vitro and in vivo. J Exp Med 165: 302-319

Kawamura H, Rosenberg SA, Berzofsky JA (1985) Immunization with antigen and interleukin-2 in vivo overcomes Ir gene low responsiveness. J Exp Med 162: 381-386

Kirkman RL, Barrett LV, Gaulton GN, Kelley VE, Ythier A, Strom TB (1985) Administration of anti-interleukin-2 receptor antibody prolongs cardiac allograft survival in mice. J Exp Med 162: 358-362

Kupiec-Weglinski JW, Diamantstein T, Tilney NL, Strom TB (1986) Therapy with monoclonal antibody to interleukin-2 receptor spares T suppressor cells and prevents or reverses acute allograft rejection in rats. Proc Natl Acad Sci USA 83: 2624-2627

Landolfo S, Gariglio M, Gribaudo G, Jemma C, Giovarelli M, Cavallo G (1988) Interferon-γ is not an antiviral, but a growth-promoting factor for T lymphocytes. Eur J Immunol 18: 503-509

Lehtonen L, Vainio O, Toivanen P (1986) Mechanisms of transplantation tolerance in B-cell-chimeric chickens: impairment of tolerance by T cell growth factor. Transplantation 42: 184-191

Loveland B, Hunt R, Malkovský M (1986) Autologous lymphoid cells exposed to recombinant interleukin-2 *in vitro* in the absence of antigen can induce the rejection of long-term tolerated skin allografts. Immunology 59: 159-161

Malkovský M (1987) Is T cell help involved in establishment of tolerance? Theory and experiment. In: Matzinger P, Flajnik M, Nemazee D, Rammensee HG, Rolink T, Stockinger G, Nicklin L (eds) Tolerance workshop 1986, Editiones Roche, Basle pp 73–79

Malkovský M, (1989) The relativity of immunological information. In: Aiuti F, Bonomo L, Danieli G (eds) Topics in immunology, Il Pensiero Scientifico, Roma, pp 1–7

Malkovský M, Medawar PB (1984) Is immunological tolerance (non-responsiveness) a consequence of interleukin-2 deficit during the recognition of antigen? Immunol Today 5: 340–343

Malkovský M, Sondel PM (1987) Interleukin-2 and its receptor: structure, function and therapeutic potential. Blood Rev 1: 254–266

Malkovský M, Asherson GL, Stockinger B, Watkins MC (1982) Nonspecific inhibitor released by T acceptor cells reduces the production of interleukin-2. Nature 300: 652–655

Malkovský M, Doré C, Hunt R, Palmer L, Chandler P, Medawar PB (1983) Enhancement of specific antitumour immunity in mice fed a diet enriched in vitamin A acetate. Proc Natl Acad Sci USA 80: 6322–6326

Malkovský M, Medawar P, Hunt R, Palmer L, Doré C (1984) A diet enriched in vitamin A acetate or in vivo administration of interleukin-2 can counteract a tolerogenic stimulus. Proc R Soc Lond [Biol] 220: 439–445

Malkovský M, Medawar PB, Thatcher DR, Toy J, Hunt R, Rayfield LS, Doré C (1985) Acquired immunological tolerance of foreign cells is impaired by recombinant interleukin-2 or vitamin A acetate. Proc Natl Acad Sci USA 82: 536–538

Malkovský M, Brenner MK, Hunt R, Rastan S, Doré C, North ME, Aherson GL, Prentice HG, Medawar PB (1986) T-cell depletion of allogenic bone marrow prevents acceleration of graft-versus-host disease induced by exogenous interleukin-2. Cell Immunol 103: 476–480

Malkovský M, Loveland B, North M, Asherson GL, Gao L, Ward P, Fiers W (1987) Recombinant interleukin-2 directly augments the cytotoxicity of human monocytes. Nature 325: 262–265

Malkovský M, Philpott K, Dalgleish AG, Mellor AL, Patterson S, Webster ADB, Edwards AJ, Maddon PJ (1988) Infection of B lymphocytes by the human immunodeficiency virus and their susceptibility to cytotoxic cells. Eur J Immunol 18: 1315–1321

Pestka S, Langer JA, Zoon KC, Samuel CE (1987) Interferons and their actions. Annu Rev Biochem 56: 727–777

Tomonari K (1988) Downregulation of the T-cell receptor by a mitogenic anti-Thy-1 antibody. Eur J Immunol 18: 179–182

van Noesel C, Miedema F, Brouwer M, de Rie MA, Aarden LA, van Lier RAW (1988) Regulatory properties of LFA-1 α and β chains in human T-lymphocyte activation. Nature 333: 850–852

Genetic Requirements for Interactions Between Cells for Murine Islet Allograft Rejection.
Class I and Class II Antigens in Mouse Islet Rejection

V. Hauptfeld-Dolejsek

Since I came to the United States I have been working on the *H-2* system, the major histocompatibility complex (MHC) of mouse. I was very fortunate to start in the center of activity, in Jan Klein's laboratory. It fills me with a special pride and joy that it was during my stay in his laboratory that we were one of several groups to discover immune response-associated (Ia) antigens. The finding of Ia antigens, later named class II antigens, presented us with enormous research opportunities.

In the following years I broadened my horizons by crossing the entire United States from the far north, Ann Arbor, Michigan, to the deep south, Dallas, Texas – where I received the greatest joy of all, my daughter. I finally settled in the Midwest, on the Mississippi River, so well known to me from Tom Sawyer's adventures. And it is Saint Louis, the symbolic gate to the west, where I have spent the last 10 years.

During these years I have pursued the goal of helping to define the structure and function of the *H-2* complex gene products. Many a year has been spent producing new intra-*H-2* recombinants, a powerful tool in helping to answer these questions. The antisera, produced by the use of these recombinants, were basically used in three different ways. First, to characterize all new strains and draw a more precise map of the *H-2* complex. Second, to correlate the presence of MHC molecules on the surface of cells with their known function. Third, to investigate the presence, or equally importantly the absence, of MHC molecules on individual cells, tissue, and organs, especially those of importance in transplantation. It is the results of this third group of experiments which are described here.

The two types of genes within the MHC are the immune response genes coding for dimeric polypetides (I-A and I-E, class II) and the genes coding for the single-chain glycoprotein transplantation antigens (K and D class I). Both classes of antigens are important in transplantation immunity and in immune response in general.

Many attempts had been made to transplant organs such as kidney, heart, thyroid, pancreas, islets of Langerhans, skin, etc. Many of these tissues had defied attempts to transplant them even though a variety of pretreatments had been tried to prolong allograft survival. There are basically two kinds of pretreatment. One is of the recipient, using a wide variety of agents such as antilymphocytic serum (ALS), immunossuppressive drugs, and, lately quite successfully, lymphokines. The other type of pretreatment is of donor or the graft. One of the most successful pretreatments of the graft tissue was devised by Lafferty et al. (1975) for thyroid and con-

Table 1. Effect of pretreatment of islets with antibody directed to Ia determinants on islet allograft survival

Group	Donor-recipient	Islet treatment	Individual transplant survival[a] (days)
1	B6–B6	None	>200, >200, >200, >200, >200
2	B10.BR–B6	None	5, 5, 6, 6, 8, 12, 135, 139, >200, >200
3	B10.BR–B6	$\alpha I^k + C$	>200, >200, >200, >200, >200
4	B10.BR–B6	$\alpha I^s + C$	6, 8, 10, 28, >200

[a] Transplant survival was determined by plasma glucose levels. Rejection of transplanted islets was considered to have occurred when individual serum glucose levels were >250 mg/100 ml for three consecutive bleedings.
C, complement.

sists in culturing the tissue in vitro for several days in the presence of high levels of oxygen. This method was applied to pancreatic islet transplants with equal success by Lacy's group. The marked prolongation of survival achieved by this treatment across the MHC barrier was attributed to the diminished amount of passenger lymphocytes.

Since lymphocytes bear class I and the majority of them also class II antigens, and we also know that the MHC antigens play a crucial role in the allograft rejection, we set out to investigate what, if any, MHC-encoded antigens are on cells of Langerhans, namely on β cells.

Islets were isolated from the pancreas by collagenase, separated from other tissue on a Ficoll gradient and hand picked. A single-cell suspension was obtained by treatment with Dispase (Godo Shusei Ltd., Tokyo, Japan) and allowed to recover for 6–24 h prior to testing.

Three strains were used to investigate the presence of MHC molecules: A/J, B10.AKM and BALB/c. By cytotoxicity test, class I antigens, K and D, were readily detectable, whereas the anti-Ia sera remained negative. After ruling out the possibility that the lack of Ia expression might be due to Dispase treatment, we came to the conclusion, that β cells of Langerhans do not bear class II antigens. This finding defined a completely new approach for the transplantation of islets.

As mentioned before, results from Lafferty et al. (1975) and Lacy's group made us believe that passenger lymphocytes are those responsible for the graft rejection. Since β cells do not carry class II antigens, we treated freshly prepared islets with anti-Ia serum and complement to remove Ia$^+$ cells. The results are summarized in Table 2. B6 mice were made diabetic by injection of streptozotocin and, when their plasma glucose levels were about 400 mg/dl, they were transplanted with 550–750 B10.BR islets into the portal vein. Mice transplanted with syngeneic islets (group 1) and with anti-Ia^k plus complement-treated islets (group 3) became normoglycemic and remained that way for the observation period of 200 days. The majority of the animals which received untreated islets (group 2) or islets treated with irrelevant serum (group 4), acutely rejected the allograft. Surprisingly, in both control groups one to two mice did not reject their grafts. We attributed this to the picking and repicking of islets under the green light, therefore eliminating the lymph nodes from the preparation.

Table 2. Effect of RBC pretransplant immunizations on islet allograft survival

Group	Pretransplant Treatment	B10.BR($H-2^k$) transplant survival in B6($H-2^b$)[a] (days)
1	RBC $H-2^{k^b}$	16, 16, >100 (×10)
2	RBC $H-2^s$	7, 7, 7, 13, >100
3	Whole blood $H-2^k$	2, 2, 2, 2, 2, 3, 3, 3, 5
4	None	5, 5, 6, 6, 8, 12, 35, 39, >100, >100

[a] See Table 1.
[b] Erythrocytes were obtained by treating the whole blood with anti-Ia^k (group 1), anti-Ia^s (group 2) plus complement.

Our success in the transplantation of grafts after eliminating Ia-bearing cells without the need to immunosuppress the recipient was very encouraging, especially because the ultimate goal is to apply the procedures to humans.

Although we were quite sure that the acceptance of the graft was due to the elimination of Ia-bearing cells rather than some alteration of the β cell surface, we wanted to prove it. We took two mice with an accepted islet allograft, one at 80 days and one at 100 days post-transplantation and injected them with 10×10^6 splenocytes of the donor haplotype. The blood glucose levels went up a little bit, fluctuated, and went down again. However, the second injection of 50×10^6 splenocytes initiated the rejection of the islets. Therefore, the islets bearing class I antigens, although incapable of stimulating the allograft rejection by themselves, serve as a target for ongoing response.

What was really surprising was the large dose that was needed to elicit the rejection, more than 10×10^6 lymphocytes, whereas very few lymphocytes are sufficient to cause rejection when transplanted simultaneously with islets. This result points toward an active mechanism in graft acceptance, probably by acquired tolerance through active suppression.

To test our conclusion, we decided to try to induce the tolerance by injection of class I-bearing, class II nagative cells to see if this treatment would permit the successful transplantation of fresh, untreated islets. B6 recipients received three injections, prior to transplantation of islets, of either RBC, where whole blood was treated with anti-Ia serum and complement or whole blood. As seen in Table 2, injection of RBC of the same haplotype as the islet transplant assured the islet survival for more than 100 days. Mice which received an injection of RBC from an irrelevant haplotype (B10.S, group 2), rejected the graft with the same speed as control mice (group 4). The immunization with whole blood resulted in sensitization of the recipient and accelarated islet allograft rejection. Apparently, the immunization with class I-bearing cells rendered mice tolerant.

To investigate if mice are tolerant in a haplotype-specific manner we challenged those mice which remained normoglycemic for more than 200 days with two skin grafts - one of the islet donor haplotype, B10.BR, and one of a third haplotype, B10.S (Table 3). All ten mice bearing established islet allografts (group 1) expressed markedly prolonged survival (18-23 days) of donor skin grafts, but promptly rejected the third party, B10.S, skin grafts. Six of the ten mice

Table 3. Effect of established islet allografts[a] on skin allograft rejection

Group (B6 recipients)	n	Transfusion with RBC (B10.BR)[b]	Transplantation with donor islets (B10.BR)	Skin graft survival		Islet graft survival 23 days after skin graft[c]
				B10.BR (days)	B10.S (days)	
1	10	+	+	> 23	12	Survived
				> 23	13	Survived
				> 23	12	Survived
				> 23	12	Survived
				> 23	18	Survived
				> 23	11	Survived
				23	12	Rejected
				22	15	Survived
				20	10	Rejected
				18	11	Rejected
				mean > 22,2	12.8	
2	5	+	0	10.2	ND	
3	7	0	0	10.9	ND	
4	5	0	0	ND	13.0	
5	7	0	0	12.9	12.9	

[a] Animals used for skin grafts were more than 200 days after islet transplantation.
[b] see Table 2.
[c] Serum glucose at 23 days after skin graft; survived = 81–205 mg/dl; rejected = 433–501 mg/dl.
ND, not determined.

showed no signs of rejection of either skin or islet B10.BR grafts. However, four mice rejected the skin grafts and three of them also rejected islet grafts. All the mice with long-term survival failed to produce donor-specific B10.BR antibodies. Thus, it appears that, in some animals, donor skin grafts are capable of stimulating delayed allograft rejection responses, and, when these responses are stimulated, both islets and skin are usually rejected. It also seems that the presence of the islet allograft is very important in the development or maintenance of the tolerance, as the only group which received an islet graft after the RBC injection had prolonged skin graft survival (group 1 vs. group 2).

Our results were in agreement with other reports that stable, long-term transplants specifically prolong the survival of a secondary graft of the same donor strain. However, one report seemingly contradicted our findings. Bach's group in Wisconsin (Morrow et a. 1983a) used intra-*H-2* recombinants to address the question regarding the influence of class I and class II antigens in the rejection of a mouse pancreatic islet allograft. They found that disparities in K alone or D alone as well K + D were sufficient to elicit graft rejection. On the other hand, grafts from animals differing in the I region were accepted in the vast majority of cases. They, too, decided to ask the question regarding the mechanism by which an allograft is accepted.

Using intra-*H-2* recombinants as in the original study, they pretreated islets with anti-Ia antibody. About 100 days after successful transplantation, recipients were challenged with a skin graft of the donor haplotype. They found an acceleration of skin graft rejection in all groups, which in many cases was accompanied by rejection of the established islet allograft. The major difference between our experimental protocol and that of Morrow et al. (1983b) was the duration that the islet allografts resided in the host. Tolerance was not seen in their animals bearing allografts for 100 days, but was clearly evident in our mice that had allografts for 200 days. In addition, they did not use complement in conjunction with the antibody. It is quite feasible that there were Ia$^+$ cells remaining, not enough to trigger cytotoxic response alone but, judging from a second set kinetics of skin graft rejection, the immune response had already been initiated, or at least helper T (T_H) cells had been activated.

Our observations that class I antigens are not sufficient to generate allograft response were not only in disagreement with the results of Morrow et al., but also with the well-known fact that one can generate mixed lymphocyte reaction (MLR) as well as cell-mediated lympholysis (CML) against class I antigens. So, what is the difference? In our system, using islet transplants after anti-Ia antiserum and complement treatment, we do not have any class II antigens. Therefore we conclude that class II antigens, whether syngeneic to a recipient or not, present class I.

To investigate the genetic requirements for interactions between class I and class II molecules in the initiation of islet allograft rejection, we used our experimental protocol, i.e., elimination of Ia-bearing cells with anti-Ia plus complement. Donor B10.BR (H-2^k) islets were treated with anti-Ia^k serum (A.TH anti-A.TL) plus complement and implanted into the portal vein of C57BL/6J (H-2^b) recipients that had previously been made diabetic by treatment with streptozotocin. At 21 days, normoglycemic, allograft-bearing mice were challenged with splenocytes from various intra-H-2 recombinant haplotypes selected in such a way as to share different regions of the H-2 complex with the H-2^k islet allografts. The challenge dose which would be sufficient to cause rejection of the islet grafts at 21 days was determined with B10.BR cells. The dose chosen was 10×10^6, although 5×10^6 B10.BR cells was sufficient to initiate rejection (Table 4, group 1). Cells from the B10.BR (H-2^k) strain and from H-2^k recombinant strains B10.AM (K^k, A^k, E^k, D^b) initiated rejection of previously accepted B10.BR islet allografts (Table 4, groups 1, 3). Cells from B10.MBR (K^b, I^k, D^q; group 4) and B10.TBR3 (K^s, A^k, E^b, D^b; not shown) had no effect on the survival of the graft. However, as we expected, B10.OL (K^d, A^d, E^d, D^k) cells initiated the rejection of B10.BR islets.

The findings allow us to draw several conclusions. First, β cells of Langerhans, which lack class II antigens, do not alone initiate a cellular response against the class I (K/D) antigens which they carry. Second, to supply cells bearing donor class II antigens without the proper (donor) class I antigens is not sufficient to initiate an immune response. This is clearly demonstrated by the inability of B10.MBR (K^b, I^k, D^q) cells to initiate rejection of H-2-K^k or H-2-D^k target cells. Third, cells bearing *any* class II antigens with appropriate (graft donor) class I will initiate an anti-class I-specific response as seen with B10.OL cells (K^d, I^d, D^d), which will cause rejection of an appropriate class I-bearing graft. Thus, class I antigens are the molecules which serve as targets in this system.

The question remains as to what the target molecule is in the case in which intra-H-2 recombinants differing only in the I region are chosen as the recipient-donor combination. Results obtained from such experiments vary greatly depending

Table 4. Effect of injection of splenocytes or erythrocytes 21–24 days after successful islet transplantation on subsequent islet allograft survival: (B10.BR) [H-2^k] to B6 [H-2^b]

Group	Splenocyte injection	Individual survival after challenge (days)
1	1×10^7 B10.BR	14, 14, 17, 21, 49
2	No splenocytes	$7 \times >200$
3	B10.AM (K^k, A^k, E^k, D^b)	14, 14, 14, 23, 36
4	B10.MBR (K^b, A^k, E^k, D^q)	$5 \times > 150$
5	B10.OL (K^d, A^d, E^d, D^k)	45, 48, 89, 140
6	5×10^7 B10.BR erythrocytes (K^k, D^k)	$>200, >200$
7	1×10^7 B10.BR erythrocytes (K^k, D^k)	$>185, >185, >158, >158, >158$
8	Control mice transplanted with untreated allogeneic islets	5, 6, 8, 10, 22, 38, $>100, >100$

In groups 3–5 recipients received 1×10^7 cells. In groups 6, 7 the whole blood was depleted of Ia-bearing cells by a treatment with anti-Ia^k and complement.

on the organ chosen as well as the haplotype combination. If class II antigens do not serve as a target, then these differences might be explained by varying tissue distributions of class I antigens, including class I other than classical K/D in different organs. The involvement of class I antigens other than K/D would explain results by Okazaki et al. (1981), in which they were unable to induce tolerance to skin grafts across KI region differences with purified erythrocyte populations. Erythrocytes carrying K/D antigens could induce tolerance to K/D antigens, but not to any other antigens involved in the skin graft rejections.

Our success in the induction of tolerance for β cells of Langerhans by erythrocytes or ultraviolet-irradiated splenocytes (Agostino et al. 1984) indicates that β cells do not carry any class I antigens that erythrocytes do not.

Okazaki et al. (1981) induced tolerance toward skin grafts by injecting whole blood. Their success in initiating tolerance might be more proof that, in the case of whole blood-skin graft combinations, only one of two required antigens was present (Ia$^+$ K/D$^-$) to initiate an immune response. Recent data by Caughman et al. (1986), showing that murine epidermal dendritic (Langerhans) cells are quite deficient in K/D expression, support this notion and suggest that we should look more broadly at the mechanisms involved in interactions between class II and class I antigens, e.g., Qa, that lead to immune response or tolerance.

Reflections. When I first went to the Institute of Experimental Biology and Genetics of the Czechoslovak Academy of Sciences in 1965, I was a student from Charles University looking for a place to do my PhD thesis. The director of the Institute was Professor Milan Hašek, an outstanding scientist, whose work on transplantation tolerance was well known throughout the world. As I learned later, it was through his efforts that the Institute of Experimental Biology and Genetics was founded. His enormous energy and enthusiasm were felt everywhere. It seems almost incomprehensible that he was able to attend all seminars and progress reports, even those given by numerous students. Although he was world-renowned scientist, he never had a word of harsh criticism or expression of depreciation toward a student, a total novice in the field.

His reputation attracted many bright young people, and soon the Institute became internationally renowned by its most distinctive contributions in immunology, particularly in transplantation immunology. Beside the pioneering work on immunological tolerance by Hašek, Lengerová, and Hraba, many prominent geneticists and immunologists were emerging. The Institute of Experimental Biology and Genetics, recently renamed as the Institute of Molecular Biology, became known for the progressive work in the production of mouse strains, inbred dog strains, pioneering work in the transplantation of kidneys in dogs as well as in tumor immunology, to name but a few well-known projects. I am very proud that I was able to receive my scientific training in the Institute in which everything was so much influenced by the spirit of Milan Hašek. I hope that some of that enthusiasm and dedication to the work has rubbed off on me.

Acknowledgement. We wish to thank Evelyne Dye, Susan Bassett-Chu, and Pat Talley for their excellent technical assistance and Valerie Mays for expert typing of the manuscript. The research part of this communication was performed together with Denise Faustman, Reiji Terasaka, Paul E. Lacy (Department of Pathology), J. M. Davie (Department of Microbiology), and Donald C. Shreffler (Department of Genetics). The work was supported by NIH grants AI 12734 and AM 01226.

References

Agostino M, Prowse SJ, Lafferty KJ (1984) Induction of tolerance using ultraviolet-irradiated cells. Transplantation Proceedings XVI: 959–960
Caughman SW, Sharrow SO, Shimada S, Stephany D, Mizuochi T, Rosenberg AS, Katz Si, Singer A (1986) Ia$^+$ murine epidermal Langerhans cells are deficient in surface expression of the class I major histocompatibility complex. Proc Natl Acad Sci USA 83: 7438–7442
Lafferty K, Cooley M, Woolnough J, Walker K (1975) Thyroid allograft immunogenicity is reduced after a period in organ culture. Science 188: 259–261
Morrow CE, Sutherland DER, Steffers MW, Najarian JS, Bach FH (1983a) H-2 antigen class: effect on mouse islet allograft rejection. Science 219: 1337–1339
Morrow CE, Sutherland DER, Steffers MW, Najarian JS, Back FH (1983b) Lack of donor-specific tolerance in mice with established anti-Ia-treated islet allografts. Transplantation 36: 691–694
Okazaki H, Maki T, Wood ML, Jones S, Monaco AP (1981) Prolongation of skin allograft survival in H-2 K and I region-incompatible mice by pretransplant blood transfusion. Transplantation 32: 111–115

Chicken Major Histocompatibility Complex and Its Role in Disease

K. Hála

Introduction

I have the privilege of being one of the most recent emigrés of our group. I left the Prague Institute of Molecular Genetics (the successor of the Institute of Experimental Biology and Genetics) in August 1980, just a few hours before the 12th anniversary of August 1968. I had two reasons for my late farewell party. First, I (intentionally) missed the train in 1968 as I was hoping that the old atmosphere at the Institute would stay for ever. It took 1 or 2 years after a sabatical year in Copenhagen to realise that I was naive. Secondly, it took me many years to get out with my whole family.

O tempora, o mores. The first time I met Milan was in 1955, when I was a young student in my fourth semester at the biological faculty. At the beginning of our meeting, he asked Mrs. Zikesova, his secretary, for two coffees. The second shock was that Milan discussed with me a book about genetics written by my faculty professor of genetics. He had received this book for review and at the time he was very critical of some of the genetic concepts put forward in the book. I was very impressed to be able to participate, as a student, in an afternoon's discussions.

Under Milan's supervision I prepared the work for my diploma which was about tolerance to red blood cells, and my dissertation about chicken inbred lines and MHC. Milan was my teacher, my friend, and later my director. All those years when I was together with Milan are still in my memory, the time in the department, the exponential growth of the Institute and at the end the chain of changes culminating in the changed name of the Institute with a new director. This is not nostalgia for a youth that is nearly gone, but recognition of the special time in our old Institute. Milan, many thanks!

Chicken MHC and Its Role in Disease

Structure of Chicken MHC

Chicken MHC, first described as a blood group system by Briles et al. (1950), is composed of at least three (B) regions, which code for the corresponding F, L and G antigens or antigenic complexes. Class I is represented by the B-F antigen, present on the majority of somatic cells and all peripheral blood lymphocytes

(PBL) and erythrocytes (RBC). The class II antigen is B-L, which is present on the majority of bursal cells, bursa-dependent PBL and cells of the monocyte-macrophage series and activated T lymphocytes. The B-G antigen is unique to the chicken and is restricted to the membrane of RBC and their progenitors (Hála et al. 1981). The presence of class III antigens in chicken MHC is still very controversial.

The molecular weight and biochemical characteristics of class I and II antigens are very similar to mammalian MHC antigens (Pink et al. 1977; Wolf et al. 1984).

The genetic organisation of chicken MHC was elucidated in 1976 with the first description of a recombination event (Hála et al. 1976). In this and subsequent recombinants (for review see Hála et al. 1988), the recombination events have taken place between the B-G region on one hand and the B-F/B-L regions on the other hand or within the B-G region (in so-called Briles recombinants). With the aid of molecular biological methods it was shown that the B complex does not contain well-defined class I and class II regions since B-F and B-Lβ genes are tightly linked with unrelated genes. Out of four DNA clusters covering 320 kb chicken MHC, which contained class IIβ genes, in two clusters B-Lβ genes were closely linked to class I genes and in one DNA cluster to the nucleolar organiser region (Guillemot et al. 1988). This might explain why the search for recombination between B-F and B-L regions has so far been unsuccessful, even when using serological typing together with additional methods such as in vitro mixed lymphocyte reaction (MLR) and restriction fragment length polymorphism (RFLP) (Hála et al. 1988).

The Expression of MHC Antigens During Ontogenesis and Functional Analysis of MHC Antigen-Bearing Cells

The B-G antigen can be detected on RBC from day 6 of embryonal life, and the level remains constant throughout the life of the chicken. The B-L antigen is present on cells of the bursa of Fabricius as early as the 10th day of embryogenesis (Hála et al. 1981). The B-F antigen is first detected after hatching. The percentage of B-F-positive PBL and bursa cells increases up to 9 days after hatching. By 2 weeks after hatching almost 100% of the RBC, PBL and bursa cells were positive, whereas the thymus showed only 20% positive cells. These were found mainly in the medulla, the cortex was negative. The graft-versus-host reaction (GVHR) of these subpopulations of thymus cells was compared after sorting by the fluorescence-activated cell sorter (FACS). The splenomegaly in MHC-incompatible embryos was associated primarily with the B-F positive cell population. Double staining studies with peanut agglutinin and monoclonal antibody anti-B-F proved that the peanut-negative thymocytes were identical with B-F-positive thymocytes (Sgonc et al. 1987).

Nomenclature of Chicken MHC Haplotypes

With the development of different inbred lines and detailed characterization of a few special lines it was possible to change the nomenclature. Formerly the name of the haplotype was based on the reactivity of RBC with the panel of alloantisera.

The new nomenclature for chicken MHC, the result of the workshop held at the Institute for General and Experimental Pathology (Innsbruck, Austria) has been established on the basis of reference populations (Briles et al. 1982). The reference strain designations are intended to guard against possible future ambiguity in haplotype nomenclature. Therefore inbred or particularly well-studied lines have been selected for reference where possible. The additional aims of the workshop were to compare the MHC haplotypes present in chicken flocks in different parts of Europe and North America. Altogether 27 distinct haplotypes were accepted and defined by the standard or reference chicken strains.

Function of MHC

The role of chicken MHC for immunology has recently been reviewed (Toivanen and Toivanen 1987); therefore, we will limit ourselves to two specific points: MHC and spontaneous autoimmune thyroiditis, and regression of Rous sarcoma virus (RSV)-induced tumours.

Spontaneous Autoimmune Thyroiditis (SAT) in Obese Strain (OS) Chickens

The OS chicken is a good animal model for human Hashimoto thyroiditis. The first phenotypically "obese", i.e. clinically hypothyroid, chickens of small body size with subcutaneous fat deposits and long silky feathers were identified in 1956 by Cole at Cornell Veterinary College, Ithaca, New York, within a closed colony of the Cornell C strain (CS) of White Leghorns. After 14 generations of selective breeding, the OS was established with more than 99% animals (both males and females) developing autoantibodies to thyroglobulin (Tg-AAb) as well as mononuclear infiltration of the thyroid gland. At present, quantitative differences in the onset of the infiltration, in the degree of SAT, and in the titre of Tg-AAb are being observed (for review see Wick et al. 1981, 1982, 1987).

As in humans and mice, there is a close association between the MHC type and the development of SAT disease. Bacon et al. (1974) first observed a correlation of the severe SAT with the B^{13} haplotype in the OS, while the B^5 haplotype was associated with very mild disease. However, in our colony of OS, which had been separated from the America OS animals for at least 5 years (Wick et al. 1979), the B^5 haplotype, together with B^{13}, was also associated with severe SAT (Table 1), whereas the B^{15} haplotype was associated with very mild disease.

Table 1. Association between the haplotype of MHC and severity of SAT[a]. (Partly from Wick et al. 1982)

Haplotype nomenclature (Briles et al 1982)	Lines	Bacon et al. (1974)	Bacon (1976)	Bacon et al. (1977)	Wick et al. (1979)
B^{13}	OS	+ + + +	+ +	+ + + +	+ + + +
B^{15}	OS	NT	+ + + +	NT	+
B^5	OS	+	±	+[b]	+ + + +

[a] Arbitrary grading of severity of thyroiditis (±, +, + +, + + +, + + + +).
[b] Occasional B^4B^4 chicks developed severe (+ + + +) thyroiditis.
NT, not tested.

By mean of serological analysis and GVHR only three haplotypes, namely B^5, B^{13} and B^{15}, were shown to be segregating within OS chickens. Histocompatibility and blood group antigens were used as the criteria for genetic heterogeneity of OS animals. From the results obtained, we conclude that chickens of our own OS colony segregate in at least some histocompatibility loci (mean survival time of transferred skin grafts was 18.5 days, 4.3 ± SD) and in most blood group loci. Selection for SAT apparently does not render them homozygotic in histocompatibility and blood group loci (Hála 1988).

The genetic background of the disease was analysed by means of cross-breeding experiments. From previous work by other authors it can be assumed that the development of SAT is under the control of several genes which segregate within healthy populations of normal White Leghorns, but with such a low frequency that the probability of their accumulation in one single animal, with resulting disease, is very low. Since there are at present no means of identifying these genes directly, we could only detect their effect via the assessment of the disease. To avoid complications due to undetectable differences between animals from different families and generations, we selected the inbred line CB as a reference line. From the analysis of F1 and F2 hybrids and animals from backcross generations with both CB and OS parental lines, we concluded that SAT is a multigenic trait regulated by about five genes (Neu et al. 1985, 1986).

In summary, two important results emerge from our experiments:

1. The existence of animals with a high titre of Tg-AAb but without significant lymphoid infiltration of the thyroid. These animals are healthy and show no symptoms of autoimmune disease (Neu et al. 1986).
2. It was possible to induce lymphoid infiltration of the thyroid glands by passive transfer of Tg-AAb in a certain number of animals of the backcross generation (OS × CB) F1 hybrids with OS (Neu et al. 1985).

These results indicate that we are dealing with two independent events, the reactivity of the immune system against autoantigens regulated by one family of genes and the susceptibility of the target organ(thyroid) to the attack of an autoreactivity of the immune system, coded by a second gene family. According to our concept, there are qualitative differences among genes controlling SAT. Genes that are an absolute prerequisite for the development of the disease are called "major genes". Those which are not able to induce the disease themselves but under special conditions are capable of modulating the action of the major genes are called "minor genes" (Fig. 1). These genes are especially important in animals with an incomplete set of major genes. MHC genes play an important role in outbred populations, but they are not a prerequisite for the development of the disease. Fully developed, early onset SAT is only seen in an animal where all major genes are present. Further analysis is, however, needed to confirm this assumption.

Regression of RSV-Induced Tumours
RSV-induced tumours in chickens, using subcutaneous inoculation of virus, either progress and kill the host or grow for some weeks and than regress. Progression and regression are under the control of one or more genes associated with the MHC. Because the mechanism of regression is immunological, we have examined

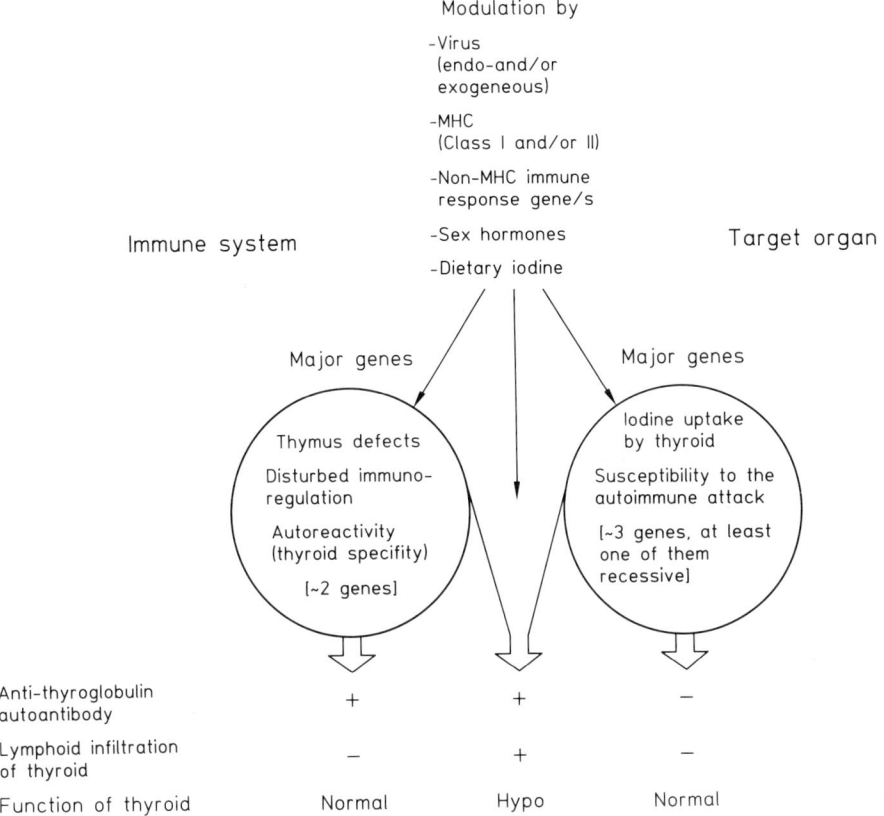

Fig. 1. Reactivity of the immune system against autoantigens and susceptibility of the target organ to the attack of an autoreactivity of the immune system

the cells within Rous sarcomas for the expression of B-L antigens that are coded for by chicken MHC class II genes regulating immune response to some antigens.

For the analysis we used direct or indirect immunofluorescence on unfixed cryostat sections from regressing and progressing Rous sarcomas. For the test we used monoclonal antibodies to B-L that react with a common nonpolymorphic epitope of that antigen and alloantisera to B-L4 and B-L12 antigens, expressed in the congenic lines CB and CC.

Altogether 40 9-week-old chickens were inoculated with 100 focus-forming units of virus in the left wing web. Tumours were visible about 10 days after inoculation and they continued to progress for about 4 weeks in all the chickens. Thereafter, tumour growth was progressive in all CC animals and in four CB chickens. In the remaining 24 CB chickens the tumours regressed completely by the 8th week (Table 2). Sarcoma cells in regressing tumours expressed B-L antigens both in the vicinity of foci of mononuclear infiltrates, but also in uninfiltrated areas. The tumour cells from progressing sarcomas were negative (Powell et al. 1987).

Table 2. Relationship between regression of RSV-induced tumours and expression of class II antigens

Line	n	RSV-induced tumours			
		Regression		Progression	
		Class II antigen		Class II antigen	
		+	−	+	−
CB	28	24	0	0	4
CC	12	0	0	0	12

It is not clear which factor/s are responsible for induction of B-L antigen expression on tumour cells from regressing Rous sarcoma or whether the appearance of the antigen precedes, follows or is a coincidence with the extensive lymphoid infiltration in these tumours.

Working and Living Abroad

This is a difficult question for me, for the simple reason: that coming from Prague to Vienna ist not going abroad. The last few centuries of joint development brought the same architecture (National Museum), the same culture (Kokoschka and Kafka), the same inventors (Ressl) and scientists (Mendel) and of course the same food (including *Knödel*) to both nations. Almost the only difference, especially for my generation raised during the war, is language because German is a foreign language for us.

And my experiences at my new permanent address? It was a dream, as I did not expect such a level of solidarity. For instance, the director of Charitas was happy to use money in Austria instead of sending it to Africa. The Catholic Church and, last but not least, all our colleagues at the Institute helped us in the beginning. And in all these things, the gesture of human solidarity was more important than the financial aspects.

Most of the difficulties we have are got with respect to our attitude in daily life. From a country with socialism, where even bread has no worth, we had to learn the value of money. Sitting on a pendulum, you have to be careful. My grandmother once told me that money is important but does not mean everything in life. We are happy to be here.

Acknowledgements. The work discussed here was supported by the Austrian Ministry of Science and Research, project "Chicken Major Histocompatibility Complex", the Austrian Scientific Research Fund (project No. 4423); the Austrian Cancer Research Fund; and the Austrian Research Council (project No. S-41/05). The results are the outcome of cooperation with my colleagues and coauthors of the papers quoted. I am grateful to my three teachers: to Milan Hašek for introducing me to chickens and to tolerance, to Morten Simonsen for introducing me to alloreactivity and to George Wick for introducing me to autoimmunity. I wish to thank R. L. Boyd and K. N. Traill for improvement of the English in this manuscript.

References

Bacon LD (1976) Thyroiditis in (OS×CS) F1 chickens. Fed Proc 35: 713

Bacon LD, Kite JH, Rose NR (1974) Relation between the major histocompatibility (B) locus and autoimmune thyroiditis in obese chickens. Science 186: 274–275

Bacon LD, Sundick RS, Rose NN (1977) Genetic and cellular control of spontaneous autoimmune thyroiditis in OS chickens. In: Benedict AA (ed) Avian immunlogy. Plenum New York, pp 305–315

Briles WE, McGibbon WH, Irwin MR (1950) On multiple alleles affecting cellular antigens in the chicken. Genetics 35: 663–652

Briles WE, Bumstead N, Ewert DL, Gogusev J, Hala K, Koch C, Longenecker BM, Nordskog AW, Pink JRL, Schierman LW, Simonsen M, Toivanen A, Toivanen P, Vainio O, Wick G (1982) Nomenclature for the chicken major histocompatibility (B) complex. Immunogenetics 15: 441–447

Guillemot F, Billault A, Porquié O, Béhar G, Chaussé AM, Zoorob R, Kreibich G, Auffray C (1988) A molecular map of the chicken major histocompatibility complex: the class IIβ genes are closely linked to the class I genes and the nucleolar organizer. EMBO J 7: 2775–2785

Hála K (1988) Hypothesis: immunogenetic analysis of spontaneous autoimmune thyroiditis in Obese strain (OS) chickens: a two-gene family model. Immunobiology 177: 354–373

Hála K, Vilhelmova M, Hartmannova J (1976) Probable crossing-over in the B blood group system of chickens. Immunogenetics 3: 97–103

Hála K, Boyd R, Wick G (1981) Chicken major histocompatibility complex and disease. Scand J Immunol 14: 607–616

Hála K, Wick G, Boyd RL, Wolf H, Böck G, Ewert DL (1984) The B-L (Ia-like) antigens of the chicken. Lymphocyte plasma membrane distribution and tissue localisation. Dev Comp Immunol 8: 673–682

Hála K, Chaussé AM, Bourlet Y, Lassila O, Hasler V, Auffray C (1988) Attempt to detect recombination between B-F and B-L genes within the chicken B complex by serological typing, in vitro MLR and RFLP analyses. Immunogenetics 28: 433–438

Neu N, Hála K, Dietrich H, Wick G (1985) Spontaneous autoimmune thyroiditis in obese strain chickens: a genetic analysis of target organ abnormalities. Clin Immunol Immunopathol 37: 397–405

Neu N, Hála K, Dietrich H, Wick G (1986) The genetic background of spontaneous autoimmune thyroiditis in the obese strain (OS) of chicken studied in hybrids with an inbred line. Int Arch Allergy Appl Immunol 80: 168–173

Pink JRL, Droege W, Hála K, Miggiano VC, Ziegler A (1977) A three-locus model for chicken major histocompatibility complex. Immunogenetics 5: 203–216

Powell PC, Hála K, Wick G (1987) Aberrant expression of Ia-like antigens on tumor cells of regressing but not progressing Rous sarcomas. Eur J Immunol 17: 723–726

Sgonc R, Hála K, Wick G (1987) Relationship between the expression of class I antigen and reactivity of chicken thymocytes. Immunogenetics 26: 150–154

Toivanen A, Toivanen P (eds) (1987) Avian immunology: basis and practice. CRC Press, Boca Raton, Florida

Wick G, Gundolf R, Hála K (1979) Genetic factors in spontaneous autoimmune thyroiditis in OS chickens. J Immunogenet 6: 177–183

Wick G, Boyd RL, Hála K, deCarvalho L, Kofler R, Müller PU, Cole RK (1981) The obese strain (OS) of chickens with spontaneous autoimmune thyroiditis. Curr Top Microbiol Immuol 91: 109–128

Wick G, Boyd RL, Hála K, Thunold S, Koflar H (1982) Pathogenesis of spontaneous autoimmune thyroiditis in obese strain (OS) chickens. Clin Exp Immunol 47: 1–18

Wick G, Krömer G, Neu N, Fässler R, Zimiecki A, Müller RG, Ginzel M, Béládi I, Kühr T, Hála K (1987) The multi-factorial pathogenesis of autoimmune disease. Immunol Lett 16: 249–258

Wolf H, Hála K, Boyd RL, Wick G (1984) MHC- and non-MHC-encoded surface antigens of chicken lympoid cells and erythrocytes recognized by polyclonal xeno-, allo- and monoclonal antibodies. Eur J Immunol 14: 831–839

Tolerance, the Thymus, and H-Y

L. Jerabek

Introduction

I was hired as a technologist at the Institute of Experimental Bilogy and Genetics in the Czechoslovak Academy of Sciences in the summer of 1962 after attending the School of Medical Technology in Prague. In the beginning, I worked with Dr. Pavol Ivanyi and did not have much direct contact with Milan Hašek, the director of the Institute. It was only later that I realized what a valuable experience it was to work there. Hašek's position allowed him to travel all over the world and to communicate with scientists in the most progressive institutions in Europe and America. He made it possible for other scientists at the Institute to travel and learn as well – an opportunity one was hard pressed to find in Czechoslovakia at that time. When the young and already well-known geneticist Jan Klein recommended me for a position at Stanford University, it was a dream come true. Technicians such as myself were not usually offered such rare opportunities. Milan Hašek approved my professional passport and sent me on my way to California.

I arrived at Stanford University on July 11, 1968. I knew this once-in-a-lifetime chance would be my ticket to a better life than I could have expected otherwise, but I never knew how far it would end up taking me. I was going to learn English, experience a new culture, meet new people, gain a new perspective on life, and of course, learn a lot of science. I thought I would return to Prague to my husband and 2-year-old daughter after 1 year. Needless to say, what happened in August 1968 in Czechoslovakia just 5 weeks after my departure from Prague significantly changed my plans.

I last saw Milan Hašek in 1968 during his visit to Stanford. He returned to Czechoslovakia, while many of the scientists from the Institute emigrated. I will never forget his encouragement, his optimism, and his love of life – the infectious spirit that touched the lives of everyone around him. That same spirit did not die with Hašek, but continues to flourish today among the many scientists following in his footsteps. July 11, 1988 was my 20th anniversary at Stanford University. Working with Professor Irving Weissman, upon whose guidance and friendship I could always rely, I have been able to realize the dream that began in Milan Hašek's Institute in Prague.

Tolerance, the Thymus, and H-Y

In 1968, when I joined the Weissman laboratory, two major parallel research themes were already ongoing: first, what is the role of the thymus in the development of immune responsiveness? And second, how does transplantation tolerance to the H-Y antigen work on a mechanistic level? I helped in studies which showed that not only could tolerance be induced to the H-Y antigen by injection of male spleen cells as late as 15 days after birth (Weissman 1966), but also that long-lasting immune deficiency to H-Y (but not *H-2* or SRBC) could be induced by thymectomy until 10–15 days of age (Weissman 1970; Klein et al. 1974). These two facts would make sense if the first significant numbers of anti-H-Y thymocytes appeared at ~ 10–15 days after birth, and if these cells were selectively susceptible to transplantation tolerance induction during their development.

At that time, Weissman had just had a paper on H-Y tolerance transfer rejected that he had been trying to publish since 1964. I worked on the subject of the paper upon my entry into the laboratory in 1968, and, oddly enough, twice again in 1976 and then in 1986. The question we first approached was whether tolerance induced in neonatal females by injection of male spleen cells was due to clonal abortion (Burnet 1957) or the persistance of some agent or agents which actively maintain the tolerant state (Weissman and Lustgraaf 1961). We tested these two models by investigating a phenomenon we called "transfer of tolerance". Transfer of tolerance occurs when spleen cells from tolerant adult females are transferred into neonatal females; when they grow up, a high proportion of them are also tolerant of the H-Y antigen (Weissman 1973). We wanted to know whether the tolerance was due to male cells persisting in the spleen at a level sufficient to induce tolerance or if something other than or in addition to the male antigen might be responsible for this tolerance transfer. To assess the amount of male specific antigen in tolerant female spleens, we established dose-response assays for tolerance induction in newborn females and accelerated graft rejection (sensitization) in

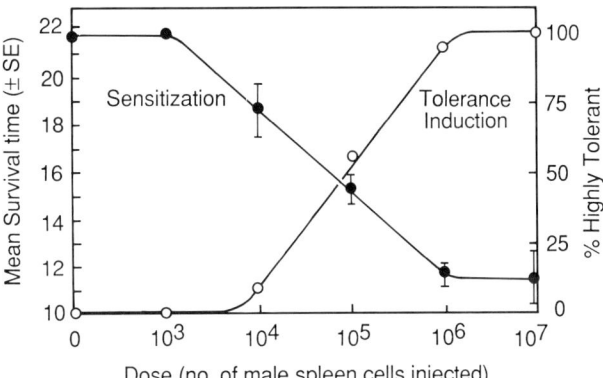

Fig. 1. Similar numbers of male spleen cells are required to sensitize syngeneic female adults and induce tolerance in syngeneic female newborns. The indicated number of adult (BALB/c × C57Bl/Ka)F$_1$ male spleen cells were injected subcutaneously into adult syngeneic females 3 weeks prior to grafting with syngeneic male tail skin, or intraperitoneally into newborn syngeneic females 4–8 weeks prior to grafting

adult females, both following injection of adult male spleen cells. As shown in Fig. 1, these two assays, remarkably, have very similar dose-response characteristics. For example, injection of 10^4 male spleen cells induces very little tolerance in newborn females and very little sensitization of adult females to subsequently applied male skin grafts. Injection of 10^6 spleen cells is just as effective in inducing full tolerance in newborn females as are 10^7 cells; and similarly, 10^6 cells sensitize adult female hosts to accelerated graft rejection (it reduces the mean survival time of subsequently applied male tail skin grafts from ~22 to ~11 days) equally as well as 10^7 cells. For both assays about 50% of the sensitization level and about 50% induction of tolerance occur when 10^5 cells are injected.

We then asked what would happen if we took the tolerant female spleen cells, as shown in Fig. 2, and transferred them in graded doses to neonatal females to test for tolerance transfer, and to adult females to assess the number of sensitizing male H-Y antigen antigenic spleen cells. The answer was a complete surprise. In

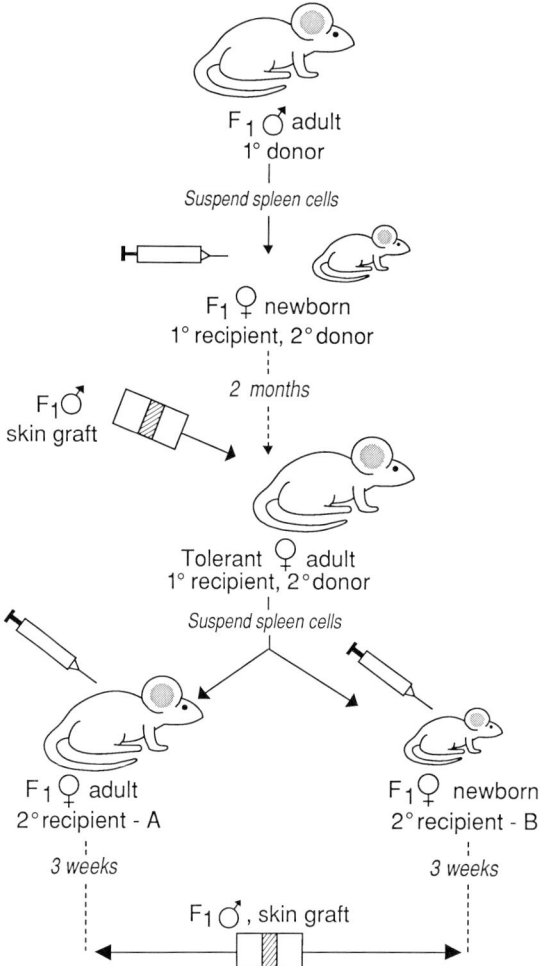

Fig. 2. The method for assessing persistence of sensitizing male cells (F_1 *female adults secondary recipient - A)* or tolerogenic cells *(F_1 female newborn secondary recipient - B)* in female mice made tolerant by injection of male spleen cells at birth

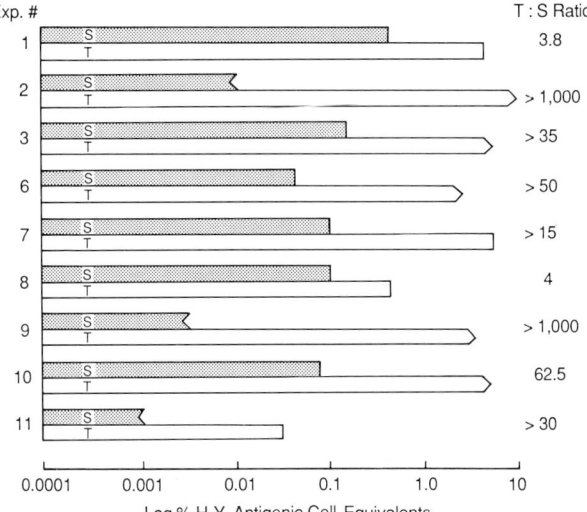

Fig. 3. In tolerant female spleens, the level of tolerizing H-Y is always greater than the level of sensitizing H-Y

Fig. 3 we show that the number of spleen cells that was necessary to transfer tolerance, in many cases, was 1000-fold less than the amount of male spleen cells indicated to be present as determined by the adult female sensitization assay. In all cases, the number of cells assessed by the tolerance induction assay was at least fourfold greater than the number assessed by the adult sensitization assay. However else one may wish to interpret these data, it was quite clear that immunological tolerance in this case was not just a lack of reacting cells, as would be expected from strict clonal abortion hypotheses. At that time (1968) we had two models that could have explained the phenomenon: (a) perhaps male cells or male antigen (tolerogen) persisted in tolerant female spleens in a form which was very efficient at tolerance induction, but inefficient at sensitization; or (b) perhaps among the female spleen cells a group of what we called "repressor" cells (Weissman and Lustgraaf 1961) – now called "suppressor cells" (Gershon and Kondo 1971) – might be present. With the addition of some of the new data we had generated, the manuscript was resubmitted and accepted in 1972.

Just 4 years later, we entered the game again. By this time techniques useful for separating T and B lymphocytes were available, and we wondered if we could test whether or not the mouse spleen cells used in these studies contained subsets of cells which were particularly efficient at inducing tolerance. We began a series of experiments to determine whether subsets of T or B cells could induce (or transfer) tolerance. We therefore initially separated the male spleen (and/or lymph node) cells into populations highly enriched with or depleted of T cells or B cells. The separation of cells from the initial mouse spleen provided a striking and totally unexpected answer (Weissman et al. 1984). Whereas both T and B cells from male donors sensitized adult female hosts with equal efficiency (Table 1), T cells, *but not B cells,* were sufficient to induce tolerance in neonatal females (Tables 2 and 3). In fact, in these experiments Lyt2$^+$ (CD8) T cells alone were capable of inducing active immonological tolerance with high efficiency; and most remarkably,

Table 1. Both T cells and B cells express sensitizing H-Y antigen

Lymphoid cell population injected	Mean survival time of male skin grafts ($X \pm SD$)	n
Female lymph node cells	22.3 ± 3.8	6
Male lymph node cells	16.7 ± 1.7	4
Male lymph node cells: B cell enriched	15.7 ± 1.1	14
Male lymph node cells: T cell enriched	17.0 ± 0.00	5
Male lymph node cells: CD8 T cells depleted	16.1 ± 1.3	9
Male lymph node cells: CD8 T cell enriched	15.7 ± 1.5	6

Table 2. Transplantation tolerance to H-Y antigen is induced by male T cells, but not male B cells or macrophages

Cells Injected	T (%)	B (%)	Mø (%)	Expected percentage tolerant if all cell types tolerogenic (%)	Expected percentage tolerant if only T cells are tolerogenic (%)	Observed tolerant (%)	Tolerant / Total (n)
Lymph node	59	35	2	90–100		82	14/17
Lymph node: T cell enriched	90	7	NT	80–85	70–75	72	21/29
Lymph node: B cell enriched	5	82	NT	80–85	20–30	25	14/55
Peritoneal exudate macrophages	NT	NT	70	35–40	?	0	0/32
None	–	–	–	0	0	0	0/3

Mø, macrophage; NT, not tested.

Table 3. Both major T cell subsets are tolerogenic

Cells injected	B220 (%)	Thy-1 (%)	$CD8^+$ (%)	$CD8^-$ ($CD4^+$?) (calculated)	Tolerant (%)	Tolerant / Total (n)
Lymph node	23	63	30	43	NT	NT
Lymph node: T cell enriched	15	89	NT	NT	83	5/6
Lymph node: CD8 depleted	7	76	19	70	75	6/8
Lymph node: CD8 enriched	<3	98	91	7	89	8/9
None					–	0/4

NT, not tested.

Table 4. A cytotoxic male T cell clone is tolerogenic

Cells injected[a]	Tolerant (%)	Tolerant/Total
Clone B12.5.4[b] (CD8+)	57	4/7
None	0	0/2

[a] A total of $2-5 \times 10^6$ cells injected per host
[b] Clone B12.5.4 is a male C57Bl/6 anti-H-2^d cytotoxic clone that is dependent on T cell growth factors in vitro.

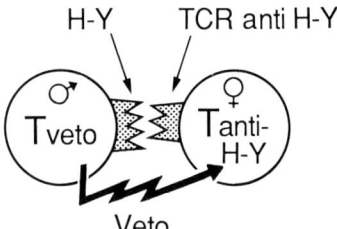

Fig. 4. Model of how T veto cells inhibit (or kill) T cells that are anti-H-Y

a male antigen-bearing cytotoxic T cell clone (which was alloreactive) also efficiently induced tolerance (Table 4). At that time, Miller and his colleagues had begun a series of experiments wherein they found a set of cells which they called "veto" cells, because they could veto the activity of antigen-specific cells responsible for cell-mediated immunity (Miller and Phillips 1976). We proposed that the induction of tolerance by T cells represented a veto-like phenomenon, and that such veto cells survived selectively in tolerant female spleens (Weissman 1973). Conceptually, that model is shown in Fig. 4. In that model a male T cell (designated T veto) expresses on its surface MHC-restricted H-Y antigen – presumably MHC plus the H-Y peptide. Conjugated to that H-Y antigen (via its T cell receptor complex) is an effector T cell of female origin which, upon conjugation, is the subject of a back reaction from the veto cell, vetoing the activity of that T effector cell. The result is clonal abortion, but clonal abortion that requires persistence of male T veto cells.

Thus we felt that we were dealing with a veto phenomenon, and that a T cell was the effector cell. As we implied above, there was a striking correlation in the developing neonatal mouse of susceptibility to tolerance induction, and the appearance of thymus-dependent immune competence to H-Y antigens (Weissman and Lustgraaf 1961). Was it possible that H-Y antigen-positive veto cells were not only present in the spleen, but could be involved in self-tolerance and/or experimentally induced tolerance at the level of thymic production of anti-H-Y T cells? When Fink was in the laboratory she had demonstrated unequivocally that allo-sensitization in the periphery can result in alloreactive peripheral T cells arriving in the thymus (Fink et al. 1984); and that tolerance to minor histocompatibility antigens had a particular cross-specific deletion or tolerance induction bias that implied an intrathymic involvement of veto cells (Fink et al. 1983).

If the thymus is the site of tolerance to H-Y by a veto-induced clonal abortion, or by any other means, the deletion of those cells might be directly demonstrated

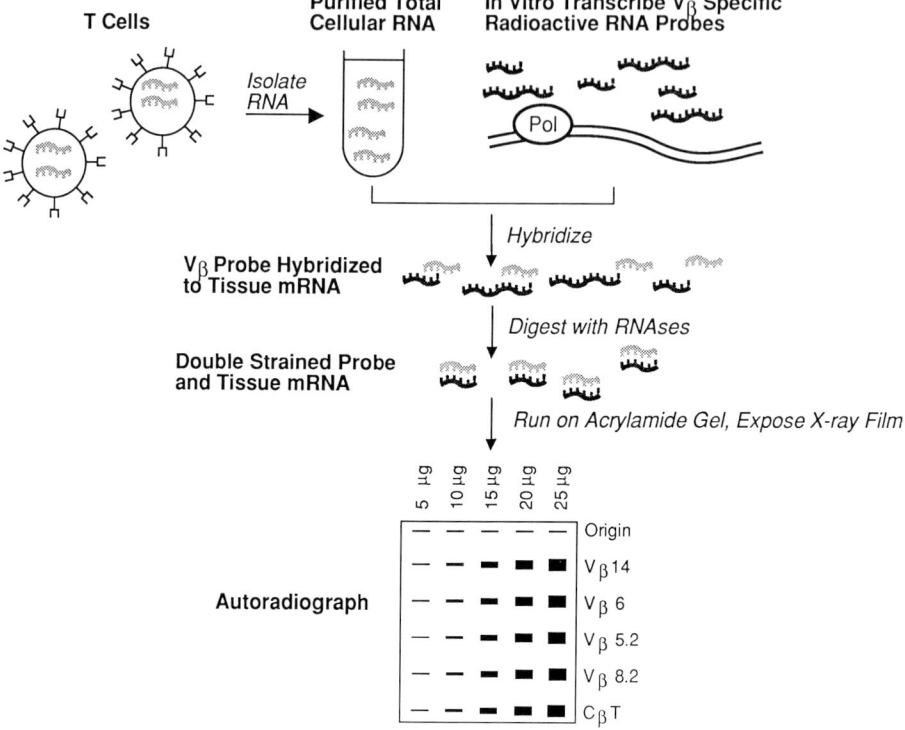

Fig. 5. The technique for assessing the level of T cell receptor $V\beta$ transcripts

on the basis of the specificity of the T cell receptor they express. In a brilliant series of experiments, Marrack and Kappler, and then others, demonstrated that tolerance of I-E and also Mls antigens appears to be via clonal elimination of cells within the thymus (Kappler et al. 1987, 1988; McDonald et al. 1988). This phenomenon could be studied only because the particular $V\beta$ chain of the T cell receptor complex that is expressed on a cell correlates, in some instances, with the specificity of the immune response of that cell. There are only 20–30 $V\beta$ chains in mice. Thus we had hoped to test whether tolerance of H-Y antigens would result in a reduction, or clonal elimination, of T cells bearing any particular $V\beta$ chain. We did not test directly whether cloned anti-H-Y cells used any particular $V\beta$ gene segment, but instead chose to develop a technique (Okada et al., in preparation) to assess the level of mRNA expression for a large number of $V\beta$ receptor gene segments for which we could obtain probes. We compared the level of expression of these gene segments in thymocytes (most of which had not yet undergone maturation and selection) versus peripheral T lymphocytes. In Fig. 5 we show our method: we used $V\beta$ antisense probes in a RNAse protection assay to quantify the amount of mRNA expressed for each $V\beta$ family member. As expected, in I-E$^+$ strains $V\beta$ 5.2 was expressed in thymus, but not in the periphery. This $V\beta$ gene was expressed in both the thymus and the periphery of peripheral I-E$^-$ strains (Okada et al., in preparation). Thus we had in place a system which could detect the de-

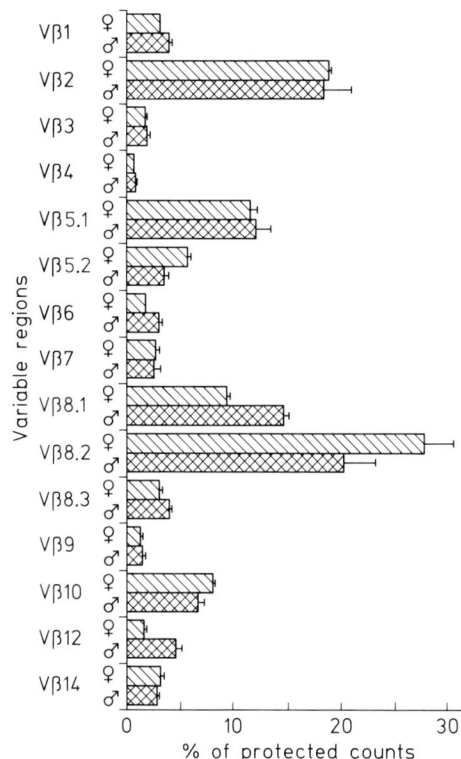

Fig. 6. The levels of T cell receptor Vβ transcripts in peripheral lymphoid organs of male vs. female mice

pletion of a subset (or all the members of a family) of Vβ gene segments as the result of a clonal deletion process upon recognition of a self or tolerizing antigen.

We wished to test whether the anti-H-Y immune response by T cells might be predominantly associated with any particular Vβ family member. The first and most obvious test was to compare the thymus mRNA with periphery T cell mRNA from C57BL/Ka males and females (C57BL is a high responder to H-Y transplantation antigens [Eichwald et al. 1958]). We were seeking, especially, Vβ gene segments expressed in females at approximately equal levels of mRNA in thymus and in the periphery, but in males at a higher level in the thymus than in the periphery. Thus we would expect that in males those T cells bearing Vβ regions that recognized H-Y antigens would be deleted and would be underrepresented in the peripheral T cell mRNA pool. As shown in Fig. 6, our first, preliminary experiment indicated that gene segment Vβ 5.2 and possibly Vβ 8.2 fulfills these criteria. There is a significant difference in the expression of Vβ 5.2 between peripheral lymphocytes of males and females – it is expressed at higher levels in the females. Also, when comparing the thymus to the peripheral lymphoid tissues of C57BL/Ka males, there is a higher level of expression in the thymus than in the periphery. This is evidence in favor, but not proof, of the hypothesis that some cells using the Vβ 5.2 gene segment might be able to react with H-Y antigens in C57BL/Ka mice.

Where do we go from here? First, we must verify that a subset of $V\beta$ 5.2 genes is indeed deleted in males but not females of all mouse strains which are immune responsive to H-Y transplants. Second, we should test, in addition, those strains which are unresponsive, to see whether the unresponsiveness in any way relates to this somatic alteration of the expressed T cell receptor repertoire. Third, and most importantly, we shall test whether females tolerant of the H-Y transplantation antigen following injection at birth with male spleen cells or male T cells also show this deletion, and determine whether the deletion is expressed in that subset of thymic cells which are mature, or if it is only expressed in the periphery. Thus we shall be able to compare self-tolerance and experimentally induced transplantation tolerance in a system which has natural congenic strains differing only at the Y chromosome.

Who would have thought that, 35 years after the observations, experiments, and ideas concerning self-tolerance and experimentally induced tolerance by that illustrious group of thinkers and experimentalists (Hašek, Burnet, Jerne, Medawar, and Owen), we would still be working on this system, still trying to understand how it works; and still trying to find a way to apply it to transplantation in man?

Epilogue

For a long time, "home" meant that country thousands of miles away, where my mother, father, and brothers lived, where a foreign power had subdued the spirit of the people. No doubt I considered myself fortunate to have slipped away with my husband and daughter, but to call my new country "home" seemed like breaking my spiritual commitment to my people and their struggle. I felt guilty.

There was little time to dwell on my feelings, however, during those early years when we struggled to assimilate ourselves into a new culture and become accustomed to a new style of life. My work in Irv Weissman's laboratory afforded me a measure of release from the more mundane concerns of life and allowed me not only to stretch my mind, but also to interact with budding scientists from all walks of life. The special camaraderie that developed in the Weissman laboratory grew richer with each new postdoctoral researcher and medical student who cleared a space for him- or herself on an already crowded laboratory bench. I often wondered how I would manage the influx of people and projects, but the enthusiasm and scientific curiosity of both the new additions and the old hands – and a bit of logistical maneuvering – assured that there was always room for one more.

Friendship and teamwork flourished amid our frequently hectic, yet always stimulating, research environment, sustained by a tireless and devoted Irv Weissman. Aside from his commitments to teaching, writing, and traveling, not to mention keeping abreast of all of the progress within his own laboratory, Irv found time to guide and advise me both inside and outside of the laboratory. He became one of my most trusted friends and confidants. It was as though I had found a new brother, someone I could turn to in good times and bad, someone who helped me fight the estrangement and loneliness that threatened to plague me in my new world.

A few years ago, I caught myself answering the question "Where are you from?" with "I'm from California, near Stanford University" – not with "I'm from Czechoslovakia" or with "I'm from Prague," but with a response, however unconsciously formulated, that embodied a journey ended, a realization attained. I knew that I had not forsaken a commitment to my native country or my family there, but rather I had opened the door to a new and better life for myself and made a new commitment to my own family and to the people I had grown to love. I had set out into the world and carved a niche for myself, and I knew I was home.

References

Burnet FM (1959) The clonal selection theory of acquired immunity. Cambridge University Press, London
Eichwald EJ, Lustgraaf EC, Weissman I, Strainer M (1958) Attempts to demonstrate sex-linked histocompatibility genes. Transplant Bull 5: 387
Fink PJ, Weissman IL, Bevan MJ (1983) Haplotype-specific suppression of cytotoxic T cell induction by antigen inappropriately presented on T cells. J Exp Med 157: 141
Fink PJ, Bevan MJ, Weissman IL (1984) Thymic cytotoxic T lymphocytes are primed in vivo to minor histocompatibility antigens. J Exp Med 159: 436
Gershon RK, Kondo K (1971) Infectious immunological tolerance. Immunology 21: 903
Kappler JW, Roehm N, Marrack P (1987) T cell tolerance by clonal elimination in the thymus. Cell 49: 273
Kappler JW, Staerz U, White J, Marrack PC (1988) Self tolerance eliminates T cells specific for Mls-modified products of the major histocompatibility complex. Nature 322: 35
Klein J, Livnat S, Hauptfeld V, Jerabek L, Weissman I (1974) Production of H-2 antibodies in thymectomized mice. Eur J Immunol 4: 41
McDonald HR, Schneider R, Lees RK, Howe RC, Acha-Orbea H, Festenstein H, Zinkernagel RM, Hengartner H (1988) T-cell receptor Vβ use predicts reactivity and tolerance to Mls^a enclosed antigens. Nature 323: 40
Miller RG, Phillips RA (1976) Reduction of the in vitro cytotoxic lymphocyte response produced in vivo exposure to semiallogeneic cells: recruitment or active suppression. J Immunol 117: 1913
Weissman I (1966) Studies on the mechanism of split tolerance. Transplantation 4: 565
Weissman I (1970) The role of the thymus and extrathymic factors in the development of immune competence. In: Šterzl J, Řika I (eds) Development aspects of antibody formation and structure, vol 1. Academia, Prague, p 55
Weissman I (1973) Transfer of tolerance. Transplantation 15: 265
Weissman I, Lustgraaf EC (1961) Antibody formation and repressor systems. Transplant Bull 28: 134
Weissman IL, Jerabek L, Greenspan S (1984) Tolerance and the H-Y antigen: male T cells, and not B cells are required to induce tolerance. Transplantation 37: 3

Autologous Mixed Lymphocyte Culture: Immunoregulatory Aspects

F. Pazderka

Introduction

It is well established that the autologous mixed lymphocyte reaction (AMLR) represents an immunologic response of T cells to surface antigens on autologous non-T cells. Autologous mixed lymphocyte culture (AMLC) has been shown to possess two main attributes of immune responses: immunologic specificity and memory. AMLC stimulation may result in a variety of effector and immunoregulatory activities. We were interested predominantly in the latter aspects, namely, generation of suppressor cells in AMLC. The critical role in stimulating AMLC response belongs to class II MHC antigens, and any cells expressing class II antigens (B cells, monocytes, and activated T cells) are able to stimulate AMLC reactivity. Cells responding to AMLC stimulation are T lymphocytes, and recent investigations have demonstrated that the cells predominantly proliferating in AMLC are T4 lymphocytes (Engleman et al. 1981). Isolated T8 cells are unable to proliferate in AMLC, presumably, because of lack of interleukin 2 (IL-2) production by these cells. Ability of T8 cells to proliferate in AMLC is restored if T4 cells (as the source of Il-2) or exogenous IL-2 are added to the culture (Romain et al. 1984). Nevertheless, even under these circumstances, the relative contribution of T4 cells to the proliferative response in AMLC is much greater than that of T8 cells (Kotani et al. 1984). In this communication, we describe the activity of suppressor cells generated in AMLC and attempt to analyze cellular interactions involved in that phenomenon, at the level of functionally heterogeneous subpopulations within major T cell subsets.

Results and Discussion

Our experimental design was as follows: peripheral blood lymphocytes (PBL) were separated into T and non-T cells using 2-aminoethylisothio-uronium bromide hydrobromide (AET)-treated sheep red blood cell (SRBC) rosetting. T cells were then cocultured with mitomycin C-treated or irradiated (2000 R) non-T cells for 7 days. After incubation, cells harvested from AMLC were added to a fresh (indicator) culture composed of autologous responders and allogeneic stimulators at a ratio of responders:stimulators:putative suppressor cells 1:1:0.5.

In the indicator culture, the activity of suppressor cells was assessed by their

Table 1. Effect of AMLC-activated cells on cytotoxic and proliferative responses of autologous responders in MLC

Experiment	Cells added to MLC	CML		MLC	
		Cytotoxicity (%)	Inhibition (%)	SI	Inhibition (%)
1	–	43.4		17.6	
	AMLC-activated	23.6	45.6	9.4	46.6
	AMLC-activated$_m$	42.4	2.8	22.1	−25.6
2	–	34.1		20.0	
	AMLC-activated	7.6	77.7	2.1	89.5
	AMLC-activated$_m$	28.4	16.7	6.4	68.0
3	–	31.2		28.9	
	AMLC-activated	9.3	70.2	11.5	60.2
	AMLC-activated$_m$	22.6	27.6	29.5	− 2.1

T cells were cultured for 7 days in the presence of autologous (non-T)$_m$ cells and then added, after or without mitomycin C treatment, to a second culture containing autologous responders and allogeneic stimulators. Proliferation and cytotoxic activity (against allogeneic phytohemagglutinin (PHA) blasts) were measured in indicator culture after 6 days of incubation.
SI, stimulation index, calculated as: cpm in experimental culture/background cpm.

effect on the amount of proliferation and on the activity of cytotoxic cells (CTL) generated in this culture.

The techniques of these assays were described in detail in our previous communication (Pazderka et al. 1983). Table 1 illustrates the results of several initial experiments where the effect of AMLC-induced suppressor cells was tested with respect to both cytotoxic and proliferative responses. As can be seen from the table, both responses are significantly suppressed. It also demonstrates mitomycin C and, as established in our subsequent experiments, radiation sensitivity of suppressor cells. Mean percentage of suppression of cytotoxic activity as observed in 17 experiments was 75.3 ± 22.4; percentage suppression of proliferation was 60.6 ± 18.2.

Kinetic studies of suppressor cell generation are summarized in Fig. 1. Suppression becomes apparent after 3 days of incubation in AMLC; peak activity is reached on day 6. In all our subsequent experiments we used cells harvested after 6–7 days of incubation in AMLC; in assessing their suppressive activity we concentrated on a cell-mediated lympholytic (CML) assay only.

In order to separate autoreactive (or autoactivated) cells from nonactivated ones, we performed Percoll density gradient centrifugation following the procedure of Kozak et al. (1982). Table 2 illustrates the composition of different Percoll fractions in terms of lymphoblasts and small cells as determined by microscopic examination. As can be seen from the table, the majority of blasts are concentrated in fraction I, suggesting the enrichment of this fraction with autoactivated cells. When tested for proliferative activity ([^{3}H]thymidine incorporation), cells collected from fraction I showed most proliferation, while virtually no thymidine incorporation was observed in fractions of small cells (fractions III and IV). Fraction II showed intermediate values.

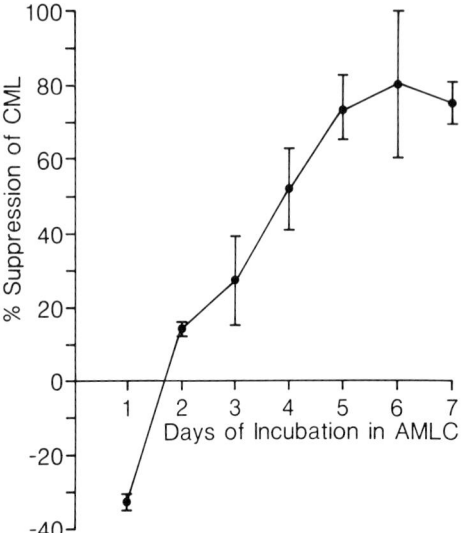

Fig. 1. Kinetics of generation of suppressor cells in AMLC. AMLC-stimulated T cells were harvested at various time intervals after initiation of AMLC and added to indicator culture (A/Xx) at a ratio 1:1:0.5. *Points* and *bars* represent mean ± standard error obtained in three independent experiments

The results of 18 independent experiments are summarized in Fig. 2. As can be seen from Table 2 and Fig. 2, both parameters (blastogenesis and tritiated thymidine incorporation) indicate the highest amount of activation following AMLC in fraction I. Fraction IV shows minimal, if any, evidence of activation. In our subsequent experiments, fraction I cell activities were compared to those of fraction IV, as representing autoactivated and nonactivated cells, respectively.

Further evidence of autoactivation in fraction I was provided by the experiments involving restimulation of cells harvested after primary AMLC using autologous or allogeneic stimulators. The results of a representative experiment are shown in Fig. 3. A similar trend was observed in three additional independent experiments. As can be seen from Fig. 3, both unfractionated cells and cells from fraction I showed secondary kinetics of proliferative response to autologous but not to allogeneic stimulators. In contrast, fraction IV cells showed virtually no response to autologous stimulators, both at day 3 and day 7. Their response to allogeneic stimulation showed typical primary kinetics. These results are in agreement with assumption that, indeed, fraction I represents cells activated in primary AMLC, while fraction IV contains predominantly AMLC nonactivated cells. Cells harvested from fractions I and IV were analyzed in terms of their suppressor activity and T cell phenotypes as established by indirect fluorescence using T subset-specific monoclonal antibodies.

Table 3 shows T subset composition of AMLC-stimulated T lymphocytes. While unfractionated cells were composed of 79.3% Leu3 (T4) and 20.7% Leu2 (T8) cells, the percentage of Leu3 cells in fraction I was increased to 86.9%, and Leu2 decreased to 13.0%. In the fraction of AMLC nonactivated cells, the percentage of Leu3 and Leu2 cells was 72.3% and 27.7%, respectively. These results illustrate enrichment of AMLC-activated fraction with Leu3-positive cells. Accordingly, these changes are reflected in Leu3/Leu2 ratios in various fractions: the ratio of

Table 2. Cell recovery and percentage of lymphoblasts in various density fractions of AMLC-stimulated T cells

Experiment	Cell recovery Fractions				Blasts Fractions				
	I (%)	II (%)	III (%)	IV (%)	I (%)	II (%)	III (%)	IV (%)	Unfractionated (%)
1	33.3	19.7	16.0	30.9	81.5	18.7	0	4.0	33.3
2	33.3	22.9	31.2	12.5	68.7	9.1	0	0	27.5
3	29.0	23.2	23.2	26.1	87.2	6.2	3.3	8.1	40.7
4	32.9	25.0	26.3	15.8	78.0	13.2	2.5	0	18.7
5	40.6	25.0	18.7	15.6	83.0	15.6	0	0	38.5

Purified T cells were stimulated by autologous non-T cells for 7 days and then fractionated on Percoll density gradients. Fraction numbers correspond to the following Percoll density interfaces: I = 40%–50%; II = 50%–55%; III = 55%–60%; IV = 60%–70%.

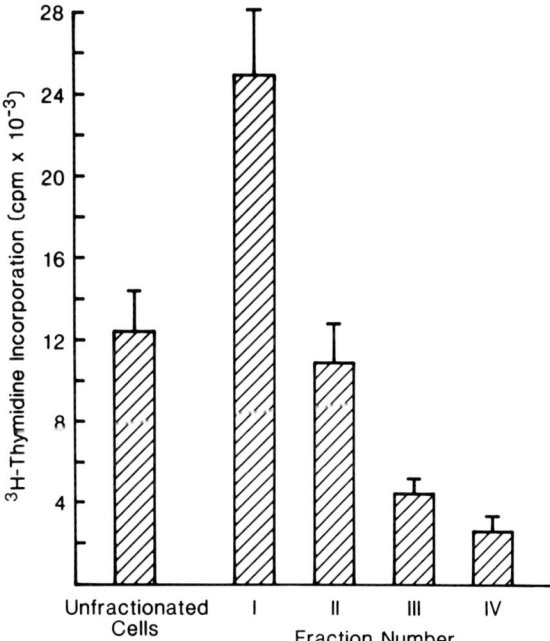

Fig. 2. [^{3}H]thymidine incorporation by various density T cell fractions after stimulation in AMLC. T cells were stimulated in culture by autologous non-T cells for 7 days and then fractionated on discontinuous Percoll density gradients. Cells from each fraction (1×10^5) were transferred into wells of round-bottomed microtiter trays (in triplicates) and labeled with [^{3}H]thymidine (1 μ Ci/well). Cells were harvested 16–18 h later, and radioactivity was measured in a liquid scintillation counter. Each *bar* represents mean counts per minute ± standard error based on 18 experiments

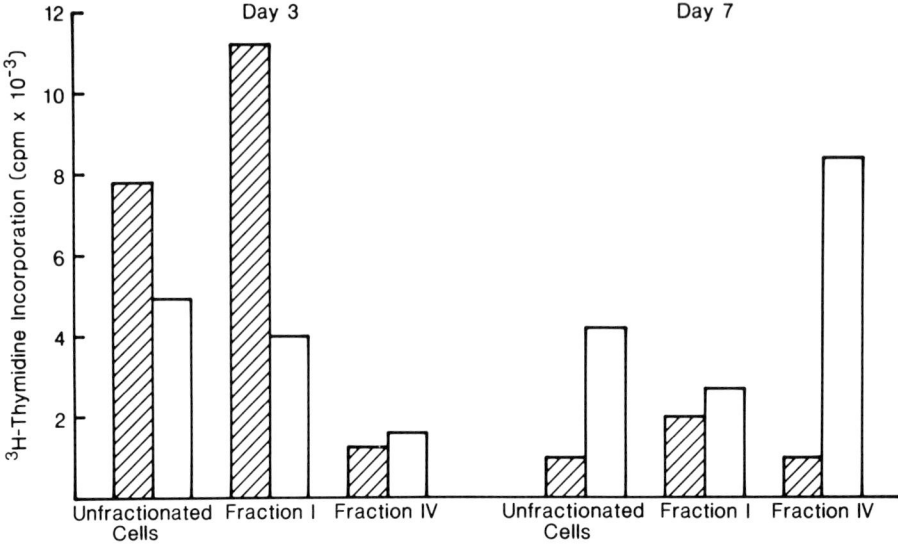

Fig. 3. Proliferation of AMLC-stimulated cells upon stimulation with autologous and allogeneic stimulators in a secondary MLC. T cells were cocultured with autologous non-T cells for 7 days. Cells collected after cultures were fractionated on Percoll density gradients and restimulated, in microculture, with autologous non-T cells and allogeneic peripheral blood lymphocytes (PBL), using 1×10^5 cells as responders and an equal number of cells as stimulators. Proliferation was measured on day 3 and day 7. Results are expressed as median counts per minute. Background counts were 500 cpm. *Shaded bars*, autologous stimulation; *open bars*, allogeneic stimulation

Table 3. Phenotypes of AMLC-stimulated T cells

Cells	Phenotypes (percentage of Leu4)		Leu3/Leu2 ratio
	Leu3	Leu2	
Unfractionated	79.3 ± 8.4[a]	20.7 ± 8.4	4.5 ± 2.0
Fraction I	86.9 ± 6.8	13.0 ± 6.8	8.3 ± 4.2
Fraction IV	72.3 ± 7.5	27.7 ± 7.5	3.0 ± 1.6

[a] Mean and standard deviation (six experiments).
After 7 days of stimulation in AMLC, T cells were collected, fractionated on Percoll density gradients, and stained for indirect immunofluorescence.

4.5 observed in unfractionated cells was increased to 8.3 in fraction I and decreased to 3.0 in fraction IV, the difference between fraction I and fraction IV being statistically significant ($p < 0.02$).

Suppressor cell activity exerted by various fractions is compared in Table 4. The mean percentage of suppression caused by unfractionated cells was 60.1%. Suppression exerted by fraction I cells was 78.1%. Cells from fraction IV caused very little suppression (24.8%). The difference in suppressor cell activity between AMLC-activated and nonactivated cells was statistically significant ($p < 0.001$). Thus, AMLC activation as assessed by the functional study and phenotypical analysis of Percoll gradient-separated fractions appears to result in (a) an increase

Table 4. Suppressor activity of T cells after stimulation in AMLC

Cells added to second culture	Suppression of CTL induction in second culture (%)
Unfractionated	60.1 ± 26.5[a]
Fraction I	78.1 ± 9.7
Fraction IV	24.8 ± 32.9

[a] Mean and standard deviation (eight experiments).
After 7 days of stimulation in AMLC, T cells were collected, fractionated on Percoll density gradients, and added to indicator culture. After 6 days of incubation, cells from the second culture were harvested and assayed in CML against allogeneic stimulators (PHA blasts).

in the proportion of Leu3$^+$ cells; and (b) an increase in suppressor cell activity as compared to unfractionated cells.

This observation led to a further series of investigations directed at the following questions: (a) is suppression exhibited by the blast cell fraction mediated by Leu3 or Leu2 blasts; (b) if Leu3 cells are responsible for suppression, do they act as functional suppressors or inducers of suppression; (c) if the predominant role of Leu3 cells is to induce suppression by Leu2 cells, is this effect exerted during AMLC or by acting on fresh Leu2 cells present in the indicator culture; (d) is the suppression by autoactivated cells simply due to exhaustion of IL-2 in a second culture through binding of lymphokine to IL-2 receptors expressed on activated T cells.

To answer these questions, separation of T4 (Leu3) and T8 (Leu2) cells was performed at various stages of experimental procedure, and their effect on CTL development in a second culture was assessed separately. To estimate the possible effect of IL-2 exhaustion in indicator culture, exogenous IL-2 was added at different concentrations in an attempt to reverse the suppression.

In order to evaluate the role of T4 vs. T8 blasts in AMLC-induced suppression, we separated AMLC-stimulated T cells and their Percoll fractions into major T cell subsets using the technique of cytotoxic elimination with monoclonal antibodies (MAb) and complement (Miyawaki et al. 1982). The results of a representative experiment are shown in Table 5. Leu3 blasts were 95.0% suppressive, while Leu2 blasts caused only 3.8% suppression. Both Leu3 and Leu2 cells isolated from fraction IV were virtually nonsuppressive. To assess functional involvement of T cell subsets in AMLC-induced suppression further, we analyzed the activity of isolated subsets.

In one series of experiments, separation was performed before using T cells as responders in AMLC. Although it is known that isolated T8 cells do not proliferate in response to autologous non-T cells, it is not clear what the functional consequence of their exposure to autologous non-T cells is.

The results of five experiments are summarized in Table 6. As can be seen from the table, maximal suppression is exhibited by Leu3 cells stimulated by autologous non-T cells: 68.2% ± 25.6%; suppression by similarly stimulated Leu2 cells is negligible (7.0% ± 29.4%). In the second series of experiments, cytotoxic elimination of T cell subsets was performed after 7-day AMLC. The results summa-

Table 5. Suppressive effect of T cell subsets isolated by cytotoxic elimination after Percoll fractionation of AMLC-stimulated T cells

Fraction	T cell subset	Suppression (%)
I	Unseparated T	71.1
	Leu3	95.0
	Leu2	3.8
IV	Unseparated T	23.8
	Leu3	7.4
	Leu2	−13.8

After 7 days in AMLC, T cells were harvested and fractionated on Percoll density gradients. After that, cells of fractions I and IV were treated with MAb (OKT4 and OKT8) and complement. The suppressive effect of isolated subsets and untreated T cells from the same fractions was assayed by adding them to indicator culture (see footnotes for Table 4).

Table 6. Suppressive effect of T cell subsets separated before activation in AMLC

Subset	Suppression (%)
Unfractionated/non-T cells$_x$	65.0 ± 21.6[a]
Leu3/non-T cells$_x$	68.2 ± 25.6
Leu2/non-T cells$_x$	7.0 ± 29.4

[a] Mean and standard deviation (five experiments).
Purified T cells were treated with MAb and complement and then used as responders in AMLC. After 7 days of incubation, cells were harvested and tested for suppressor activity upon addition to indicator culture (see footnotes to Table 4).

rized in Table 7 show that Leu3 cells were significantly more efficient in mediating suppression than Leu2.

Our further approach to the analysis of the phenomenon of AMLC-induced suppression involved evaluation of functionally heterogeneous subpopulations within major subsets of T cells by means of two-color fluorescence. Leu3$^+$ Leu8$^+$ cells are known to function as inducers of suppression (Gatenby et al. 1982), while Leu2$^+$ Leu15$^+$ cells represent functional suppressors (Clement et al. 1984).

We have followed the effect of AMLC stimulation on a proportion of these subpopulations. As can be seen from Table 8, AMLC stimulation results in significant increase of Leu3$^+$ Leu8$^+$ (suppressor-inducer) cells as compared to nonstimulated cells. A proportion of Leu2$^+$ Leu15$^+$ cells shows a slight increase; however, the difference is not statistically significant. Furthermore, no significant correlation was found between proportions of Leu3$^+$ Leu8$^+$ and Leu2$^+$ Leu15$^+$ cells harvested from the same AMLC, indicating that only a small amount of activation of functional suppressors of Leu2 lineage takes place during AMLC; this observation is in agreement with the results of functional tests (Table 7) and with the observations of Romain et al. (1984) and Reinberz et al. (1982) that demonstrated preferential activation of suppressor-inducer cells in AMLR using different sets of MAbs.

Table 7. Suppressor activity of T cells and their subsets separated after activation in AMLC

Subset	Suppression (%)	p
Unfractionated	52.7 ± 24.9[a]	
Leu3	59.5 ± 25.2	<0.01
Leu2	22.2 ± 16.8	

[a] Mean and standard deviation (nine experiments).
T cells harvested after 7 days in AMLC were treated with MAb and complement and then added to an indicator culture.

Table 8. Proportion of suppressor-inducer and suppressor-effector T cells before and after stimulation in AMLC

Subpopulation	Resting T cells (%)	AMLC-stimulated T cells (%)	p
Leu3+ Leu8+	10.2 ± 7.7	28.1 ± 15.7	<0.05
Leu2+ Leu15+	6.7 ± 6.7	10.3 ± 11.3	NS

Samples of purified resting T cells were stained for two-color fluorescence and flow cytometry. Remaining cells were stimulated in AMLC and, after 7 days of incubation, harvested and stained for fluorescence-activated cell sorter (FACS) analysis. Proportions of cells showing double fluorescence are expressed as percentage of total numbers of T (Leu4) cells.

To test the assumption that AMLC-activated suppressor-inducers might act during the second culture through activation of suppressor-precursors of Leu2 lineage, we correlated the proportions of Leu3+ Leu8+ cells added to the second culture with (a) proportions of Leu2+ Leu15+ cells in indicator culture; and (b) the percentage suppression observed in this culture. In both cases, the correlation was moderate ($r = 0.50$ and 0.31, respectively) and did not reach the level of statistical significance. This suggests that although a certain amount of suppressor cell induction is taking place in indicator culture, this mechanism cannot be solely responsible for the total suppressive effect.

The remaining possibility is that AMLC stimulation results in the activation of not only suppressor-inducers, but functional Leu3 suppressors as well, as demonstrated by Thomas et al. (1982) in a different experimental model. However, this possibility is difficult to test directly since (a) MAb marking of functional suppressors among Leu3 cells is not available at the present time; and (b) in our experimental system, the assay is based on the measurement of cytotoxic activity of Leu2 cells in indicator culture and, thus, the possibility of interaction between these two subpopulations cannot, at this point, be entirely excluded.

So far, our evidence concerning the role of functional suppressors of Leu3 lineage in the AMLC-induced suppression phenomenon is rather indirect. It is based on our findings of a strong correlation between the percentage of Leu3 cells and the percentage of suppression in indicator culture: $r = 0.78$; $p < 0.01$ (Fig. 4) in the absence of such a correlation with Leu3+ Leu8+ (data not shown). Figure 4 also shows the absence of a significant correlation between the suppression and the numbers of Leu2+ Leu15+ cells ($r = -0.34$; not significant).

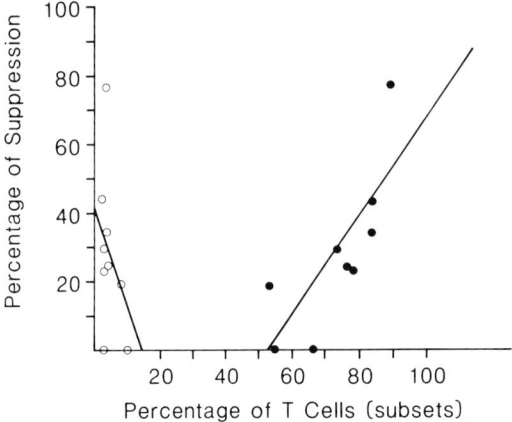

Fig. 4. Correlation between percentage of suppression and proportion of Leu3 cells in indicator culture. AMLC-stimulated T cells were added to the indicator culture and, after 6 days of incubation, effector cells harvested from the second culture were stained for fluorescence and flow cytometry. The percentage of suppression observed in each experiment was plotted against the percentage of the Leu3 subset *(solid circles)* and Leu2$^+$ Leu15$^+$ cells *(open circles)* detected in this experiment. Correlation with suppression was as follows: Leu3: $r=0.78$; $p<0.01$; Leu2$^+$ Leu15$^+$: $r=-0.34$; not significant

We are aware of the possibility of an alternative explanation of this phenomenon, namely, the one suggested by Orosz and Ferguson (1985): responder cell dilution by the progeny of suppressive lymphocytes as observed by these authors in an allo-mixed lymphocyte culture-induced suppressor system. However, this explanation seems unlikely as applied to our experimental model, since the mean percentage of Leu3 cells in unsuppressed culture is not significantly lower than that in suppressed cultures (data not shown).

Finally, to address the question of whether the suppression could have resulted from IL-2 exhaustion in the indicator culture, we attempted to reverse the suppression by adding exogenous IL-2 to a second culture. IL-2 was added, in graded amounts, to indicator culture along with unfractionated AMLC-stimulated T cells or their subsets. The results of nine experiments are summarized in Table 9. As can be seen from the table, no significant reversal of the suppression could be observed at any dose of IL-2, thus indicating that exhaustion of IL-2 is not the factor responsible for the suppressive effect of autoactivated T cells.

In conclusion, our results show that the main functional consequence of AMLC is activation of T cells exerting suppressor activity. This activity is preferentially expressed in a fraction of autoactivated blasts which are simultaneously enriched for Leu3 cell subset. Leu3 but not Leu2 blasts are characterized by maximal suppressive activity. As far as functional subpopulations within major T cell subsets are concerned, AMLC results in a significant increase of Leu3$^+$ Leu8$^+$ (suppressor-inducer cells) and only a marginal increase of Leu2$^+$ Leu15$^+$ (suppressor-effectors). Suppressor-inducer cells exert a moderate effect on Leu2 suppressor-precursors both at the level of the inducing culture (AMLC) and in the indicator culture. In addition to suppressor-inducer cells, functional suppressors of

Table 9. Suppressive effect of AMLC-stimulated cells in the presence of exogenous IL-2 in the indicator culture

Cells added to indicator culture	IL-2 added (units/ml)	Suppression (%)
T (unfractionated)		57.0 ± 23.1[a]
	5	51.0 ± 24.6
	10	57.6 ± 21.1
	20	58.6 ± 30.2
Leu3		59.0 ± 24.8
	5	53.6 ± 26.9
	10	51.8 ± 16.0
	20	N.D.
Leu2		30.2 ± 21.6
	5	44.0 ± 22.5
	10	39.4 ± 32.7
	20	N.D.

[a] Mean and standard deviation (nine experiments).
T cells, harvested after 7 days of AMLC, were separated into subsets by MAb and complement and added to indicator culture in the presence of graded amounts of IL-2 (lectin-free CR interleukin 2, Collaborative RES., Lexington, Mass., USA). Optimal concentration of IL-2 was 10 units per milliliter as established previously using an IL-2-dependent cell line.

Leu3 lineage appear to be activated in AMLC. The total amount of suppression observed in this system represents a cumulative effect of these three contributing factors.

Complexity of cellular interactions occurring during AMLC is, perhaps, the reason why so many controversial results concerning the activity of AMLC-stimulated cells have been reported. AMLC has been described as resulting in helper (Yu et al. 1980), suppressor (Sakane and Green 1979), or dual-function (Kotani et al. 1986) autoactivated cells. Different functional consequences of T-non-T, as opposed to T-T AMLC have been outlined (Gupta et al. 1985). Although the majority of investigators agrees that AMLC represents an important self-recognition and immunoregulatory event, many questions concerning the mechanisms of AMLR still remain unanswered.

At present, our approach to the analysis of the AMLR phenomenon involves the study of various lymphokines released during AMLC both at the level of protein products and at the level of gene expression. These investigations are now in progress.

Acknowledgements. Most of the experiments were done with J. Enns and J.B. Dossetor. The work was supported, in part, by MRC of Canada and the Alberta Cancer Board Research Initiative Program. We wish to express out thanks to Dr. Philip Halloran for his criticism and helpful suggestions, Mrs. Linda Marchuk for skillful technical assistance, and Ms. Lynn Linklater for flow cytometry analysis.

References

Clement LT, Grossi CE, Gartland GL (1984) Morphologic and phenotypic features of the subpopulation of Leu2$^+$ cells that suppresses B cell differentiation. J Immunol 133: 2461–2468

Engleman EG, Benike CJ, Grumet FC, Evans RL (1981) Activation of human T lymphocyte subsets: helper and suppressor/cytotoxic T cells recognize and respond to distinct histocompatibility antigens. J Immunol 127: 2124–2129

Gatenby PA, Kansas GS, Xian CY, Evans RL, Engleman EG (1982) Dissection of immunoregulatory subpopulations of T lymphocytes within the helper and suppressor sublineages in man. J Immunol 129: 1997–2000

Gupta S, Chandy KG, Thornton M, Goldberg M (1985) Autologous mixed lymphocyte reaction in man. XIII. Characterization of the T-T autologous mixed lymphocyte reaction. J Clin Immunol 5: 187–194

Kotani H, Takada S, Ueda Y, Murakawa Y, Suzuki N, Sakane T (1984) Activation of immune regulatory circuits among OKT4$^+$ cells by autologous mixed lymphocyte reactions. Clin Exp Immunol 56: 390–398

Kotani H, Mitsuya H, Jarrett RF, Yenokida GG, James SP, Strober W (1986) An autoreactive T cell alone that can be activated to provide both helper and suppressor function. J Immunol 136: 1951–1959

Kozak RW, Moody CE, Staiano-Coico L, Weksler ME (1982) Lymphocyte transformation induced by autologous cells. XII. Quantitative and qualitative differences between human autologous and allogeneic reactive T lymphocytes. J Immunol 128: 1723–1727

Miyawaki T, Nagaoki T, Yokoi T, Yachie A, Uwadana N, Taniguchi N (1982) Cellular interactions of human T cell subsets defined by monoclonal antibodies in regulation B cell differentiation: a comparative study in Nocardia water-soluble mitogen- and pokeweed mitogen-stimulated culture systems. J Immunol 128: 899–903

Orosz CG, Ferguson RM (1985) Suppression of in vitro CML generation by alloactivated lymphocytes: analysis of antigen-nonspecific suppressive mechanisms. J Immunol 134: 45–50

Pazderka F, Angeles A, Kovithavongs T, Dossetor JB (1983) Induction of suppressor cells in autologous mixed lymphocyte culture (AMLC) in humans. Cell Immunol 75: 122–133

Reinherz EL, Morimoto C, Fitzgerald KA, Hussey RE, Daley JF, Schlossman SF (1982) Heterogeneity of human T4$^+$ inducer T cells defined by a monoclonal antibody that delineates two functional subpopulations. J Immunol 128: 463–468

Romain PL, Morimoto C, Daley JF, Palley LS, Reinherz EL, Schlossman SF (1984) Reactivity of inducer cells subsets and T8-cell activation during the human autologous mixed lymphocyte reaction. Clin Immunol Immunopathol 30: 117–128

Sakane T, Green I (1979) Specificity and suppressor function of human T cells responsive to autologous non-T cells. J Immunol 123: 584–589

Thomas Y, Rogoazinski L, Rothman P, Rabbani LE, Andrews S, Irigoyen OH, Chess L (1982) Further dissection of the functional heterogeneity within the OKT4$^+$ and OKT8$^+$ human T cell subsets. J Clin Immunol 2: 8S–14S

Yu DTY, Chiorazzi N, Kunkel HG (1980) Helper factors derived from autologous mixed lymphocyte cultures. Cell Immunol 50: 305–313

Immunogenetics (MHC)

Mickey, Hugo, and Eve: A Study in the Evolution of the Major Histocompatibility Complex

J. Klein

> Mother to Miloš:
> "You must do your best, and make sure that the trains don't collide."
>
> Jiří Menzel and Bohumil Hrabal: *Closely Watched Trains*

The Switchman

There are moments in one's life that resemble a switch in a railroad yard. Lift one lever and the train is sent off in the direction of Paris, pull another one and it travels to Amsterdam.

Such a moment occurred in my life in October 1961. I was the train pulling into a station and Milan Hašek, the switchman who had the train's destination, if not its destiny, in his hands. The moment remains deeply embedded in my memory. It was the first time I came face-to-face with Milan, and although I knew how much was at stake in this interview, I was not nervous. Already the handshake, firm and long, with direct eye-to-eye contact, made you forget the awesome reputation and the myth that surrounded this tall, handsome man. The interview was candid and to the point. It seemed that Milan was not interested so much in the circumstances that brought me into his office, as in my disposition to these circumstances. It was as if he was probing not my life, but my mind; not what I had made of my life, but why. I realized right then and there that there was no way of bluffing while he was probing you, an impression that I later had many opportunities of reinforcing. He saw right through you and would immediately ridicule any pretensions. Halfway through the interview, he seemed to have made up his mind: he apparently trusted his instincts more than the particulars of my curriculum vitae. There was no evasive "We will let you know" to postpone the necessity of making a decision; the issue was settled right there and then. Despite my complete lack of credentials, despite the absence of a single letter recommending me for scientific work, he took the risk of accepting me as his student. The lever was pulled and the train headed off in a new direction. Goodbye to dreams of becoming a world expert on Violacea and welcome to the H-2 cabal! For the subject I was going to work on was also decided in that interview, which did not last more than half an hour. The way this decision was reached was characteristic of Milan.

"As for the topic of your PhD work ....," a pause and a few puffs of his pipe, then a flicker in his eyes as if he had just hit on a mischievous idea ..., "have you heard of George Klein and his work on *H-2* heterozygous tumors?" I shake my head.

"No, of course not, it has nothing to do with beans" (a reference to my previous interest). Then follows a brief discourse on the ideas George and Eva Klein were pursuing in their studies, which I naturally comprehend only dimly. The sparkle returns to his eyes and a wicked grin spreads over his face: "Let's confuse everyone a bit and have a third Klein working on H-2 tumor variants! Yes, that's a splendid idea!" Then with finality: "You will work on *H-2*." And so I did, and still do. Before entering his office, I did not know that something called "the *H-2* locus" even existed, and now it was to become my destiny, my luck, my karma, my kismet.

O Fortuna, velut luna statu variabilis.

A closely watched train pulling out of the station.

Actually, the train was not closely watched at all. The next time Milan heard of the progress I was making with the topic he had assigned to me was at my PhD defense 2 years later. (No, I am exaggerating slightly.) It suited me perfectly that he paid so little attention to my work because it made me learn immunogenetics the hard way, and that was good for me.

The Train's Stops

From studying somatic tumor variants to becoming fully engrossed in the *H-2* complex was only a small step which I did not hesitate to take at the first opportunity. But since few know about somatic tumor variants these days, perhaps I had better explain.

Tumors are rejected when transplanted from the inbred strain in which they arose to a congenic strain which differs from the donor at the *H-2* complex only. This is so because the H-2 molecules act as potent antigens stimulating both cellular and humoral immune response. Tumors are also rejected when transplanted from an F_1 hybrid of two such strains to either of the parental strains. The recipient recognizes the H-2 antigens of the opposite parent expressed by the *H-2* heterozygous tumor and mounts an immune response against them. From time to time, however, such F_1-derived tumors throw off variants that become fully compatible with one of the two parental strains, and in some of the variants it could be demonstrated that they had lost the H-2 antigens of the opposite parent while retaining the antigens of the recipient to which they became adapted (Klein and Klein 1958). The question was: by what mechanism did the variants arise? Good evidence could be put forward that the mechanism had a genetic basis, and there was therefore hope that the variants would provide a means of studying the genetic organization of the *H-2* complex in somatic cells as an alternative to the conventional way based on methods involving formal genetics.

I did not, I must admit, bring the problem any closer to a solution than the Stockholm group did (Klein 1966), and sometimes I toy with the idea of returning to the project in order to find out what was really going on in those tumor cells that suddenly lost a whole set of H-2 antigens. I had, however, learned a lot about *H-2* during this work and I became so fascinated by this genetic region that for the next 25 years I let it dominate my scientific life.

In those 25 years, the scenery around me changed at approximately 5-year intervals, as the train pulled into various stations along the route: Prague, Stanford, Ann Arbor, Dallas, Tübingen, Miami. ... The work, too, acquired new twists, for the *H-2* complex provided a great selection of topics to study. Are you immunologically inclined? The *H-2* will provide a perfect diving board from which you can jump into this particular swimming pool. All you have to do is to ask how the *H-2* complex controls the immune response, and before you know it, you become a cellular immunologist. Or do you get particular pleasure from studying the behavior of genes in populations? The *H-2* is a wonderful model system, ideally suited for such work. It suffices merely to interest yourself in the *H-2* polymorphism, and soon you are swimming in a completely different pool. Do you get a special kick out of deciphering the organization of gene complexes? There are few chromosomal regions more suited to appeasing your craving than *H-2*.

I could go on like this because the possibilities (and temptations) offered by the *H-2* complex are many. I have explored several of them and enjoyed them all. Here, I would like to discuss the one that has occupied me lately and that has taken me perhaps furthest away from my original destination.

Mickey's Ancestors

While trying to understand the origins of the *H-2* polymorphism, it occurred to me that there might be a different way of considering it from that adopted by immunologists and geneticists until then (Klein 1980). Previously, it had been taken for granted that the polymorphism arose after speciation and therefore in a relatively short time (in geological terms). Take mice as an example. The ancestors of the common house mouse, from which the laboratory mouse with all its inbred strains is derived, probably lived somewhere in present-day Pakistan, or at least on the Indian subcontinent (Klein et al. 1988a, b). They constituted a single, probably very large population, living completely independently of humans and of other primates. Then, between 1 and 2 million years ago, the single gene pool somehow split into two, between which gene exchange was no longer possible. Perhaps as a result of climatic changes, the Iranian plateau and the bordering mountains became temporarily hospitable, and the mouse population spread via the southern part of the Soviet Union into China. Later, when harsh conditions returned to Iran, the Chinese mouse population could no longer communicate with the Pakistani population, and the two began to evolve in separate ways. At the time the barrier arose between them, both populations were of considerable size, adding up to millions of individuals. Both populations contained a large pool of *H-2* alleles, probably no less than 100 at each of the functional loci, just like mouse populations do today. At the start of the separation period, the allelic endowment at the *H-2* loci was more or less the same in both populations; it began to differentiate only after the separation. After 1 million years, the populations had acquired a sufficient number of differences to prevent free interbreeding when they eventually met in central Europe. Their encounter was most likely a direct consequence of the neolithic agricultural revolution that took place some 8000–6000 years ago in the "fertile crescent" and in China.

Storing of grain by humans amounted to a direct invitation to mice (for which grain was the main food resource) to move into human dwellings, or at least their close vicinity. The mice, of course, accepted this invitation unconditionally and found the arrangement so congenial that when humans got the migratory itch and began to colonize the entire Earth, mice spread with them, first to Europe, and then to the rest of the world. There may have been two different sources of mice spreading into Europe, corresponding to the two populations that became separated 1–2 million years ago. From China, an eastern form spread, perhaps in a single, continuous wave, via the Soviet Union into eastern Europe. From the Middle East, a western form spread, probably for the most part by ships in multiple, discontinuous, quantal jumps via ancient trading routes in the Mediterranean region and then into western Europe. The two forms met on an imaginary line crossing Europe from north to south from the Jutland peninsula to the Adriatic coast (Sage et al. 1986a). The fact that they were different forms became apparent at this imaginary line. Although some of the eastern mice mate with the western mice, the hybrids in the narrow "hybrid zone" are often infertile. The two forms apparently became, since their separation more than 1 million years ago, different species or "almost-species" (taxonomists have not reached an agreement on this point): the eastern form is *Mus musculus* and the western form is *Mus domesticus*.

The sterility of some of the *M. musculus* × *M. domesticus* hybrids from the hybrid zone is a consequence of the two species accumulating genetic differences, some of which influence reproductive behavior (Ivanyi et al. 1969). There may, however, also be other reasons why the two species hold their lines and do not intermix freely, such as subtle adaptation to a particular climate (the hybrid zone lies in a region of transition between Atlantic and continental climates; see Klein et al. 1988a, b), a different degree of dependency on humans for food and shelter, or a different parasite load (Sage et al. 1986b).

The remarkable thing about the two species is that they hardly differ in their *H-2* alleles. Most of the alleles found in *M. domesticus* (wild or laboratory) also occur in *M. musculus*. Whether they are exactly the same alleles, we are not certain, but they are indistinguishable serologically and in some instances also by tryptic peptide mapping of the H-2 molecules (Arden and Klein 1982). To be sure, there are differences in frequencies of the individual alleles in the two species, but such differences also exist among populations within a given species. Moreover, thorough analysis will probably show that a few alleles present in one species are either missing or under-represented in the other species. On the whole, however, it is difficult to differentiate the two species as far as the *H-2* complex is concerned.

It seemed to me inconceivable that all the *H-2* polymorphism arose independently in the two species in the last 1 million years. If this were so, many differences in *H-2* alleles between the two species should be found, identical alleles in these species should not occur (it is extremely unlikely that convergent evolution would achieve in 1 million years more than 50 identical nucleotide substitutions in two genes, no matter how strong the selection on the genes were), and the *H-2* genes would have to evolve at an incredibly rapid speed. It seemed more logical to postulate that the lack of any great differences between *H-2* polymorphism of *M. musculus* and *M. domesticus* was a reflection of the mode in which the two species arose (Klein 1980). Neither species started from a single pair or from very few individuals, but from a large population in which the *H-2* polymorphism was as great as in the ancestral population before it split. As the two populations began to evolve their separate ways, each of them could fall back on a rich endowment of *H-2* alleles that they had inherited from the common ancestral population. During their separate evolution, they of course enriched this endowment by slowly adding (not at a faster pace than is common to many genes) mutational differences to the alleles that they had inherited, and the two species thus began gradually to drift apart also at their *H-2* loci. However, the differences now, after 1 million years, are still too small to be easily detected by serological methods. In other words, the bulk of the existing *H-2* polymorphism predates speciation.

Hugo's Legacy

In an attempt to verify the trans-species hypothesis of *MHC* polymorphism, my co-workers and I turned to another taxonomic group, the primates. Mice are good to work with if one is interested in populations, immune response, or gene organization. On the other hand, very little is known about their evolution, and so arguments about the origin of *MHC* polymorphism usually fall on deaf ears when one begins to discuss *M. musculus* and *M. domesticus*. "They are not even real species, only a few experts can tell them apart, and they interbreed in the laboratory" is an argument that one hears frequently. Nobody, on the other hand, questions the fact that chimpanzees are a different species from humans, and so we turned from mice to these primates.

The particular chimpanzee we worked with goes by the name of Hugo and his home is the Primate Center at Rijswijk, Netherlands. Several years ago, a serological analysis of Hugo's white blood cells revealed that he carries a ChLA antigen (ChLA-A108) very similar to the human HLA-A11: the cells reacted with most of the HLA-A11-specific human antisera (Balner et al. 1978). This observation could have reflected a chance occurrence of the same epitope between two distantly related molecules, but it could also have signaled a close evolutionary relationship between alleles in chimpanzees and humans. To choose between these two possibilities, we isolated Hugo's gene coding for ChLA-A108 antigen and sequenced it (Mayer et al. 1988). The sequence demonstrated unambiguously that the *ChLA-A108* allele is indeed closely related to the *HLA-A11* allele, much more than *HLA-A11* is related to certain other *HLA-A* alleles. This result is to be expected under the assumption of the *HLA* polymorphism predating the separation of humans and chimpanzees from a common ancestor, a process that is now estimated to have begun more than 5 million years ago. Sequencing of other chimpanzee class I and class II genes revealed similar affinities between other *ChLA* and *HLA* alleles, indicating that the *ChLA-A108/HLA-A11* homology is not some weird exception but an example of a general trend.

The Eve Myth

Although the original motivation for studying *MHC* polymorphism in different species was to search for proof of the trans-species hypothesis, it did not escape my attention that there is a totally different lesson to be learnt from such a study. If we accept that the bulk of the *MHC* polymorphism predates speciation, we should be able to make inferences from the degree of polymorphism about the speciation process itself, in particular about the size of the population from which a given species began. If it were true, as many biologists still believe, that most species are founded by a single pair of individuals, no more than four *MHC* alleles could be transmitted trans-specifically. Actually, in such a case *no* polymorphism would be transmitted in this way because during the phase of extremely small population size ("bottleneck"), random drift would probably eliminate three of the four alleles and fix only the fourth one. By following this logic, we should be able to estimate, from the extent of the present-day *MHC* polymorphism in each species, how large the founding population of this species was. The one species that interests us most in this regard is our own, *Homo sapiens*.

Until recently, very few scientists took the Judeo-Christian myth seriously, according to which all humanity descends from a single male, Adam, who gave rise to the first female, Eve, by a sort of vegetative propagation. In 1987, however, a study was published (Cann et al. 1987) which was widely interpreted by the press, and by some scientists as well, as providing support for the Judeo-Christian myth. According to this study, based on the analysis of human mitochondrial DNA, all humanity originates from a single female, promptly dubbed as Eve, who lived in Africa some 200 000 years ago. The analysis of the *HLA* polymorphism, however, tells a different story.

If we take the nucleotide sequence difference between *ChLA-A108* and *HLA-A11* as a measure for the trans-species origin of alleles, we can estimate which of the *HLA* alleles already sequenced must have been present in the founding population of the human species. (These alleles have, of course, since accumulated additional mutations, but this fact does not influence our considerations.) From the sequenced alleles, we can then make inferences about the rest of the *HLA* alleles, defined thus far only serologically. (Strictly speaking, serology defines only antigens, but each antigen in the WHO table of HLA specificities must be controlled by a separate allele, so that the table is at the same time a minimal list of alleles. This list does not include the antigens that have been split, but these should not have been left in the table, anyway.) From the available information, I estimate that at least 20 of the present-day *HLA-A* alleles and probably an even larger number of the present-day *HLA-B* alleles already existed in the founding human populations (not, however, in the present-day form). One can make simple computer simulations to determine how large the founding population would have to be (and what could have been the smallest bottleneck at any time afterwards) to assure that all these alleles would be passed on through all the generations to the present-day population without any of them being lost by random drift. Such simulations are still in progress but preliminary results indicate that the founding population could not have consisted of anything less than many thousands of individuals. There is certainly no way that we could all be descended from a single couple at any time during the last 5 million years, the time of our separation from a common ancestor with the chimpanzee. The Eve hypothesis therefore remains a myth.

In fact, the Eve hypothesis is based on a misunderstanding and upon the confusion between an ancestral gene and an ancestral individual. We may all derive our mitochondrial DNA from a single female, but that does not mean that this female was the only one alive at that time or that we derive all of our other genes from her. Mitochondrial DNA does not recombine and so it can be regarded as a single gene. It is a well-known fact of population biology that every gene at a particular locus could be traced back to a single ancestral individual, but it is equally obvious that genes at different loci trace back to different ancestral individuals. The identification of an ancestor of all of our mitochondrial DNA therefore does not mean that this individual begat the human race.

On the positive side, however, the study of the *MHC* polymorphism offers the opportunity not only of uprooting myths, but also of making positive statements about the process of speciation and migration. The study should allow, for example, the calculation of the smallest bottlenecks in human history and prehistory, the size of the human population that colonized the Americas 10000–15000 years ago, and the minimal number of humans that colonized Australia more than 30000 years ago, as well as to answer many interesting questions about the evolution of a great number of animal species. The switchman of the particular train 25 years ago could not have had any idea about all this, nor about the many exotic places the train would pass through. Perhaps his only concern then, like that of Miloš' mother, was not to let the trains collide. . . .

Acknowledgment. I thank Ms. Lynne Yakes for editorial assistance. The current research described in this communication was supported in part by a grant from the National Institutes of Health, Bethesda, Maryland. The Latin quote is from Carl Orff's *Carmina Burana.*

References

Arden B, Klein J (1982) Biochemical comparison of major histocompatibility complex molecules from different subspecies of *Mus musculus:* Evidence for trans-specific evolution of alleles. Proc Natl Acad Sci USA 79: 2342–2346

Balner H, van Vreeswijk W, Roger JH, D'Amaro J (1978) The major histocompatibility complex of chimpanzees: Identification of several new antigens controlled by the A and B loci of ChLA. Tissue Antigens 12: 1–18

Cann RL, Stoneking M, Wilson AC (1987) Mitochondrial DNA and human evolution. Nature 324: 60–63

Ivanyi P, Vojtíšková M, Démant P, Micková M (1969) Genetic factors in the ninth linkage group influencing reproductive performance in male mice. Folia Biol (Praha) 15: 401–421

Klein G, Klein E (1958) Histocompatibility changes in tumors. J Cell Comp Physiol 52 [Suppl 1]: 125–168

Klein J (1966) The use of tissue incompatibility in the genetics of the somatic cell (in Czech). Academia, Praha

Klein J (1980) Generation of diversity at MHC loci: implications for T-cell receptor repertoires. In: Fougereau M, Dausset J (eds) Immunology, vol 80. Academic, London, pp 239–253

Klein J, Tichy H, Figueroa F (1988a) On the origin of mice. Anales de l'Universidad de Chile (in press)

Klein J, Vincek V, Kasahara M, Figueroa F (1988b) Probing mouse origins with random DNA probes. Curr Top Microbiol Immunol 137: 55–63

Mayer WE, Jonker M, Klein D, Ivanyi P, van Seventer G, Klein J (1988) Nucleotide sequence of chimpanzee MHC class I alleles: evidence for trans-species mode of evolution. EMBO J 7: 2765–2774

Sage RD, Heyneman D, Lim KC, Wilson AC (1986a) Wormy mice in a hybrid zone. Nature 324: 60–63

Sage RD, Whitney JB III, Wilson AC (1986b) Genetics analysis of a hybrid zone between domesticus and musculus mice (*Mus musculus* complex): hemoglobin polymorphisms. Curr Top Microbiol Immunol 127: 75–85

From Histocompatibility to Cancer

P. Demant

As for most of my colleagues, the way to biology began for me at the outset of my university studies. At the Medical School in Kosice, I became a helper and collaborator on a project at the Department of Biology on the influence of radiation on immunological tolerance. These studies were inspired by and carried out in collaboration with Milan Hašek's group in Prague. I knew this fact, but I did not pay much attention to it, though it was bound to influence my career and life profoundly in the future. At the end of my studies (which I carried out, after the first 2 years in Kosice, at the Faculty of Pediatrics of the Charles University in Prague) a possibility had arisen to work on my PhD thesis in Milan Hašek's department at the Academy of Sciences, and I became a member of Pavol Ivanyi's group. At that time Pavol was involved in his original line of research – immunogenetics in rabbits – and had also started work on human histocompatibility antigens. Those were the years of pioneering work and a team spirit when we strove to create an important center of human immunogenetic research in Prague.

My memory of Milan Hašek during the years of my PhD work is more "institutional" than personal – it is the memory of the atmosphere in his Institute, which to my knowledge, has not had a parallel anywhere else in the country. In the large building in Dejvice, housing several Institutes of Academy, behind the glass door separating the not so large corridor where Hašek's Institute has been located, a different world started, in many ways brighter and more full of promise than the one left outside. Personal freedom, enthusiasm and discovery were in the air. The scientists from Paris or New York ceased to be beings from another planet, and became just colleagues – or competitors. This feeling of being the active participant in the process of development of science has been a unique gift of Milan to so many people, and one can never stop being grateful for it.

After finishing my PhD thesis, I left to work for a year with Dr. George D. Snell at The Jackson Laboratory in Bar Harbor. That stay in 1968 was one of the most pleasant experiences in my life. The excitement about the experimental work during my stay in the United States had, however, increasingly to compete for attention with the new developments in Czechoslovakia. This culminated, for me, on August 21 at about 10.30 pm, when I was busy with journals at the library of The Jackson Laboratory (open 24 h a day – a luxury unknown in Prague). Ralph Graph, who was a summer visitor in Dr. Snell's laboratory, drove from the town to the laboratory, looking for me with the news of the day.

The decision what to do was difficult for every member of our institute at that time. Mine was motivated by the belief that the Prague institute had sufficient potential to produce excellent results. I was not wrong in this respect, at least for a certain period. My memories of Milan from this second period are much more personal. I owe him much for the help in the few remaining years when he was still the director, but I remember two things most about him – first the dignity and enthusiasm with which he returned to the experimental work after he was removed from his post, and second, the insights into his way of thinking, scientific and otherwise, which he offered me during several long walks through Prague. He had not only brilliant mind and unexhaustible energy, he liked people, and he valued originality. Certainly, this account falls short of describing my feelings for the great man, but those who knew him, his times, and the Institute he built, will understand.

These developments and events were taking place against the background of the changing situation in the country and in the Institute. Although I regretted extremely having to leave the country and my coworkers with whom we had accomplished so much in such a short time, the departure was the only right decision.

In my work at the Netherlands Cancer Institute, we first aimed to extend our results on genetics and function of the class I and class III MHC products. This work has been sufficiently published (see the list of publications at the end of this book). The interest in the problem of cancer, stimulated in the new surroundings, led to realization that the customary opportunistic joining of the MHC control of immune response and tumor biology is, in the long term, not the only, and even not necessarily the best possible approach to the understanding of the role of MHC in tumor resistance. We decided to look at the possible mechanisms of the effects of MHC on tumor susceptibility. This approach aims to elucidate the role of MHC in the biology of the tumor cell and of the tumor-host relationship, not by mechanical extrapolation of presently known functions of MHC, but by analysis of its truly relevant effects. It is being presently developed in collaboration especially with Drs. Lauran Oomen, Margriet Oudshoorn-Snoek, and Martin van der Valk, and has been aided by cooperation and discussions with Drs. A. Dux and R. van Nie.

The long-term devotion to MHC research has not prevented us from realizing that the effects of the MHC on tumor susceptibility are often relatively minor and not typical for the majority of tumor susceptibility genes. The non-MHC-linked genes very often cause 10–100-fold differences in incidence or multiplicity of tumors. No less impressive are the qualitative differences among the histological types of tumors in different inbred strains. Not surprisingly, the effort to understand genetics of tumor susceptibility has been the major driving force behind the development of inbred mouse strains, and thus behind the whole mouse genetics. Paradoxically, however, looking back to the eminently successful decades of mouse genetics, identification of tumor susceptibility genes is a conspicuously rare event – with the exception of the genes affecting viral replication, and the unexpected but avidly exploited finding of the role of MHC in tumor susceptibility. Most of the non-MHC tumor susceptibility genes remain unknown.

In view of the largely unsuccessful attempts of others to identify the tumor susceptibility genes using the available genetic methods, it could be concluded that these methods do not possess sufficient resolution power to undertake the study of tumor susceptibility genes. Therefore we generated a new genetic tool specifically for this purpose. In the next pages I will give a brief outline of our present work on MHC and non-MHC tumor susceptibility genes.

Lilly et al. (1964) revealed that the *H-2* genotype affects induction of mouse leukemia by Gross-MuLV. Subsequently, *H-2* has been shown to affect many other tumors (for review see Demant and Cleton 1980). To understand the nature of the *H-2* influence on tumorigenesis, we tested whether the *H-2* genotype affects the susceptibility to virally induced mammary tumors at the target cell level, as most tumor susceptibility genes do (Dux and Mühlbock 1968), or at the systemic level. Our results show (Dux and Demant 1987) that the latter is the case. Thus, the *H-2* effects on virally induced tumorigenesis are of a quite different nature than the effects of most tumor susceptibility genes on both virally, chemically, or hormonally induced tumors which generally tend to operate at target cell level (for references see Demant et al. 1989). Thus, the effects of *H-2* on virally induced tumorigenesis are *not typical* for most genetic effects on susceptibility to viral or chemical tumor induction. This conclusion raises two questions:

1. How do *H-2* genes affect carcinogen-induced tumors in various organs?
2. What are the "other" or "non-MHC" susceptibility genes?

MHC-Linked Tumor Susceptibility

In order to avoid the well-known influence of the MHC on immune response to viral antigens, we decided to study its role in chemical induction of tumors of epithelial origin. Research on tumorigenesis in epithelial organs is of great importance. More than 75% of human cancers are of epithelial origin, only about 8% are leukemias (Silverberg and Lubera 1986), and among the leukemias only a few are of viral etiology. However, looking at the literature on *H-2* effects on tumorigenesis, one would be lead to believe that the reverse is the case, since most of the effort is devoted to the systemic and, in essence, trivial immunological effects on virally induced leukemias. It is one of the examples of the situation where 90% of the effort goes into 10% of the problem. How do the *H-2* products affect the tumorigenesis in epithelial organs? We chose to study this question using as prototypes the lung tumors and intestinal tumors of the mouse. The *H-2* haplotypes affect prenatal and postnatal inducibility of lung tumors by various chemical carcinogens as well as their spontaneous appearance. Therefore, we hypothesized that these *H-2* effects are mediated through an influence of *H-2* on certain basic functional properties of the target cell (Demant 1986; Demant et al. 1989). We used in our studies the directly acting carcinogen mutagen *N*-ethyl-*N*-nitrosourea (ENU) in order to avoid any influence of genes connected with metabolic activation of carcinogens, rather than with the actual tumorigenic process. In mice of the strain C57BL/10 and its *H-2* congenic derivatives, essentially two types of lung tumors are found, alveolar and papillary (Oomen et al. 1983, 1988, and references therein). Both tumor types are believed to have the same origin – the alveolar type II cell (Rehm et al. 1988). The *H-2* complex affects the relative proportion of alveolar and papillary tumors, and the growth rate of papillary tumors in transplacentally ENU-treated mice (Oomen et al. 1983). In addition, these mice develop intestinal adenocarcinomas (Oomen et al. 1984). ENU administration on day 15 after birth also results in alveolar and papillary lung tumors and intestinal tumors. *H-2* genotype affects the incidence and age of appearance of the two types of lung tumors and of intestinal tumors. In addition, it affects the *location* of intestinal tumors [predominantly proximal in B10.A(2R), predominantly distal in B10.A(4R)]. *H-2* also affects development of liver adenocarcinomas in males of these strains. Several genes within the *H-2* complex are responsible for these effects (Oomen et al. 1988).

When considering the possible mechanisms of these results, we noted that the *H-2* complex affects the susceptibility of fetuses to glucocorticoid (GC)-induced teratogenesis (Demant 1985 and references therein), and that GC is the major factor regulating the differentiation and function of both lung alveolar type II cells and intestinal epithelium – which are the target cells for carcinogenesis in our experiments (Ballard 1983; Henning 1986). The *H-2* complex might affect the differentiation grade of these target cells by modifying their susceptibility to GC-induced differentiation, and the resulting *H-2*-related differences in differentiation stage might cause the differences in susceptibility of these cells to carcinogenesis. In order to test this possibility, we investigated whether there are *H-2* differences in susceptibility of lung to GC-induced lung differentiation, and whether the prenatal GC treatment can affect the prenatal induction of lung and intestinal tumors. These experiments revealed that *H-2* does indeed affect the GC-induced lung development, and that the GC treatment modifies in a haplotype-specific way both the induction of papillary lung tumors and intestinal tumors (Oomen et al. 1989). The essential features of the hormonal regulation of the development of the epithelial tissues (lung, intestine, bowel, liver, urinary tract, mammary gland) are the same, and include specific mesenchymal-epithelial interactions, some of which are mediated by soluble factors (for references see Oomen et al. 1989; Demant et al. 1989). The study of the role of *H-2* in these processes may reveal presently unknown functions of the MHC and provide an insight into the relationship of the differentiation stage of the cell and its susceptibility to neoplastic development.

In the experiments of Röpcke et al. (1987), we extended the observation of Mühlbock and Dux (1981) that *H-2* congenic strains differ in susceptibility to mammary tumor induction by hormonal stimulation from pituitary isografts (Boot et al. 1981). We found that *H-2* affects, beside the development of tumors, also the growth of the pituitary isograft and the level of estrogen receptors in the transplanted hypophysis (Röpcke et al. 1987). The relationship of these two latter phenomena to tumor susceptibility is not clear, although a larger size of hypophyseal isograft is associated with the tumor generation in resistant, but not in susceptible strains (Röpcke et al. in preparation).

Preliminary results with inbred strains other than C57BL/10 (van der Valk, Oomen, and Demant, in preparation) indicate that in these strains often quite different lung and mammary tumor types occur, or that the non-*H-2* genes also affect the proportion of alveolar and papillary lung tumors (as reported previously also by Witschi 1985; Beer and Malkinson 1985). Generally, C57BL/10 is a rather atypical mouse strain. Therefore, some aspects relevant for biology of *H-2* are likely to be missed or not completely comprehended when studied only on a C57BL/10 background. This is especially likely with tumorigenesis, which is qualitatively and quantitatively so considerably influenced by non-MHC genes. A recently completed series on new *H-2* congenic strains on an O20/A background could turn out to be a useful tool for study of the biology of the *H-2* gene complex on a completely different genetic background (Demant et al. in preparation.) However, a no less exciting question is: what are the non-MHC genes which affect tumorigenesis in mouse, and how do they accomplish their effects? Our approach to this problem is described in the next section.

Definition of Non-MHC Tumor Susceptibility Genes

Besides the MHC-linked genes, a large number of other genes also affecting tumor susceptibility exist. Their effects are often larger or at least as large as those of the MHC-linked genes. They affect mainly the susceptibility to tumorigenesis at target cell level (Demant et al. 1989).

Tumorigenesis differs among inbred strains qualitatively, rather than just quantitatively. Strains may differ in the type of tumors which arise in response to a certain carcinogenic agent. Also, tumors of the same origin may differ among the strains in the prevailing type of their differentiation or in the stage of progression. This "qualitative" aspect of tumor susceptibility genes must be kept in mind in the discussion which follows, although for practical purposes the genetics of tumor susceptibility must be treated as a quantitative trait. In most instances of strain differences in tumor susceptibility several genes are involved. The definition and mapping of the tumor susceptibility genes has turned out to be very difficult, or impossible. Therefore these genes remain largely unidentified.

Various methods of statistical analysis of such multigenic quantitative differences in segregating populations have been developed (reviewed by Roderick and Schlager 1966; Falconer 1963). A quantitative phenotype, however, cannot be established reliably in a single mouse, and it is also difficult to characterize such an ad hoc population for a sufficient number of genetic markers. Therefore, this way of establishing a linkage relationship for tumor susceptibility genes was very difficult.

Bailey (1965, 1971) recognized the need for a better analytical genetic tool and devised the recombinant inbred strains (RIS). A series of RIS has been produced, using a number of pairs of F_2 mice from a cross between two inbred strains (Fig. 1a). Each RIS received approximately half of its genes from each parental inbred strain. The set of genes inherited from each parental strain is different in each RIS. The use of the RIS provided two essential advantages when compared to previously available methods.

a) The individual RIS have been genotyped in order to establish which alleles of a particular gene were received from one parental strain and which from the other. Consequently, the strain distribution patterns in the RIS of a newly studied gene can be compared with that of all previously typed genes, greatly facilitating the finding of linkage.

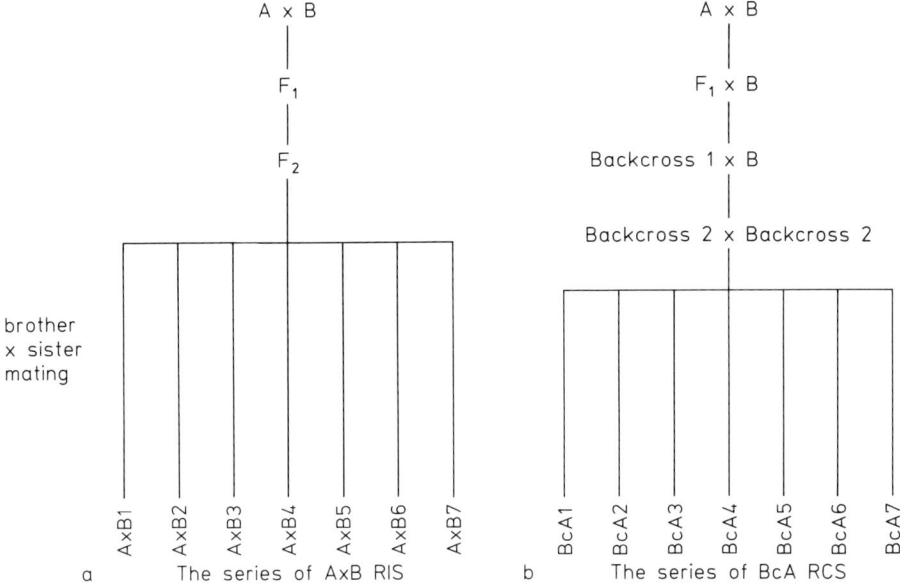

Fig. 1a, b. Production of recombinant inbred strains and recombinant congenic strains. **a** Recombinant inbred strains; **b** recombinant congenic strains

b) A quantitative phenotype, like incidence of tumors, can be established in RIS with the same certainty as in an inbred strain. Its strain distribution pattern can then be compared with that of previously typed genes in order to find evidence for linkage (Bailey 1981; Taylor 1978, 1980).

Although the gene mapping with the help of RIS has been generally very fruitful, this, unfortunately, did not turn out to be the case with tumor susceptibility genes. In most studies the phenotypes (e.g., tumor incidence) of different RIS form a continuous range of values, rather than well-defined phenotypic classes (Demant and Hart 1986). Therefore, no exact information about the genes involved and their linkage relationships could be obtained. This is primarily due to additive and nonadditive interactions among the several genes controlling tumor susceptibility. The correlation among the phenotypes of RIS and their genotypes, required for the genetic interpretation, is distorted or destroyed by such interactions, because similar phenotypes may be caused by different genotypes. A theoretical example of analysis of tumor susceptibility controlled by three nonlinked loci by a series of 16 RIS is given in Table 1A. Genetically quite different RIS strains (1, 2 versus 11, 12; and 5, 6 versus 15, 16) are phenotypically similar. The linkage indicated by the RIS is often even spurious and misleading. For example, the locus number 4 in Table 1 is not involved at all in tumor susceptibility, but exhibits the best correlation with it. The incomplete representation of all possible genotypic combinations in a series of RIS is another factor which makes the assessment of the nature of genetic control of a multigenically determined trait very difficult (Demant and Hart 1986).

Table 1. Tumor susceptibility genes analyzed with recombinant inbred strains and recombinant congenic strains – a model with three nonlinked loci

	Strains															
	1	2	3	4	5	6	7	8	9	10	11	12	13	14	15	16
A. RIS																
Locus 1	A	A	A	A	A	A	B	B	A	A	B	B	B	B	B	B
Locus 2	A	A	A	A	B	B	A	A	B	B	A	A	B	B	B	B
Locus 3	A	A	B	B	A	A	A	A	B	B	B	B	A	A	B	B
Locus 4	A	A	A	A	B	B	B	B	A	A	A	A	B	B	B	B
Incidence	90	90	100	100	20	20	40	40	60	60	80	80	0	0	10	10
B. RIS																
Locus 1	B	A	B	B	B	B	B	B	B	B	B	B	B	B	B	B
Locus 2	B	B	A	B	B	B	B	B	B	B	B	B	A	B	B	B
Locus 3	B	B	B	B	A	B	B	B	B	B	B	B	A	B	B	B
Locus 4	B	B	B	A	B	B	A	B	B	B	B	B	B	B	B	B
Incidence	10	60	80	10	0	10	10	10	10	10	10	10	40	10	10	10

Parental strains: A = tumor incidence 90%
B = tumor incidence 10%
Effects of the individual genes:
Locus 1: allele A 50%   allele B 0%
Locus 2: allele A 0%   allele B 70%
Locus 3: allele A 40%   allele B 80%
Locus 4: allele A 0%   allele B 0%

The multigenic nature of the control of tumor susceptibility is the principal obstacle in its genetic analysis using segregating populations or the RIS. Therefore, we devised a new analytic system, the recombinant congenic strains (RCS), which would transform the multigenic effect into a set of single gene effects which could be subsequently mapped and analyzed separately (Demant and Hart 1986). While each RIS received genes in equal proportions from each of the two parental strains, in the RCS the genes of one parental inbred strain (the "donor" strain) are randomly "diluted" in small proportions in the genetic background of the second parental inbred strain (the "background" strain). This is done by backcrossing repeatedly the donor strain to the background strain, and subsequent brother-sister mating (Fig. 1b). Each RCS contains a relatively small set of genes originating from the donor strain. Each of the several genes affecting tumor susceptibility in the donor strain will most likely be transferred into a different RCS. The majority of the RCS will be phenotypically identical to the background strain, but those RCS which received such genes from the donor strain will differ from the background strain in tumor susceptibility. The segregation of the tumor susceptibility genes in RIS and RCS and the resulting phenotypes, using a theoretical situation with three unlinked loci, are given in Table 1B. As the RCS become genotyped, the strain distribution of each new trait/gene can be compared with that of the previously typed genes to obtain indication of linkage.

What are the relative merits of the use of RCS (or RIS) on the one hand, and transgenic mice on the other? Transgenic mice have turned out to be a very useful tool in analysis of biological effects of specific genes which were cloned and in many instances also coupled with a desired promoter/enhancer element, or otherwise mutated. Therefore, the transgenic mice represent a *unigenic analytic system*. On the other hand, the RCS and RIS represent *coordinate* or *correlational* analytic systems, because they use the available information about the distribution of alleles of the genes of the two parental strains a set of coordinates with which one can correlate any new genetic trait. With the coordinate/correlational system a virtually unlimited number of polymorphic genes can be analyzed by a single set of 20–25 RIS or RCS. With a unigenic system, on the other hand, for each gene a separate strain of transgenic mice is needed.

Presently, three series of RCS are being produced in our laboratory: C3HcB10, 020cB10.020 and BALBccSTS, with the background and donor strains C3H/Sn and C57BL/10Sn, 020/A and B10.020/Dem, and BALB/cHe and STS/A, respectively. These strains are suitable for studying, among others, genetics of susceptibility to lung and intestinal tumors, colon tumors, liver tumors, virally and hormonally induced mammary tumors, and virally induced leukemias. However, they can also be used to study genetics of various aspects of immune response and other functional traits.

The RCS can also lead to a better understanding of the interactions of MHC genes with genes on other chromosomes. At present little is known about such interactions, although several examples on non-MHC-linked genes affecting class I (Sutton et al. 1983; van de Meugheuvel et al. 1985; Plata et al. 1987), class II (de Preval et al. 1985), and class III (Muir et al. 1984) expression and function were reported. Using the effects of non-MHC-linked genes on the expression of the two *S*-region genes *C4* and *Slp* (Bruisten and Demant 1989) as a model system, we demonstrated that the effects of non-MHC transregulatory genes quantitatively often equal or even exceed the effects of the *cis*-regulatory elements, and that some of these non-MHC effects are haplotype- and sex-specific, indicating complex interactions between the regulatory sequences of the *C4* and *Slp* genes and the products of non-MHC genes (Bruisten et al. 1989a). The expression of the *Slp* transregulatory genes appears to be connected with the androgen regulation of *Slp* expression (Bruisten et al. 1989b).

As the transregulatory factors are known to affect expression of a variety of target genes (for review see Ptashne 1988), it is likely that these *Slp* transregulatory genes also affect other androgen-regulated genes and processes. This is particularly interesting for further analysis of the interactions between the *H-2* complex and the sex-dependent effects of glucocorticoid hormones on carcinogen-induced tumorigenesis in the small intestine (Oomen et al. 1989) and sex-dependent *H-2* effects on liver carcinogenesis (Oomen et al. 1988). The RCS produced between 020 and B10.020 may be particularly useful in identifying these non-MHC *Slp*-regulatory genes. The RCS may also aid in identification of non-MHC immune response genes and genes affecting expression of T cell receptors (Pullen et al. 1988) and their interactions with the MHC regulation of immune responsiveness.

Acknowledgement. During the work discussed here I enjoyed the critical and stimulating discussions with Drs. A. Dux, L. C. J. M. Oomen, M. Oudshoorn-Snoek, G. Röpcke, M. A. van der Valk, A. A. M. Hart, S. M. Bruisten, C. J. A. Moen, and Prof. L. F. M. van Zutphen, and their collaboration in various aspects of this work.

Many thanks are due to Mrs. A. de Moes-Bezemer, Mrs. P. van Hasselt-Elsenburg, Mrs. M. Treur-Mulder, Mrs. E. Delzenne-Goette, Mrs. M. Butzelaar and Mr. J. de Moes and Mr. H. van Vugt for creative and expert technical assistance, and Mrs. M. Sonne-Gooren for excellent secretarial work.

References

Bailey DW (1965) A search for genetic background influences on survival time of skin grafts from mice bearing gamma-linked histoincompatibility. Transplantation 3: 531–534

Bailey DW (1971) Recombinant inbred strains: an aid to finding identity, linkage, and function of histocompatibility and other genes. Transplantation 11: 325–327

Bailey DW (1981) Recombinant inbred strains and bilineal congenic strains. In: Foster HL, Small JD, Gox JG (eds) The mouse in biomedical research. Academic, New York, pp 223–239

Ballard PL (1983) Hormones and receptors in developing lung. Prog Clin Biol Res 140: 103–117

Beer DG, Malkinson AM (1985) Genetic influence of type 2 or Clara cell origin of pulmonary adenomas in urethan-treated mice. J Natl Cancer Inst 75: 963–969

Boot LM, Kwa HG, Röpcke G (1981) Hormonal induction of the mouse mammary tumors. In: Hilgers J, Sluyser M (eds) Mammary tumors in the mouse. Elsevier/North-Holland, Amsterdam, pp 117–200

Bruisten SM, Demant P (1989) Regulation of expression of mouse C4 and Slp genes by non-H-2-linked genes. Immunogenetics 29: 6–13

Bruisten SM, Skamene E, Demant P (1989a) Haplotype-specific interactions of non-H-2-linked genetic factors controlling the mouse C4 and Slp protein levels. Genetics (in press)

Bruisten SM, Demant P, Robins DM (1989b) Trans-regulatory genes affect Slp^a and Slp^o expression and act in a tissue-specific manner. Immunogenetics (in press)

De Preval C, Lisowska-Grospierre B, Loche M, Griscelli C, Mach B (1985) A trans-acting class II regulatory gene unlinked to the MHC controls expression of HLA class II genes. Nature 318: 291–293

Demant P (1985) Corticosteroid-induced cleft palate: Cis interaction of MHC genes and hybrid resistance. Immunogenetics 22: 183–188

Demant P (1986) Histocompatibility and the genetics of tumour resistance. Introductory essay. J Immunogenet 13: 61–67

Demant P, Cleton FJ (1980) Histocompatibility genes and neoplasia. In: Cleton FJ, Simons JWIM (eds) Genetic origins of tumor cells. Nijhoff, The Hague, pp 109–125

Demant P, Hart AAM (1986) Recombinant congenic strains: a new tool for analyzing genetic traits determined by more than one gene. Immunogenetics 24: 416–422

Demant P, Oomen LCJM, Oudshoorn-Snoek M (1989) Genetics of tumor susceptibility in the mouse: major histocompatibility complex and non-MHC genes. Adv Cancer Res 53: 117–179

Dux A, Demant P (1987) The influence of the MHC on resistance against C3H-MTV induced mammary tumors is predominantly systemic rather than local. Int J Cancer 40: 372–377

Dux A, Mühlbock O (1968) Susceptibility of mammary tissues of different strains of mice to tumor development. JNCI 40: 1259–1265

Falconer DS (1963) Quantitative inheritance. In: Burdette WJ (ed) Methodology in mammalian genetics. Holden-Day, San Francisco, pp 193–216

Henning SJ (1986) Development of the gastrointestinal tract. Proc Nutr Soc 45: 39–44

Lilly F, Boyse EA, Old LJ (1964) Genetic basis of susceptibility to viral leukemogenesis. Lancet 2: 1207–1209

Mühlbock O, Dux A (1981) Histocompatibility genes and mammary cancer. In: Hilgers J, Sluyser M (eds) Mammary tumors in the mouse. Elsevier/North-Holland, Amsterdam, pp 545–572

Muir WA, Hedrick S, Alper CA, Ratnoff OD, Schacter B, Wisniesky JJ (1984) Inherited incomplete deficiency of the fourth component of complement (C4) determined by a gene not linked to human histocompatibility leukocyte antigens. J Clin Inv 74: 1509–1514

Oomen LCJM, Demant P, Hart AAM, Emmelot P (1983) Multiple genes in the H-2 complex affect differently the number and growth rate of transplacentally induced lung tumours in mice. Int J Cancer 31: 447–454

Oomen LCJM, van der Valk MA, Emmelot P (1984) Stem cell carcinoma in the small intestine of mice treated transplacentally with N-ethyl-N-nitrosourea: some quantitative and histological aspects. Cancer Lett 25: 71–79

Oomen LCJM, van der Valk MA, Hart AAM, Demant P, Emmelot P (1988) Influence of mouse major histocompatibility complex (H-2) on N-ethyl-N-nitrosourea-induced tumor formation in various organs. Cancer Res 48: 6634–6641

Oomen LCJM, van der Valk MA, Hart AAM, Demant P (1989) Glucocorticoid hormone effect on transplacental carcinogenesis and lung differentiation: influence of histocompatibility-2 (H-2) complex. J Natl Cancer Inst 81: 512–517

Plata F, Langlade-Demoyen P, Abastado JP, Berbar T, Kourilsky P (1987) Retrovirus antigens recognized by cytolytic T lymphocytes activate tumor rejection in vivo. Cell 48: 231–240

Ptashne M (1988) How eukaryotic transcriptional activators work. Nature 335: 683–689

Pullen AM, Marrack P, Kappler JW (1988) The T cell repertoire is heavily influenced by tolerance to polymorphic self-antigens. Nature 335: 796–801

Rehm S, Ward JM, ten Have-Opbroek AAW, Anderson LM, Singh G, Katyal SL, Rice JM (1988) Mouse papillary lung tumors transplacentally induced by N-nitrosoethylurea: evidence for alveolar type II cell origin by comparative light microscopic, ultrastructural, and immunohistochemical studies. Cancer Res 48: 148–160

Roderick TH, Schlager G (1966) Multiple factor inheritance. In: Green EL (ed) Biology of the laboratory mouse. McGraw-Hill, New York, pp 151–164

Röpcke G, Sluyser M, Demant P (1987) H-2 and the hormonal factors in mammary tumorigenesis. In: David CS (ed) H-2 antigens: genes, molecules, and functions. Plenum, New York, pp 681–689

Silverberg E, Lubera J (1986) Cancer statistics 1986. CA 36: 9–16

Sutton VR, Hogarth PM, McKenzie IFC (1983) Description of a new QA antigenic specificity, Qa-m9, whose expression is under complex genetic control. J Immunol 131: 1363–1367

Taylor BA (1978) Recombinant inbred strains: use in gene mapping. In: Morse HC (ed) Origin of inbred mice. Academic, New York, pp 423–438

Taylor BA (1980) Recombinant inbred mice: use in genetic analysis of disease resistance. In: Skamene E, Kougsharn PAL, Landy M (eds) Genetic control of natural resistance to infection and malignancy. Academic, New York, pp 1–8

Van de Meugheuvel W, van Seventer G, Demant P (1985) A new Tla region antigen Qa-11, similar to Qa-2 and associated with B-type beta-2-microglobulin. J Immunol 134: 2507–2512

Witschi HP (1985) Enhancement of lung tumor formation. In: Mass MJ, Kaufman DG, Siegfried JM, Steele VE, Nesnow S (eds) Cancer of the respiratory tract – predisposing factors. Raven, New York, pp 147–158

HLA Antigens and Matching for Kidney Transplantation

P. T. Klouda

On a breezy afternoon during the Ninth International Transplantation Society meeting in August 1983 I met Milan Hašek again after many years. A group of us were sitting on the terrace of the Metropole Hotel in Brighton, discussing the latest trends and developments in transplant immunology. Tolerance was of course high on the agenda and so was the role of the HLA system in the new cyclosporin era which was just beginning. Milan Hašek did not hide his delight when he was commenting on the role of HLA matching in improving graft survival. Not surprisingly, since it was in 1965 that colleagues from Milan Hašek's institute in Prague, in collaboration with Professor Dausset in Paris first described the ancestor of the HLA, the Hu-1 system (Dausset et al. 1965). The Ivanyis and Dausset stood at the cradle of the newly described system of leucocyte antigens. Milan Hašek was the godfather who witnessed its birth and followed its progress over the years with great interest.

The role of HLA matching in renal transplantation has not always been undisputed. In 1971 Terasaki and Mickey suggested that HLA matching might not have as great an impact on graft survival as was hoped, but by the time of the Ninth Congress of the Transplantation Society in Brighton the role of HLA matching in improving graft survival was generally accepted. Numerous papers both from single centres and from national and international transplant registries were suggesting that HLA matching had an important role in transplantation. Since 1975, when pre-transplant blood transfusions became a common practice in most transplant centres, there has been a steady improvement in the rate of survival of cadaver kidney transplants. Apart from the blood transfusion factor, the introduction of cyclosporin played an important role in further improving the annual rate of graft survival.

Because of these improvements in graft survival, the role of HLA matching has been repeatedly questioned. Has the blood transfusion effect and Cyclosporin therapy obliterated the role of HLA matching and is HLA matching still relevant in the cyclosporin era?

Materials and Methods

The United Kingdom Transplant Service (UKTS) is a national organisation with which transplantation centres and tissue-typing laboratories throughout the British Isles cooperate. UKTS was established in 1972 to coordinate the distribution of kidneys in order to improve histocompatibility matches in patients waiting for a kidney transplant. UKTS also maintains the national waiting list and collects data on graft and patient survival, and provides an information service and biostatistical analysis of transplant survival data. The results of these analyses are used to implement policies which maximise the survival time of transplanted organs through HLA matching and any other factors identified by the analyses.

The role of HLA matching was investigated in a total of 2282 first cadaveric kidney transplants performed between 1979 and 1984. Details of the donors and recipients and the biostatistical methods used in the analyses have been described in detail by Gilks et al. (1987).

Results and Discussion

In the past it was customary to study the influence of HLA-A and -B matching and of DR matching separately. When sufficient numbers of DR-typed recipients were transplanted, the influence of matching for the three loci was usually analysed jointly with no distinction whether mismatches occurred at any one of the three loci.

With the large number of transplants on the UKTS registry it is possible to analyse the effects of mismatching at HLA-A, -B and -DR loci independently. At each locus there are three possible levels of mismatching (no mismatches, one mismatch and two mismatches). The combination of three HLA loci and three levels of mismatching at each results in 27 categories of mismatches among the recipients. Table 1 shows the 1-year graft survival rate in some of the mismatch categories.

Patients who receive grafts with no identifiable mismatches have a superior graft survival rate (93%) than patients who have received a graft with one or more HLA mismatches. However, even among patients with one single HLA mismatch, there is a difference in graft survival depending on which locus is mismatched. In the group of patients with one mismatch for HLA-A antigen the graft survival rate is 86%. Patients with one B locus mismatch have a graft survival rate of 81%. Patients with one identifiable DR locus mismatch have a graft survival rate of 67%. Graft survival in the patients in the last category is no different from graft survival in patients mismatched for two or more antigens at any one, or at different, HLA loci. The results show that patients with no more than one mismatch at A or B locus but no mismatch at DR locus enjoy far better graft survival than patients mismatched for either a single DR antigen or numerous mismatches for A, B or DR loci. Patients in the first category have been referred to as "beneficially matched". The concept of beneficial matching has been confirmed by the results of other national and international registries. In 1986 Terasaki reported a graft survival rate in

Table 1. One year graft survival and HLA matching in first cadaver graft recipients

HLA-A, -B, -DR mismatches	000	100	010	001	Total 2	Total 3	Total 4	Total 5
One-year survival (%)	93	86	81	67	73	70	71	65

excess of 90% in HLA-A, -B and -DR-matched first cadaver transplants. Patients with one mismatch at the A locus had similar graft survival, whereas mismatching for B locus or DR locus antigens resulted in a graft survival rate of 80% and 75%, respectively, with further mismatching having a minimal effect on the decline in the 1-year graft survival rates.

The statistics provide clear-cut evidence of the importance of HLA matching in graft survival and particularly the importance of transplanting with no incompatibilities. The examination of the HLA types of recipients and donors in which this degree of matching has been achieved shows a strong deviation in the frequencies of HLA antigens from those observed in the overall donor population. As expected, donors with one detected antigen at any one locus are easier to match than heterozygotes. This is particularly true for the DR locus. Kidneys from donors with conserved haplotypes are also more likely to be beneficially matched than kidneys from donors with HLA antigens which are not in strong positive linkage disequilibrium.

Among the 2282 transplants in which the beneficial matching effect was established, 68 recipients received grafts with no mismatches. Forty-nine received kidneys from donors who carried HLA-A1, -B8 and -DR3 antigens. Furthermore, 13 kidneys with no mismatches were typed as A1, B8, DR3 only.

In a further study of the effect of benefical matching, a total of 408 beneficially matched grafts were reported to UKTS during 1986 and 1987. Of those 115 (28%) were A1, B8, DR3-positive with 23 kidneys transplanted from donors homozygous for A1, B8, DR3 or at least for B8, DR3. The frequencies of other commonly occurring haplotypes in the British Isles was increased in the donors whose kidneys were beneficially matched.

This observation raises the question of whether the increased frequency of the common types and haplotypes in the group of patients with no mismatches is purely a result of the ease with which these kidneys can be matched or whether the improved graft survival observed in the group of patients is the result of genotype rather than phenotype matching. It is possible to speculate that matching for preserved haplotypes such as A1, B8, DR3; A3, B7, DR2 or A2, B44, DR7, which results in the improvement of graft survival, is equivalent to transplantation of HLA identical related individuals. Presently there are not enough beneficially matched transplants from donors who have not got identifiable haplotypes to compare their graft survival with patients beneficially matched for well-documented haplotypes. And so, after the identification of the role of beneficial matching in kidney transplantation, the question of HLA types and haplotypes which are important in improved graft survival requires further analysis.

Acknowledgements. It is customary to acknowledge the collaboration of colleagues who have been directly involved in producing the data and results presented in a report and those who helped in preparing the manuscript for print. I would therefore like to thank Professor Bradley and all my colleagues at the UKTS for their help and also my collaborators at the MRC Biostatistical Unit in Cambridge, Dr. Sheila Gore and Dr. Wally Gilks, without whose collaboration the analysis of the data would have not been possible. I would also like to thank Mrs. Anne Darch for typing this manuscript.

It is not customary to thank people who have not been directly involved in the work and analysis of results but who have left a lasting impression on the author through past collaboration. I would like to take this opportunity to thank my colleagues and friends with whom I collaborated back in the late 1960s at the Institute of Experimental Biology and Genetics in Prague who set me on the path of HLA which I have followed ever since I left the Institute, first in London, then in Geneva, Manchester and finally in Bristol. Without the friendship, stimulating discussions and help from Pavol Ivanyi, Peter Demant, Eva Ivaskova, Milena Rychlikova and many others with whom I spent numerous hours discussing the Hu-1 and later the HL-A system, this paper would have not existed. And, during these discussions and scientific disputations, we were always aware of the presence of the towering figure of Milan Hašek whose institute provided a haven for the scientific community and the intellectual milieu in which many new ideas originated.

References

Dausset J, Ivanyi P, Ivanyi D (1965) Tissue alloantigens in humans: identification of a complex system (Hu-1). In: Balner H et al. (eds) Histocompatibility testing. Munksgaard, Copenhagen, pp 51–62

Gilks WR, Bradley BA, Gore SM, Klouda PT (1987) Substantial benefits of tissue matching in renal transplantation. Transplantation 43: 669–674

Terasaki PI, Mickey MR (1971) Histocompatibility – transplant correlation, reproducibility and new matching methods. Transplant Proc 3: 1057–1071

Terasaki PI (1986) Editorial in Clinical Transplants, UCLA Tissue Typing Laboratory, Los Angeles California

HLA Subtypes

H. Mervart

> When my family moved to our new homeland Canada, it was the mention of the name Milan Hašek as both my PhD supervisor and mentor that was largely responsible for my first position. Throughout the worldwide scientific field Milan was well known and respected professionally. Those of us who were fortunate to have been associated with him will always remember his boundless energy, high spirits, and especially his friendliness that made Milan dear to everyone who worked with him.

Introduction

The major histocompativility complex (MHC) in man is known as the HLA system and has been localized to a small segment of chromosome 6. The HLA complex is the most polymorphic genetic system found in humans. It is composed of a series of at least 11 closely linked genes. Based on the most recent nomenclature report (Bodmer et al. 1988) the World Health Organization (WHO) recognizes the expressed products of seven multiallelic loci (HLA-A, -B, -C, -D, -DR, -DP, and -DQ) along with the existence of three other genes (HLA-E, -DN, and -DO).

The HLA complex plays an important and basic role in the immune response. Current concepts on the immunobiology of the human MHC have recently been reviewed in several publications (Dupont 1989; Duquesnoy and Trucco 1988; Klein 1986; Tiwari and Terasaki 1985).

Proteins encoded for by HLA genes can be divided into two major groups (designated as class I or class II) based on properties such as biochemical structure, distribution, and function.

Class I HLA molecules are heterodimeric glycoproteins composed of a polymorphic 45-kilodalton heavy chain noncovalently associated with a 12-kilodalton polypeptide. This light chain has been identified as beta-2-microglobulin (β-2-M). The heavy chains are encoded for by genes found in the HLA-A, -B, or -C loci while β-2-M is controlled by a gene present on chromosome 15. Class I antigens are found on the surface of all nucleated cells. Class I molecules are primarily involved in the recognition of foreign antigens by cytolytic or suppressor T cells.

Class II molecules are also heterodimeric glycoproteins. They are composed of a 34-kilodalton alpha chain noncovalently associated with a 28-kilodalton beta chain. They are encoded by genes present in the HLA-DR, -DP, and -DQ loci. Class II specificities are more restricted in their expression and are found on the surface of B cells, macrophages, and activated T cells. Class II antigens are primarily involved in the recognition of foreign antigens by helper T cells.

HLA Subtypes

The alleles within a single HLA locus share basic common properties such as organization and structure at both the protein and gene levels. However, it is not unusual to observe that groups of three or more antigens often demonstrate a much closer relationship to one another than to the other alleles. Within such groups usually the member that was historically defined first is called the "broad" antigen, and the others are referred to as either "subtypes," "splits," "variants," or "narrow specificities." All the members of the group react with the reagents that define the original broad specificity indicating that they share and express an identical immunological determinant. Apart from the common determinant, each subtype must also express a unique characteristic that permits it to be distinguished from the other split(s). The phenomenon of splitting an antigen into subtypes is usually the result of identification of more precise reagents or special techniques capable of recognizing the differences between variants.

Table 1. Designations for HLA-A (A locus) specificities

Recognized by WHO		Additional subtypes detected by		RFLP Unique fragments
Antigen	Subtype	Serology	ID – IEF	
A1			A1, A1[a]	A1
A2		A2 sh. (Oriental) A2 sh.a (Oriental) A2 sh.b (Oriental) A2 sh.c (Oriental)	A2.1, A2.2, A2.3 A2.4, A2.5	A2
A3		A3 Black	A3.1, A3.2	A3
A9			A23	A23, A24
	A23	A23 sh.	A24.1, A24.2, A24.3	
	A24	A24 long (Oriental)	A24[a]	A24
A10				
	A25		A25	
	A26	A26.1 (Japanese)	A26.1, A26.2, A26[a]	A25, A26
	Aw34	Aw34 sh. (South African Blacks)	Aw34.1, Aw34.2	
	Aw66		Aw66	
A11			A11.1, A11.2, A11.3	A11
Aw19				
	A29		A29.1, A29.2	
	A30	A30.1 (assoc. B18) A30.3 (assoc. B13)	A30.1, A30.2, A30.3	A30
	A31		A31	A31
	A32		A32	
	Aw33		Aw33.1, Aw33.2	
	Aw74			
A28			A28.1, A28.2	
	Aw68			
	Aw69			
Aw36			Aw36	
Aw43			Aw43	

[a] Rare variants.
sh., short.

Since the First International Histocompatibility Workshop in 1964, classical serology using the microlymphocytotoxicity procedure continues to be the most commonly employed technique for HLA typing. With the exception of the 32 cellularly defined HLA-D and -DP determinants, the remaining 116 specificities currently recognized by the WHO nomenclature committee are identified serologically. Reports for serological identification for HLA-DP specificities have been made, but the availability of reliable reagents is limited at the present time.

In recent years the use of various techniques in the study of the HLA complex has shown that this system is more polymorphic than once believed and that additional subtypes of well-defined antigens exist. This is probably best demonstrated from the results of the Tenth International Workshop held in 1987 (Dupont 1988).

This international collaboration consisted of a series of studies that examined the components of the HLA complex at different levels (cellular, protein, and gene) employing a variety of techniques. Among the methods utilized were serology using alloantisera and monoclonal antibodies, one-dimensional isoelectric focusing for class I antigens, two-dimensional gel electrophoresis for class II alpha and beta chains, T cell clones for class I and class II epitopes and restriction fragment length polymorphism (RFLP) by Southern blot analysis. The preliminary results of each study are summarized in Tables 1–5. At present, the number of

Table 2. Designations for HLA-B (B locus) specificities

Recognized by WHO		Additional subtypes detected by		RFLP Unique fragments
Antigen	Subtype	Serology	ID – IEF	
B5				
	B51		B51, B51[b]	B51
	Bw52		Bw52	
B7		B7 sh (Bpot), B7.1[a], B7.2[a]	B7.1, B7.2	
B8				B8
B12				
	B44	B44 sh	B44.1, B44.2	B44
	B45		B45	
B13		B13b (Chinese)	B13.1, B13.2	
		B13c (Thai)		
B14				
	Bw64		B14	
	Bw65		B14	
B15			B15.2, B15.3, B15.4	
	Bw62		B15.1	
	Bw63			
	Bw75	Bw75 sh (15.3)		
	Bw76			
	Bw77			
B16				
	B38		B16.1	
	B39	B39 sh	B16.2, B16.3	

Table 2. (continued)

Recognized by WHO		Additional subtypes detected by		RFLP Unique fragments
Antigen	Subtype	Serology	ID – IEF	
B17			B17.1, B17.2, B17.3	
	Bw57		B17.2	Bw57
	Bw58		B17.2	
B18			B18.1, B18.2	
B21			B21.1, B21.3	
	B49		B21.2	
	Bw50	Bw50 sh (BN21)	B21.2	
Bw22				
	Bw54		Bw22.1	
	Bw55		Bw22.3	
	Bw56	Bw56.1 (Caucasian) Bw56.2 (Japanese)	Bw22.2	
B27		B27.2[a], B27.4[a], B27.5[a], B27.6[a]	B27.1, B27.2, B27.3 B27.4, B27.5, B27.6 B27[b]	
B35			B35.1, B35.2, B35.3, B35[b]	
B37			B37	
B40		BRI, BST40		
	Bw60	Bw60a (long), Bw60b (sh)	Bw60	Bw60
	Bw61	Bw61a (long), Bw61b (sh)	Bw61	Bw61, Bw60
Bw41		Bw41.2 (sh)	Bw41.1, Bw41.2	Bw41 Bw41, Bw42
Bw42			Bw42, Bw42[b]	
Bw46			Bw46, Bw46[b]	
Bw47			Bw47	Bw47
Bw48		Bw48 sh, FU (Japanese)	Bw48	
Bw53			Bw53	
Bw59			Bw59	
Bw67			Bw67	
Bw70				
	Bw71		Bw70.2	
	Bw72	Bw72.1, Bw72.2	Bw70.1, Bw70.3	
Bw73				
Bw4				
Bw6				

[a] Also defined by cytotoxic lymphocytes (TCD).
[b] Rare variants.

Table 3. Designations for HLA-C (C locus) specificities

Recognized by WHO		Additional subtypes detected by		RFLP Unique fragments
Antigen	Subtype	Serology	ID - IEF	
Cw1			Cw1.1, Cw1.2	
Cw2			Cw2	
Cw3			Cw3.1, Cw3.2	
	Cw9	Cw9 sh		
	Cw10			
Cw4			Cw4	Cw4
Cw5			Cw5	
Cw6			Cw6	
Cw7			Cw7.1, Cw7.2	Cw7
Cw8			Cw8	
*Cw11		Cw11.2 (Japanese)		
		Cw11.3 sh (Caucasian)		
				Cw blank

Table 4. Designations for HLA-DR (DR locus) specificities

Recognized by WHO		Additional subtypes detected by			RFLP Unique fragments
Antigen	Subtype	Serology	Two-dimensional allelic gel patterns	T cell-defined determinants (TCD)	
DR1		DR1 sh	DRβ I-1.1		DR1, Dw1
					DR1, Dw20
DR2		DR2.3 (Oriental)	DRβ-b-2.1	DR2.1, DR2.2	DR2
	DRw15	DR2.4 (South African Blacks)	DRβ-a-2.2	DRw15.1, DRw15.2	DRw15, Dw12
			DRβ-a-2.12		DRw15, Dw2
	DRw16		DRβ-a-2.16	DRw16.1, DRw16.2	DRw16, Dw21
					DRw16, Dw22
DR3					
	DRw17		DRβ I-3		DRw17, Dw3
					DRw17, Dw3/24
					DRw17, Dw3/25
	DRw18		DRβ I-3	DRw18.0	
DR4		DR4.1	DRβ I-4.1		DR4
			DRβ I-4.2		DR4, DQw7
			DRβ I-4.3		DR4, DQw8
			DRβ I-(4.4[a])		

Table 4. (continued)

Recognized by WHO		Additional subtypes detected by			RFLP Unique fragments
Antigen	Subtype	Serology	Two-dimensional allelic gel patterns	T cell-defined determinants (TCD)	
DR5					
	DRw11		DRβ I-11.1 DRβ I-(11.2[a])	DRw11.1, DRw11.2 DRw11.3, DRw11.4	DRw11, Dw5 DRw11, DB2
	DRw12		DRβ I-12		DRw12
DRw6					
	DRw13		DRβ I-13		DRw13, Dw18 DRw13, Dw19
	DRw14		DRβ I-14.1 DRβ I-14.2		DRw14, Dw16
DR7			DRβ I-7		DR7 DR7, Dw17 DR7, Dw11 DR7, DB1
DRw8			DRβ I-8.1 DRβ I-8.2	DRw8.1, DRw8.2, DRw8.3	DRw8
DR9			DRβ I-9		DRw9, Dw23
DRw10			–		
			New: DRβ-[a]		
DRw52		DRw52a+c	DRβ III-1	DRw52a (Dw24)	DRw52 DRw52[a]
		DRw52R3	DRβ III-2 DRβ III-3	DRw52b (Dw25) DR252c (Dw26)	DRw52, DRw8 DRw52, Dw24 DRw52, Dw25 DRw52, Dw26
DRw53		DRw53 (Black)	DRβ IV-1	DRw53.1	DRw53
				New: DR81 DR81.1 DR82 DR83 DR84	

[a] Rare variants.

Table 5. Designations for HLA-DQ (DQ locus) specificities

Recognized by WHO		Additional subtypes detected by			RFLP Unique fragments
Antigen	Subtype	Serology	Two-dimensional allelic gel patterns	T cell-defined determinants (TCD)	
DQw1			DQα-1.2-DQβ-1.12[a]		DQw1 DQw1.1
	DQw5		DQα-1.1-DQβ-(1.1[a]) DQα-1.14-DQβ-(1.9[a]) DQα-1.2-DQβ-(1.21[a])	DQw5 DQw5 (Dw1+Dw20)	DQw5
	DQw6		DQα-1.2-DQβ-1.2 DQα-1.18-DQβ-1.12 DQα-1.18-DQβ-1.18 DQα-1.2-DQβ-1.19	DQw6 (Dw2) DQw6 (Dw2+Dw12) DQw6 (Dw18) DQw6 (Dw19) DQw6 (Dw2+Dw18)	DQw6[a] DQw6.1 DQw6.2 DQw6.3
DQw2		DQw2 sh	DQα-2-DQβ-2 DQα-3.7-DQβ-2	DQw2 (DR7)	DQw2 DQw2.3 DQw2.7
DQw3				DQw3.1	
	DQw7		DQα-3.1-DQβ-3.1 DQα-2-DQβ-3.1 DQα-3.8-DQβ-3.1	DQw7.1	DQw7
	DQw8		DQα-3.2-DQβ-3.2 DQα-3.1-DQβ-3.2	DQw8.0 DQw8.1	DQw8
	DQw9		DQα-3.1-DQβ-3.3 DQα-3.7-DQβ-3.3		
DQw4			DQα-3.8-DQβ-Wa DQα-(3.1[a])-DQβ-(Wa15[a])	DQw4.1 DQw4.2 DQw4.3 New: DQA (DR7)	

[a] Rare variants.

WHO-recognized specificities within each locus (with antigens newly accepted after the Tenth Workshop in brackets) are as follows: HLA-A 24 (1), HLA-B 52 (3), HLA-C 11 (3), HLA-D 26 (7), HLA-DR 20 (4), HLA-DQ 9 (6), and HLA-DP 6. (There was no new specificity or subtype suggested for the DP locus.)

The tables show that each technique employed was capable of demonstrating the existence of additional subtypes of previously recognized antigens as well as totally new specificities. Often the heterogeneity of a particular antigen observed with one technique was confirmed by the results observed using a different approach. However, no single method was capable of detecting each of the new entities reported in the Workshop.

Table 6. Reaction pattern of HLA-A2 panel cells with local alloantisera

Cell	Serum ID							
	60	334	7611	10547	19142	24193	24777	27082
HLA-A2 panel cells (93 donors)	+	+	+	+	+	+	+	+
HLA-A2 variants								
M.S.	+	+	+	+	+	+	−	−
M.K.L.	+	+	+	+	+	+	−	−
L.L.	+	+	+	+	+	+	−	−

Panel cells were tested with alloantisera using the standard microlymphocytotoxicity procedure. Test scores of 8 are denoted by (+) while scores of 1 are indicated by (−).

Identification of HLA Class I Subtypes by Serology and Isolectric Focusing

We provide examples of the definition of subtypes by serology and isoelectric focusing. Often the definition of serologically or cellularly defined subtypes of class I antigens can be confirmed or even extended by biochemical studies (Neefjes et al. 1986). We have employed this approach to support our serological identification of subtypes. While the biochemical results may confirm our serological findings, as in the case of A2, we have also observed the opposite (B13) or even obtained indications for the existence of an IEF variant in the absence of a serological correlate (Bw58).

A2 was the earliest HLA specificity to be described in the literature during Dausset's pioneering work in the 1950s when it was known as Mac. HLA-A2 was among the first antigens to be recognized at the 1967 International Workshop and has been clearly defined with monospecific serological reagents since 1972. However, 15 years after its official recognition, studies using cellular typing and biochemical techniques have indicated that A2 was not the homogeneous entity as earlier suggested by serology (Biddison et al. 1982).

We have demonstrated that it is possible to identify a subtype of the A2 antigen using local alloantisera. As can be seen in Table 6, it was possible to identify three donors from our cell panel who express a variant form of the A2 specificity as defined by their lack of reactivity with the antisera 24777 and 27082. These A2 variant cells all share an Oriental ethnic background.

Comparison of the biochemical properties of the antigen expressed by two of the variant donors identified above with those of eight other A2-typed panel members and an EBV-transformed cell line was performed using one-dimensional isoelectric focusing (Figs. 1 and 2). The resulting gel patterns demonstrate that the variant A2 molecule expressed by M.K.L. and M.S. possesses a more acidic isoelectric point than the antigen expressed by the other donors, thereby providing confirmation of our serological findings.

These results and the lack of reactivity of the variant cells with monoclonal antibody CR11-351 (Yang et al. 1986) suggest that the A2 subtype that we have identified serologically may be identical with the HLA-A2.3 variant which has previ-

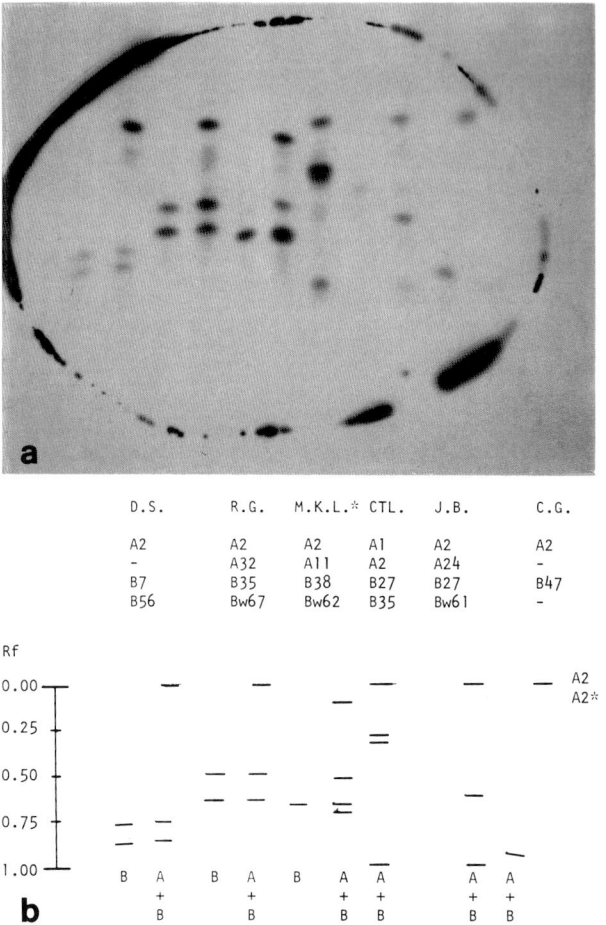

Fig. 1a, b. IEF analysis of local A2 panel cells. **a** Autoradiogram of IEF gel. **b** Schematic representation of autoradiogram. *Asterisk* denotes panel member expressing A2 subtype as defined serologically in Table 1. Samples were analyzed as described by Neefjes et al. (1986). Immunoprecipitation of class I molecules was performed using Tenth workshop reagents 4E (B locus) or w6/32 (A + B loci). *Letters beneath each lane* indicate which loci the bands are assigned to. Sample identification with their corresponding HLA-A and -B typings are shown *above the appropriate lanes.* Cathode (basic) end of gel is at the *top*

ously been detected only by cellular typing or monoclonal antibody binding studies (Russo et al. 1983).

Four principle subtypes of the HLA-A2 antigens, designated as A2.1, A2.2, A2.3, and A2.4, have been described with the A2.1 form most commonly detected, and reports of the existence of other A2 variants detected by monoclonal antibodies have recently been made (Kennedy et al. 1987). Comparison of the primary structures of the A2.1 molecule with the others shows that the differences between subtypes are few and may range from as little as one amino acid (A2.4) to four residues (A2.2) (Ezquerra et al. 1986; Hogan et al. 1988b).

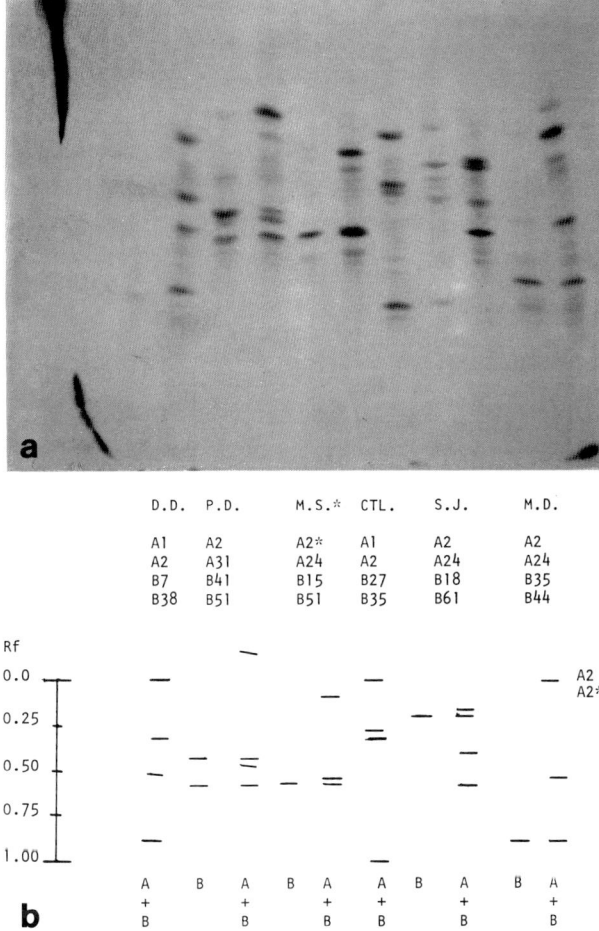

Fig. 2a, b. IEF analysis of local A2 panel cells. **a** Autoradiogram of IEF gel. **b** Schematic representation of IEF gel. *Asterisk* denotes panel member expressing A2 subtype as defined serologically in Table 1. Two other donors, P.D. and S.J., each express other biochemical subtypes of A2 antigen which are not indicated by serological results. Conditions as described in Fig. 1

Determination of the sequences of the subtypes of an HLA antigen may also provide clues to their structure-function relationships (Parham 1988). Comparison of the sequences of the A2.3 variant with the prototypic A2.1 antigen indicate that residue 149 is important for antibody reactivity, while the amino acids in positions 152 and 156 are essential for CTL reactivity (Hogan et al. 1988a).

Our experience with HLA-B13 illustrates that the definition of a class I antigen subtype by serology cannot always be confirmed by biochemistry. The HLA-B13 antigen has been well defined since the 1970 International Workshop. Although the frequency of this specificity is low, strong monospecific alloantisera have been readily available with no serological evidence of the existence of subtypes.

Table 7. Reaction pattern of HLA-B13 panel cells with local alloantisera

Cell	Serum ID					
	191	3124	10010	11372	19066	27214
HLA-B13 panel cells (eight donors)	+	+	+	+	+	+
HLA-B13 variants						
S.W.	+	+	+	−	−	−
R.N.	+	+	+	−	−	−
L.L.	+	+	+	−	−	−

Procedures were as described in Table 6.

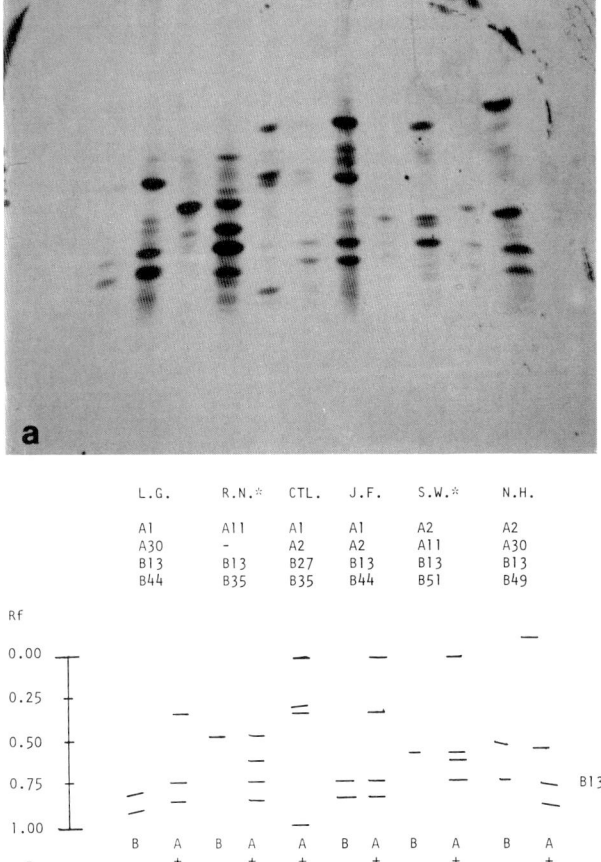

Fig. 3 a, b. IEF analysis of local B13 panel cells. **a** Autoradiogram of IEF gel. **b** Schematic representation of IEF gel. *Asterisk* denotes the two panel members who express B13 subtype as defined serologically in Table 2. Conditions as described in Fig. 1

We have identified three panel donors who express a B13 subtype using selected monospecific local alloantisera (Table 7). These three variant cells can be distinguished from other B13-typed panel members by their lack of reactivity with three of the reagents. Both the normal "long" and the variant "short" subtypes of B13 are associated with HLA-Bw4. Of the three cells which expressed the variant B13 molecule, two shared an eastern Asian origin while the third was Oriental.

Analysis of five B13 panel cells by isoelectric focusing was performed in order to determine whether or not differences between subtypes observed serologically could also be observed biochemically. We were not able to observe a significant difference in the isoelectric points of the B13 proteins expressed by the two variant cells (R. N. and S. W.) and the others (Fig. 3).

The B13 subtype that we have identified does not correspond to the Oriental form initially described by Yang et al. (1985). These researchers have shown that ethnic differences between Oriental and Caucasian B13 molecules exist, with the former being more basic in nature. The lack of any biochemical differences in our study indicates that any change in amino acids occurs within the constraints of conservative substitution.

We have also observed examples of the existence of biochemical variants in the absence of corresponding serological correlates such as in the case of HLA-Bw58. The serological analysis of Bw58-typed panel members with a selection of Tenth International Workshop reagents is shown in Table 8. Bw58 typing is assigned to any B17-positive cell that fails to react with a Bw57 monospecific reagent 483. As can be seen, all the Bw58 cells tested exhibited the identical reaction pattern.

Biochemical examination of these same cells, however, indicates that Bw58 is not the homogenous entity as suggested by serology (Figs. 4 and 5). It was possible to distinguish clearly between two distinct forms of the antigen. The more common form was present in four cells of diverse ethnic backgrounds (one Black, two Oriental, one Caucasian), while the second, more acidic version was observed in two Black panel members.

Table 8. Interaction of HLA-Bw57 and -Bw58 cells with some of the Tenth Workshop reagents

Cell	Tenth Workshop number				
	472	474	475	477	483
HLA-Bw57 panel cells (five donors)	+	+	+	+	+
HLA-Bw58					
847	+	+	+	+	−
766	+	+	+	+	−
17[a]	+	+	+	+	−
6[a]	+	+	+	+	−
15	+	+	+	+	−
26	+	+	+	+	−

[a] Cells expressing Bw58 variant on IEF gels.
Procedures were as described in Table 6.

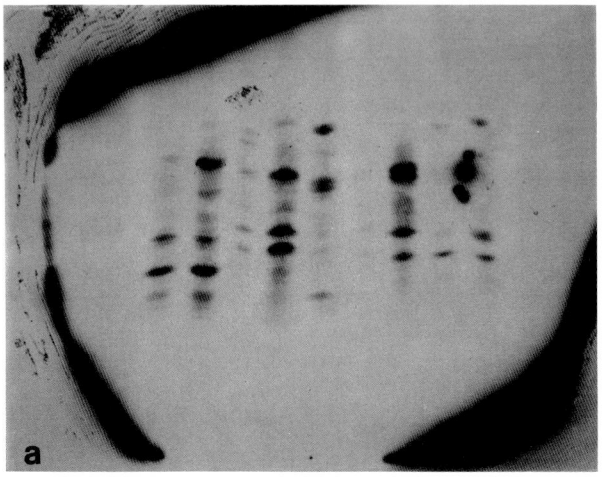

Fig. 4a, b. IEF analysis of local Bw58 panel cells. **a** Autoradiogram of IEF gel. **b** Schematic representation of IEF gel. Conditions as described in Fig. 1

One possible explanation for this type of situation is that the position of amino acid change occurs at a part of the class I heavy chain that is distinct and does not affect the serological determinant. Another possible explanation is that the reagents necessary to detect the Bw58 subtypes have not been identified as yet.

The results from our laboratory also confirm an interesting feature of HLA subtypes, namely the ethnic prevalance of the variants. For example, the A2 variant we have found was expressed only in Oriental donors, while the Bw58 split was observed only in Blacks.

Summary

The development of the HLA complex in recent years indicates that the total polymorphic nature of the system remains to be resolved. As the recent reports demon-

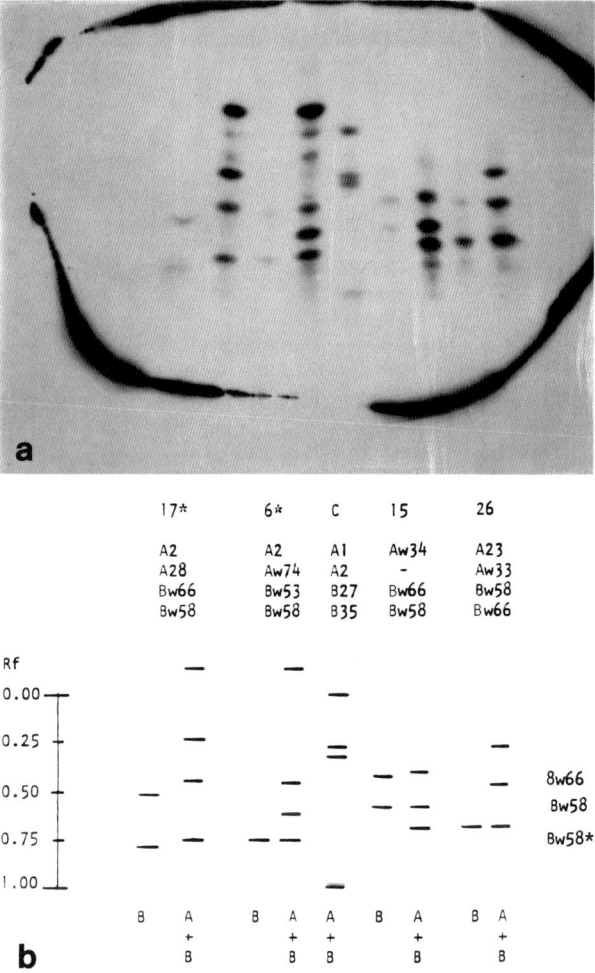

Fig. 5a, b. IEF analysis of local Bw58 panel cells. **a** Autoradiogram of IEF gel. **b** Schematic representation of IEF gel. *Asterisk* denotes the two panel members who express biochemical subtype of Bw58 (Rf = 0.77) versus more common form (Rf = 0.63). Cell 26 was included to help in the assignment of 8w66 band. Conditions as described in Fig. 1

strate almost every recognized antigen can now be split into subtypes using one method or another.

Apart from their central role as restriction elements in the immune system, HLA antigens also have other important functions such as in the determination of the success of allografts and in disease associations. With the increasing occurrence of organ and bone marrow transplants, it is becoming more critical that the accurate and precise identification of HLA specificities including subtypes be performed. Future analysis of HLA antigens and their subtypes will allow the determination of structure-function relationships of these proteins.

Acknowledgement. I would like to thank Dr. Kim Wong of the National Reference Laboratory for his help with the manuscript.

References

Biddison WE, Kostyu DD, Strominger JL, Krangel MS (1982) Delineation of immunologically and biochemically distinct HLA-A2 antigens. J Immunol 129: 730–734

Bodmer WF, Albert E, Bodmer JG, Dupont B, Mach B, Mayr W, Sasazuki T, Schreuder GMT, Svejgaard A, Terasaki PI (for the WHO Nomenclature Committee) (1988) Nomenclature for factors of the HLA system, 1987. Vox Sang 55: 119–126

Dupont B (ed) (1988) Tenth International Histocompatibility Workshop Newsletter, vol 2, no 1

Dupont B (ed) (1989) Immunobiology of HLA, vols 1, 2. Springer, Berlin Heidelberg New York (in press)

Duquesnoy R, Trucco M (1988) Genetic basis of cell surface polymorphisms encoded by the major histocompatibility complex in humans. CRC Crit Rev Immunol: 103–145

Ezquerra A, Domenach N, van der Poel J, Strominger JL, Vega MA, Lopez de Castro JA (1986) Molecular analysis of an HLA-A2 functional variant CLA defined by cytolytic T lymphocytes. J Immunol 137: 1642–1649

Hogan KT, Clayberger C, Bernhard EJ, Walk SF, Ridge JP, Parham P, Krensky AM, Engelhard VH (1988a) Identification by site-directed mutagenesis of amino acid residues contributing to serologic and CTL-defined epitope differences between HLA-A2.1 and HLA-2.3. J Immunol 141: 2519–2525

Hogan KT, Clayberger C, Le A-X, Walk SF, Ridge JP, Parham P, Krensky AM, Engelhard VH (1988b) Cytotoxic T-lymphocyte defined epitope differences between HLA-A2.1 and HLA-2.2 map to two distinct regions of the molecule. J Immunol 141: 4005–4011

Kennedy LJ, Wallace LE, Madrigal JA, Rickinson AB, Bodmer JG (1987) New HLA-A2 variants defined by monoclonal antibodies and cytotoxic T lymphocytes. Immunogenetics 26: 115–160

Klein J (1986) Natural history of the major histocompatibility complex. Wiley, New York

Neefjes JJ, Breur-Vriesendorp S, van Seventer GA, Ivanyi P, Ploegh HL (1986) An improved biochemical method for the analysis of HLA-class I antigens. Definition of new HLA-class I subtypes. Hum Immunol 16: 169–181

Parham P (1988) Function and polymorphism of human leukocyte antigen-A, B, C molecules. Am J Med 85 [Suppl 6A]: 2–5

Russo C, Ng A-K, Pellegrino MA, Ferrone S (1983) The monoclonal antibody CR11-351 discriminates HLA-A2 variants identified by T cells. Immunogenetics 18: 23–35

Tiwari JL, Terasaki PI (1985) HLA and disease associations. Springer, Berlin Heidelberg New York

Yang SY, Chang A, Olivero R, Relias V, Yunis EY (1985) IEF patterns of HLA-B13 antigens from Orientals and Caucasians. Immunogenetics 21: 125–134

Yang E, Wong KH, Ferrone S, Mervart H (1986) Recognition of a variant of HLA-A2 with a human monospecific alloantiserum. Hum Immunol 17: 145–146 (abstr)

Zeroing in on the *H-2* Complex

D. Klein

Five Snapshots

My career during the last 20 years can be likened to the zooming motion of a photographic lens, starting from a large field, taking in progressively smaller sections, and finally focusing on a single detail – zeroing in on the *H-2* complex. It was not an uninterrupted motion, for during those 20 years I have also been busy raising three children, two dogs, and one husband – in that order of difficulty. Here, instead of reviewing the entire field encompassed by my studies, I will present five stops of the zoom lens: five snapshots representing – not necessarily in chronological order – five stages in my career. They brought me exponentially ever closer to the *H-2* complex, until they landed me in the complex itself.

The First Snapshot: The Mouse

Each of us has her or his own favorite rendition of the experimental animal we work with. My favorite portrayal of the mouse is that depicted in Fig. 1 and executed by the Czech artist Ota Janeček for František Halas' delightful collection of children's rhymes *Před usnutím* (Before Falling Asleep). I first encountered the laboratory mouse at the Institute for Experimental Biology at Krč near Prague, where I worked as a graduate student. As long as the mice were caged, they looked docile enough to be handled, but once they escaped, they seemed out of control, and then we, the female staff of the laboratory, would seek refuge on the chairs and tables rather than face them on the floor. Our favorite mouse was "Fat Albert," a very old and very fat C57BL male who, because of his condition, was almost immobile.

My first project involving the laboratory mouse as an experimental animal had to do with the mapping of the *H-2* complex. At that time it was known that the *H-2* complex was linked to the loci Brachyury *(T)* and tufted *(tf)* in the linkage group IX and that these two loci were on the same side of the complex. There was no marker on the other side of *H-2* and this fact seriously hindered *H-2* mapping studies. To find such a marker, I decided to determine the position of the translocation break T138Ca, as this break seemed, from other studies, a good candidate for mapping on the other side of the *H-2* complex (Carter et al. 1955). There are two ways of testing for the presence of a translocation in a mouse – genetical (the

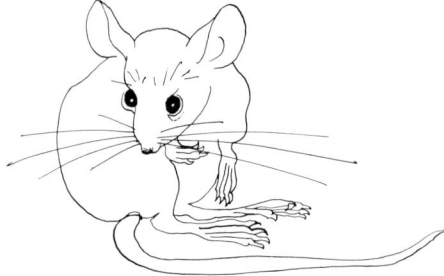

Fig. 1. *"Když probudí se hlína, je to myš"* (when a glebe wakes up, it is a mouse.) Ota Janeček's mouse for František Halas' book *Před usnutím*

translocation heterozygous females are semisterile because embryos derived from unbalanced gametes die in utero) and cytological (translocation heterozygotes are characterized by the appearance of multivalent figures at metaphase I of meiosis). I therefore set up the right crosses, dissected out a lot of uteri from pregnant females and crushed a lot of testes for cytological preparations. At the same time, I determined the *H-2* of these mice by serological typing and the Brachyury phenotype by scoring the tail length. My supposition turned out to be correct: the T138 break is indeed on what we now know to be the telomeric side of the *H-2* complex, while the *T* and *tf* loci are on the centromeric side (Klein and Klein 1972). I also observed an increased frequency of recombination in the vicinity of the translocation break - a phenomenon which, I believe, to this day remains unexplained.

The Second Snapshot: The Cell

The next level at which the zoom lens of my scientific career came to a temporary stop was that represented by the mouse tissues and cells. Twenty years ago, genetics of the *H-2* complex could be practiced only at the level of the whole mouse, which was of course time-consuming and laborious. Ways were therefore being explored of replacing the mouse with cells in culture and analyzing the *H-2* complex by methods of somatic cell genetics which, however, were then still in their infancy. The critical question was: are the H-2 molecules expressed stably on cultured cells? Obviously, if cells in culture were to lose H-2 molecules after a while, there could be no hope of ever carrying out somatic cell genetics with *H-2* genes. To answer this question, I used several cell lines that were maintained in culture for over 1 year or even longer in the laboratory of Dr. Donald J. Merchant at the Department of Microbiology, The University of Michigan, Ann Arbor, Michigan. I tested these cell lines for the expression of what now would be classified as class I H-2 molecules, using the indirect immunofluorescence technique. I was able to demonstrate that all the H-2 molecules expressed by the strains from which the cell lines were derived were present on the cultured cells and that no abnormal or unexpected expression of H-2 molecules occurred (D. Klein et al. 1970). Somatic *H-2* genetics *was* therefore possible, and later several laboratories were indeed able to make full use of this fact. My study also demonstrated that H-2 antigens could be used as markers for establishing the identity of cultured cells and heading off possible mix-ups of cell lines.

The Third Snapshot: The Chromosome

In the meantime, the identity of the chromosome bearing the *H-2* complex became known, and the expression "linkage group IX" was replaced by a more accurate idiom "chromosome 17." As the number of genes mapped to chromosome 17 steadily increased, the need arose to order them into a tidy map, particularly those close to the *H-2* complex, which were most numerous (Fig. 2). I became involved in the mapping of several *H-2*-linked genes, of which I shall mention only one – the *neuraminidase-1 (Neu-1)* locus. Neuraminidase is an enzyme that cleaves neuraminic (sialic) acid residues carried by oligosaccharides, glycoproteins, and glycolipids. Others have demonstrated that the *Neu-1* locus is probably occupied by the structural gene for the neuraminidase and that it maps close to the *H-2* complex (Womack et al. 1981). At that time, only one strain, SM/J, was known to carry a mutant allele at the *Neu-1* locus *(Neu-1^b)*, while all other inbred strains carried the wild-type *Neu-1^a* allele. With my colleagues, I was able to demonstrate the presence of the defective *Neu-1^b* allele also in certain wild-derived strains, and to show that some inbred strains carry a third allele, *Neu-1^c*, in which the level of neuraminidase activity is lower than in wild-type strains but higher than in the SM/J and related strains (Klein and Klein 1982). With the help of this third allele, we were then able to map the *Neu-1* locus more precisely than earlier investigators; it turned out that the locus resides right in the middle of the *H-2* complex, between the class II E_α and the class I *H-2D* genes (Figueroa et al. 1982; Fig. 3). The same chromosomal region is also occupied by genes coding for the complement components 2, 4, and factor B, for the enzyme 21-hydroxylase, for the tumor necrosis factor, for the repeated dipeptide, and probably for several other, as yet unidentified, genes (for a review and references, see Klein 1986).

The mapping of the *Neu-1* locus to a region within the *H-2* complex was significant in one particular respect. Until then, one could argue that the presence of complement loci in the *H-2* complex had some functional significance and that the entire chromosomal region functioned as a physiological unit. After the placement of the *Neu-1* locus in the *H-2* complex, such an argument was no longer possible (Klein et al. 1986). A much more likely explanation for the presence within the *H-2* complex of genes that clearly have nothing to do with the class I and class II *H-2* loci is that they were inserted into this region by an evolutionary accident. During the evolution of the major histocompatibility complex (MHC), many chromosomal changes occurred in the region occupied by the MHC – transpositions, inversions, insertions, deletions, and duplications. During one such change, a chromosomal segment bearing unrelated loci became integrated in the MHC and has remained in the MHC ever since. This integration may have occurred as "recently" as the rise of mammals, since birds seem to have their MHC organized in a somewhat different way (Klein 1986).

In addition to answering questions about the evolutionary origins of the MHC, the studies of linked loci provided useful information about the genetic status of common congenic strains. The *H-2* congenic strains are derived by crossing two *H-2* disparate inbred strains and backcrossing the progeny repeatedly to one of the two inbred strains, while selecting for the *H-2* haplotype of the second strain (Klein and Klein 1987). Theoretically, this procedure should transfer only the *H-2*

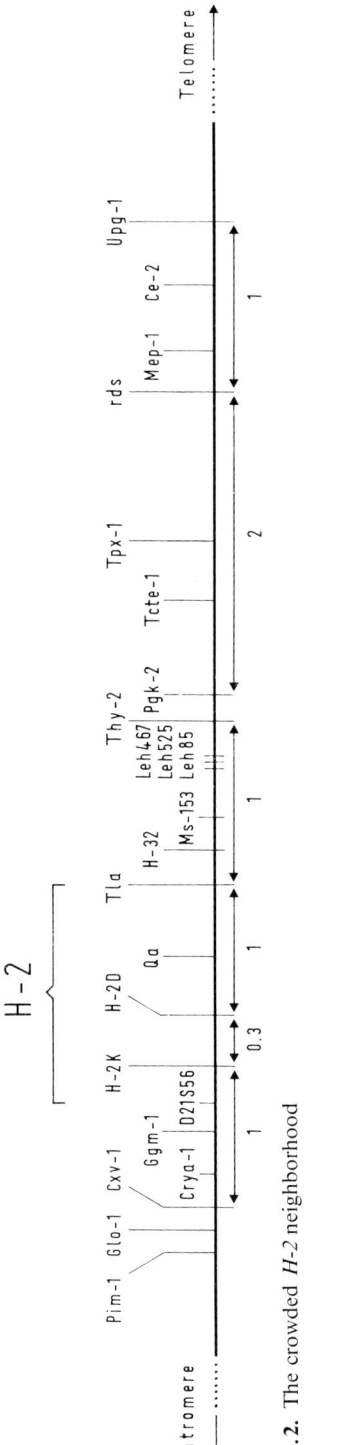

Fig. 2. The crowded *H-2* neighborhood

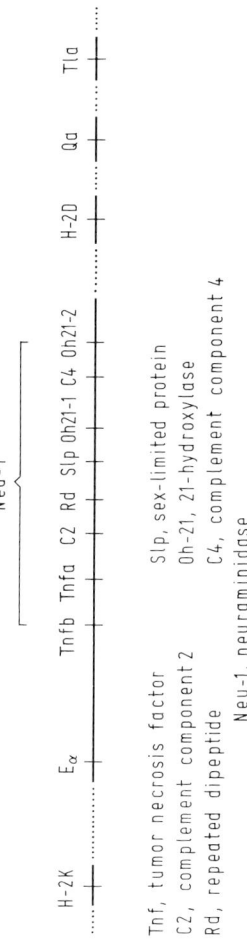

Tnf, tumor necrosis factor
C2, complement component 2
Rd, repeated dipeptide
Slp, sex-limited protein
Oh-21, 21-hydroxylase
C4, complement component 4
Neu-1, neuraminidase

Fig. 3. The insertion of unrelated loci into the *H-2* complex

complex of one of the parental strains onto the genetic background of the other strain. We wanted to know how much of the donor chromosome remains in the congenic strains in reality. We therefore typed most of the congenic strains in our collection at the Max Planck Institute for Biology in Tübingen for the linked loci. An example of the results we obtained is given in Fig. 4 (Klein et al. 1982). Clearly, it is not just the *H-2* complex that has been transferred from the donor to the background strain, but a sizeable segment of the donor chromosome 17. (It should

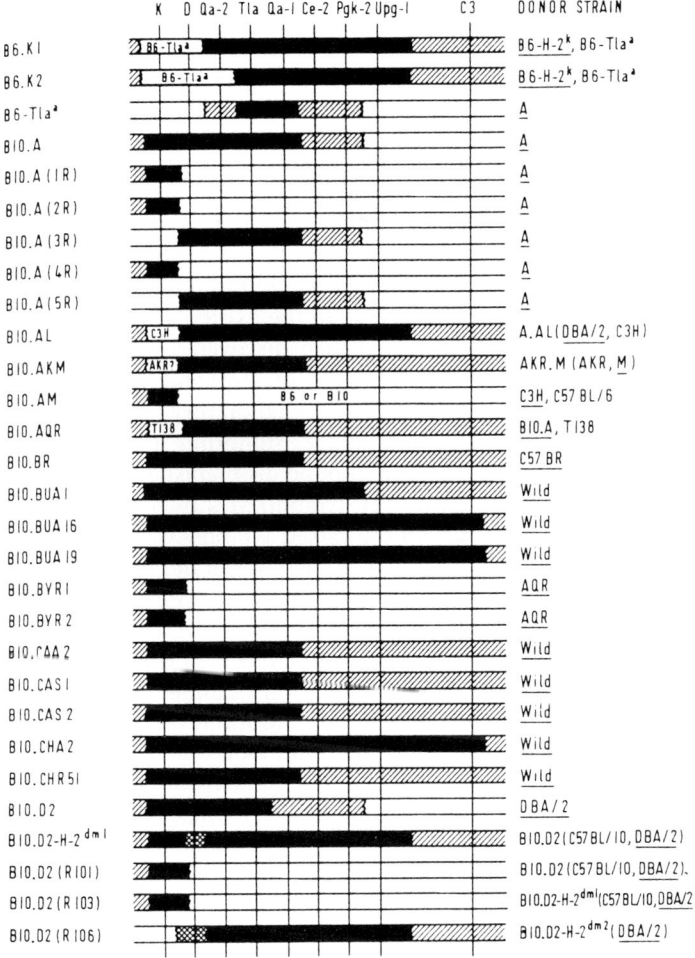

Fig. 4. The minimal length of the differential segment in the C57BL/6 (B6) and C57BL/10 (B10) congenic strains. Each *bar* represents the portion of chromosome 17 containing loci that were studied. The *solid bar* indicates the minimal length of the differential segment, the *shaded bar* the segment for which no information about its origin is available; the *open bar* indicates that this segment of the chromosome is of the inbred partner-strain origin. Some of the congenic strains are derived secondarily from other congenic strains so that the differential segment has a double origin. In such cases, an inscription indicates the strain from which this part derives; the rest of the differential segment derives from the underlined donor strain on the right. (From Klein et al. 1982)

be emphasized that the foreign segments depicted in Fig. 3 represent, in most cases, the minimal length of the donor-derived regions and that in reality these segments might be much longer than indicated.) These results not only provided a warning to all those who use congenic strains to map loci to the *H-2* complex (the strains do *not* prove that a locus is part of *H-2* or that it is even closely linked to *H-2*), but, on the more positive side, they also showed that the congenic strains could be used for ordering loci on chromosome 17. This latter use can only now be fully appreciated when a large number of anonymous DNA segments have been assigned to chromosome 17. One way of ordering these segments in a genetic map will be by testing the congenic strains carrying donor segments of various lengths.

The Fourth Snapshot: The Complex

Perhaps the most exciting phase of my career was the time my colleagues and I were working out the organization of the *H-2* complex itself. In the early 1970s only the class I genes (as they are now referred to) were known. There were, however, a number of hints pointing to the existence of a new class of *H-2* genes that had something to do with the then discovered immune response *(Ir)* genes. We were trying to identify the new class of *H-2* genes with the help of two *H-2* recombinants, one (AQR) produced in our laboratory (J. Klein et al. 1970), and another [B10.T(6R)] produced by Dr. Jack Stimpfling (Stimpfling and Reichert 1970). These two recombinants could not be distinguished serologically by any of the anti-H-2 sera then available. Yet, lymphocytes of one strain responded to lymphocytes of the other strain in the mixed lymphocyte culture (Bach et al. 1972), and the two strains also responded differently to the immunization by synthetic polypeptides such as (T,G)-A--L, (H,G)-A--L, and (Phe,G)-A--L (McDevitt et al. 1972).

To find serological differences between these two strains, we immunized one strain against cells of the other strain and then tested the antisera in the cytotoxic and immunofluorescence tests. It soon became apparent that some sort of antibodies were produced by these immunizations but these antibodies appeared to be "weak" in comparison with other antibodies we were using until then. It took us some time to convince ourselves that the reactions were "real" (and not some kind of serological artifacts) and to realize that what we originally considered as weak reactivity was in fact a strong reactivity but only with a subpopulation of cells (Hauptfeld et al. 1973). After some initial confusion as to the identity of this positive subpopulation, it eventually became clear that we were dealing with antibodies detecting a new class of H-2 antigens, which we named Ir antigens (because they were unseparable from the *Ir* locus as defined by the response to synthetic polypeptides). This designation was later changed to Ia and later still to class II antigens. In 1973, we were thus able to demonstrate that the *H-2* complex consisted of two classes of loci, class I coding for all the classically defined antigens, and class II coding for the new antigens expressed only on a subpopulation of lymphocytes (Hauptfeld et al. 1973). The existence of class II antigens was also demonstrated simultaneously but independently of our group by Dr. Chella David and his co-workers in the laboratory of Dr. Donald C. Shreffler (David et al. 1973).

Subsequently, several other laboratories reported similar findings in the mouse and also in other mammalian species, in particular humans (reviewed by Klein 1975, 1986).

The Fifth Snapshot: The Gene

In 1975, Köhler and Milstein discovered a way of producing monoclonal antibody and thus ushered in a new era which affected serologies of all sorts, including H-2 serology. The new type of reagents held the promise of simplifying the interpretation of serological results, thus allowing the use of antibodies for studies that could not be carried out with polyclonal antibodies. It became possible to study the direct relationship between the *H-2* genes and their products to an even greater extent than before.

Our laboratory adapted the Köhler-Milstein technique for the generation of hybridomas producing H-2-specific antibodies. Over the years we have produced more than 100 such hybridomas and have characterized the monoclonal antibodies secreted by these hybridomas (Figueroa et al. 1981; Klein et al. 1987). Some of the hybridomas and antibodies have been distributed to laboratories all over the world and have been used in a variety of studies, ranging from identification of restriction molecules in in vitro responses (reviewed in Klein and Nagy 1982) to mapping of epitopes on the H-2 molecules themselves (e.g., Landais et al. 1986).

We have used the monoclonal antibodies for studying the *H-2* polymorphism among wild mice and for the characterization of the immune response to certain antigens. It is not possible, in this short paper, to review all these studies; one example must suffice (Nižetić et al. 1984). Linked to the *H-2* complex is the *t* complex, which is a set of genes controlling the transmission of chromosome 17 into male gametes, and held together by at least two inversions (reviewed in Klein 1986). Because the inversions suppress crossing-over in the proximal one-third of the chromosome, the *t* chromosomes can be regarded as a kind of genetic fossil that has changed very little from the time of its origin. They accumulate mutations, of course, and some of these then become responsible for the lethality of the *t/t* homozygotes, but otherwise most of the genes locked in by the inversions remain in the same constellation as they were more than 2 million years ago when the *t* complex presumably arose. The *H-2* complex, which is included in one of the two inversions, provides – with its extensive polymorphism – an opportunity to trace the history of the *t* chromosomes. Using the H-2-specific monoclonal antibodies produced in my laboratory, this project proved to be possible. A genealogical tree of the *t* chromosomes could be constructed, and it was demonstrated that all the chromosomes are derived from a single ancestral chromosome which must have existed before the separation of the original mouse populations into two species, *Mus domesticus* and *Mus musculus*. At the same time, these studies demonstrated that, contrary to the expectations of many immunologists, the *H-2* genes have changed very little during those 2 million years after the two species separated from the common ancestor and hence that there is no evidence for a rapid evolution of the MHC polymorphism. But that is yet another story.

The actual *H-2* genes – the DNA of these genes – have become the focus of my attention only recently. This new interest will bring the zoom lens of my career to a final stop, and I will then have utilized its full potential – from the organism to the molecule.

References

Bach FH, Widmer MB, Segall M, Bach ML, Klein J (1972) Genetic and immunological complexity of major histocompatibility regions. Science 176: 1024–1037

Carter TC, Lyon MF, Phillips RJS (1955) Gene-tagged chromosome translocations in eleven stocks of mice. J Genetics 53: 154–166

David CS, Shreffler DC, Frelinger JA (1973) New lymphocyte antigen system (Lna) controlled by the *Ir* region of the mouse *H-2* complex. Proc Natl Acad Sci USA 70: 2509–2514

Figueroa F, Davis WC, Klein J (1981) Ten monoclonal antibodies detecting antigenic determinants on class I H-2 molecules. Immunogenetics 14: 177–180

Figueroa F, Klein D, Tewarson S, Klein J (1982) Evidence for placing the *Neu-1* locus within the mouse *H-2* complex. J Immunol 129: 2089–2093

Hauptfeld V, Klein D, Klein J (1973) Serological identification of an Ir-region product. Science 181: 167–169

Klein D, Klein J (1982) Polymorphism of the *Apl (Neu-1)* locus in the mouse. Immunogenetics 16: 181–184

Klein D, Merchant DJ, Klein J, Shreffler DC (1970) Resistance of H-2 and some non-H-2 antigens on long-term cultured mouse cell lines. JNCI 44: 1149–1160

Klein D, Tewarson S, Figueroa F, Klein J (1982) The minimal length of the differential segment in *H-2* congenic lines. Immunogenetics 16: 319–328

Klein D, Zaleska-Rutczynska Z, Davies WC, Figueroa F, Klein J (1987) Monoclonal antibodies specific for mouse class I and class II Mhc determinants. Immunogenetics 25: 351–355

Klein J (1975) Biology of the mouse histocompatibility-2 complex. Springer, Berlin Heidelberg New York

Klein J (1986) Natural history of the major histocompatibility complex. Wiley, New York

Klein J, Klein D (1972) Position of the translocation break T(2;9)138Ca in linkage group IX of the mouse. Genet Res Camb 19: 177–179

Klein J, Klein D (1987) Mouse inbred and congenic strains. Methods Enzymol 150K: 163–196

Klein J, Nagy ZA (1982) Mhc restriction and *Ir* genes. Adv Cancer Res 37: 233–317

Klein J, Klein D, Shreffler DC (1970) H-2 types of translocation stocks T(2;9)138Ca, T(9;13)190Ca and an H-2 recombinant. Transplantation 10: 309–320

Klein J, Klein D, Figueroa F (1986) Should the *neuraminidase-1* locus be considered as part of the major histocompatibility complex? Hum Immunol 15: 396–403

Köhler G, Milstein C (1975) Continuous cultures of fused cells secreting antibody of predefined specificity. Nature 256: 495–497

Landais D, Beck BN, Buerstedde JM, Degraw S, Klein D, Koch N, Murphy D, Pierres M, Tada T, Yamamoto K, Benoist Ch, Mathis D (1986) The assignment of chain specificities for anti-Ia monoclonal antibodies using L cell transfectants. J Immunol 137: 3002–3005

McDevitt HO, Deak BD, Shreffler DC, Klein J, Stimpfling JH, Snell GD (1972) Genetic control of the immune response. Mapping of the *Ir-1* locus. J Exp Med 135: 1259–1278

Nižetić D, Figueroa F, Klein J (1984) Evolutionary relationships between the *t* and *H-2* haplotypes in the house mouse. Immunogenetics 19: 311–320

Stimpfling, JH, Reichert AE (1970) Strain C57BL/10ScSn and its congenic resistant sublines. Transplant Proc 2: 39–47

Womack JE, Yan DLS, Portier M (1981) Gene for neuraminidase activity on chromosome 17 near H-2: pleiotropic effects on multiple hydrolases. Science 212: 6–65

Of Men and Mice

M. Pla

I have a drawer full of unsent letters – confessions, outbursts of anger, personal secrets. Some contain tender lines, others hard words. Among them there is one addressed to Milan Hašek:

Paris, December 26, 1983

Dear Milan,

It is more than a month now since we first met. I shall never forget the last few minutes at the station just before your train arrived. I was pacing up and down the platform feeling very nervous at the idea of finally meeting the famous M. H. I was not even sure that I would be able to recognize you. At last the train arrived. You got off and started to walk along the platform in the midst of a sea of people. Straight away I knew it just had to be you.

During your stay, when I had the opportunity of meeting and talking with you, you were always ready to listen to what I had to say. You would listen to me as if I had something to teach you. Your mind seemed so amazingly active. You are like a radar, always awake and on the lookout, forever receptive to everything around you. And what's more, you have that magical gift of being able to get things moving around you, wherever you may be. Now I find it almost impossible to believe that I could have felt so intimidated on that first day.

I hope that you and Marta spent a happy Christmas together and for the coming year I wish you nothing but nice surprises.

Marika

On the platform at the station, just before parting, he said something to me in his deep cello-like voice which has engraved itself on my memory: "Keep your pecker up"!

My first encounter with immunogenetics was during my stay (1972–1973) in the laboratory directed by Pavol Iványi at Institute of Experimental Biology and Genetics (Prague). By that time Milan Hašek was no longer director of the Institute. While I was there I heard a lot about him, but I never really got an opportunity to talk to him. A little later, the possibility arose to participate at the International Training Course in Molecular Biology, sponsored by UNESCO and held at the Biological Research Center in Szeged (Hungary). I spent some 3 years there. Later I got married and, because my husband is a French citizen, Paris has become my home city since 1977. I joined J. Colombani's group in the laboratory directed by J. Dausset (U93 INSERM, Hôpital Saint Louis). After reorganization of this laboratory in 1985, I was put in charge of the Mouse Immunogenetics Group. In this laboratory I have had the privilege to be in frequent contact with J. Dausset and benefit from his infectious enthusiasm. This laboratory has also provided a stimulating environment enabling fruitful interaction between research conducted in parallel on human and mouse MHC systems.

It was finally in this laboratory, and not in the corridors of Institute of Experimental Biology and Genetics, that what I had so far only imagined about Milan Hašek came true when he was invited by J. Dausset for a 1-month stay at the Collège de France. At that time I had only recently obtained a permanent position at INSERM. Having to cope with a new country, a new language, and a new research environment had been difficult. Milan Hašek came precisely at the moment when his sense of humor and his very real enthusiasm for science were able to give me the strength I needed to overcome the difficulties. He was one of the people who endowed me with the confidence necessary to start in this new life. Although I had until then never met him nor worked with him, he was for me as a true scientific director should be, an experienced guide who helped me find my way towards the new paths I was later to take. This was, in fact, my only encounter with Milan Hašek. But during the meeting in Ommen, I felt several times that it was like being with him again: so strong was his influence on those who had worked with him that he seemed to radiate from their very being.

Transgenic Mice: A Dream and a Tool

The revolution of recombinant DNA technology and advances in the manipulation of mouse embryo have made possible experiments only dreamt of before – the ability to isolate and sequence genes, engineer them in specific ways, modulate their expression, and even introduce the foreign DNA sequences into the germ line of mice. These DNA sequences (termed transgenes), once inserted into germ line, are stably transmitted from generation to generation. The benefits of transgenic technology will initially be in areas of fundamental science, and studies on transgenic mice will surely contribute to most areas of mammalian biology. These mice provide a means of exploring the complex molecular biologic effects of a gene in a living animal. The introduction of foreign DNA into both somatic and germ cells has made possible the analysis of the regulatory sequences that mediate the tissue-specific, developmental, and physiologic regulation of gene expression or the analysis of the physiologic consequences to the whole organism of the inappropriate or altered expression of normal or mutated gene products. Out of such fundamental studies will later emerge the potential for a more practical application of transgenic technology to medicine, biotechnology, and agriculture.

Very recently, the technology of production of transgenic mice by microinjection of cloned DNA into fertilized one-cell eggs has been introduced in our laboratory. It has been, for me, the most exciting period in my scientific career. Our first transgenic mice have just been born, and their characterization is in progress.

HLA-Transgenic Mice. Twenty-seven new transgenic mouse strains have been established in our laboratory by crosses of 27M TGM [transgenic mice with HLA-

Table 1. Principal characteristics of the transgenic mouse strains developed in our laboratory

Transgene(s)	Strain designated	Genetic background	H-2 haplotype
HLA-B27.2	27 B10	C57BL/10	b
	27 B10.D2	C57BL/10	d
	27 B10.BR	C57BL/10	k
	27 B10.P	C57BL/10	p
	27 B10.G	C57BL/10	q
	27 C3H.B10	C3H	b
	27 C3H.NB	C3H	p
	27 C3H.Q	C3H	q
	27 A.BY	A	b
Human β2-microglobulin	M B10	C57BL/10	b
	M B10.D2	C57BL/10	d
	M B10.BR	C57BL/10	k
	M B10.P	C57BL/10	p
	M B10.G	C57BL/10	q
	M C3H.B10	C3H	b
	M C3H.NB	C3H	p
	M C3H.Q	C3H	q
	M A.BY	A	b
HLA-B27.2 and human β2-microglobulin	27M B10	C57BL/10	b
	27M B10.D2	C57BL/10	d
	27M B10.BR	C57BL/10	k
	27M B10.P	C57BL/10	p
	27M B10.G	C57BL/10	q
	27M C3H.B10	C3H	b
	27M C3H.NB	C3H	p
	27M C3H.Q	C3H	q
	27M A.BY	A	b

B27.2 (abbreviated 27) and human β2-microglobulin (M) genes] with $H\text{-}2^b$ (B10, C3H.B10, and A.BY), $H\text{-}2^d$ (B10.D2), $H\text{-}2^k$ (B10.BR), $H\text{-}2^p$ (B10.P and C3H.NB) and $H\text{-}2^q$ (B10.G and C3H.Q) mice. The original transgenic breeders (27 and M TGM) were kindly provided by Drs. A. Berns and H. Ploegh (Netherlands Cancer Institute, Amsterdam). Table 1 summarizes the principal characteristics of these new transgenic mouse strains.

Cell Surface and Serum Expression of Transgenic B27 Protein and Human β2-Microglobulin. We have tested the ability of the HLA-B27 genes to be expressed in the transgenic mice by cytofluorometric analysis or microlymphocytotoxic test using peripheral blood and spleen lymphocytes as target cells. The level of cell membrane expression of HLA-B27 molecules in transgenic mice is dependent on the presence of human β2-microglobulin. However, a monoclonal antibody isolated from nontransgenic mice immunized with cells from mice carrying only B27 transgenes was able to detect on the cell surface HLA-B27 heavy chains associated with mouse β2-microglobulin. The human β2-microglobulin transgenic mice have a detectable level of human β2-microglobulin in their sera and express to various degrees on their cell surface the mouse class I heavy chains in association with human β2-microglobulin.

Alloantigenic Function of HLA-B27 on Transgenic Cells. Skin grafts from 27 and 27M transgenic mice were found to be rejected by normal *H-2*-matched mice, suggesting that the foreign HLA antigen is recognized as a functional transplantation antigen. Antibodies could be induced by both single (27) and double (27M) TGM lymphocytes in nontransgenic *H-2*-matched recipients, and anti-TGM monoclonal antibodies (around 50) were isolated. All of these monoclonal antibodies were HLA class I specific with various reaction patterns on human cells. Fifty percent of them displayed a monomorphic pattern of reactivity, the others a polymorphic one which varied from very broad (e.g., Bw4-specific) to rather narrow. These antibodies are presently characterized in detail.

Cell-mediated cytotoxicity assays were performed to determine whether normal mice could generate a cytotoxic T lymphocyte (CTL) response against HLA-B27-expressing transgenic spleen cells. CTL were generated in vitro in unidirectional mixed lymphocyte cultures using spleen cells from B10 mice as responder cells and irradiated spleen cells from *H-2*-matched 27M transgenic mice as stimulator cells. After 5 days, the CTL generated in these primary bulk cultures were tested in the ^{51}Cr-release assay on human Epstein-Barr virus (EBV) cell lines and Con A blasts from nontransgenic or 27M transgenic mice. The CTL exerted a significant killing of Con A blasts from 27M transgenic mice and they were also capable of killing B27-expressing human EBV cell lines. The B27-negative cell lines as well as Daudi cells (a human cell line which fails to express cell surface HLA molecules) were not killed. The availability of 27M transgenic mice carrying different *H-2* haplotypes, recently developed in our laboratory, allows us to test the *H-2*^{b} anti-*H-2*^{b} B27 CTL on the panel of Con A blasts from 27M transgenic and nontransgenic *H-2*-matched and -mismatched mice. Only target cells expressing HLA-B27 molecules were significantly lysed, whether they were *H-2*-matched (*H-2*^{b}) or mismatched (*H-2*^{d}, *H-2*^{k}, *H-2*^{p}, *H-2*^{q}). Interestingly, a low level of lysis was observed on nontransgenic allogeneic *H-2*^{d} and *H-2*^{p} target cells. The results indicate that HLA-B27 expressed on spleen cells from 27M transgenic mice can serve as an immunogenic element and that a significant portion of anti-B27 CTL response involved in recognition of HLA-B27 is unrestricted by *H-2*. Lysis of human targets and the *H-2*-mismatched B27-positive mouse cells indicate that B27 molecule on the immunizing transgenic spleen cells is recognized as a major histocompatibility antigen. At present there are insufficient experimental data to allow us to decide whether *H-2*-unrestricted anti-HLA CTL recognize a membrane-bound form of HLA molecules or HLA peptide(s) presented by these molecules.

HLA-Transgenic Mice: From a Dream to a Tool. Undoubtedly, HLA-transgenic mice provide a unique way of investigating in vivo HLA gene expression and function. Although appropriate tissue culture systems exist, only limited perspectives can be derived from such in vitro experiments. HLA-transgenic mice allow the study of HLA gene function and expression within the complexity of the whole organism.

Thus, the introduction of HLA genes into the germ line of mice provides 1001 experimental ways to investigate HLA and disease associations. However, such studies are subject to several caveats. Mouse and man are different species, leading different lives (e.g., horizontal vs. vertical position), and coping with different environmental conditions. The etiology and physiopathology of diseases may also be different and often involve various other genes and factors besides MHC genes. Nevertheless, HLA-transgenic mice allow, for the first time, the in vivo evaluation of the influence of isolated HLA genes on immune responses and their potential effects at the level of the whole organism.

HLA-transgenic mice offer completely new ways of producing the HLA-specific monoclonal antibodies. Reliable HLA typing antibodies have so far been obtained mostly from multiparous women or polytransfused individuals, and monoclonal antibodies have been produced in mice immunized with human cells or isolated HLA gene products. Most antibodies obtained after such immunizations recognize human proteins, including HLA antigens, in a monomorphic manner. HLA-transgenic mice thus represent a very interesting system, because they allow the production of HLA-specific antibodies in a quasi-allogeneic situation. HLA-transgenic mice can be immunized with lymphocytes from other transgenic mice expressing different HLA genes or with mouse cells transfected with HLA genes (intact or modified by genetic engineering). In our laboratory we have immunized HLA-B27.2 transgenic mice with *H-2*-matched cells transfected with the HLA-B27.5 or B7 genes or with constructs recombining both genes. We have obtained about 30 monoclonal antibodies, which are now being characterized in detail. All are HLA class I specific and display a polymorphic pattern of reactivity: several are broadly cross-reactive on human cells, while others show a very narrow specificity. Interestingly, some of these monoclonal antibodies cross-react with mouse cells, on which they recognize *H-2* class I molecules in a polymorphic manner. Such studies are only just beginning. Obviously a lot of work has to be done before solutions of enigmas of HLA and disease associations will be within reach.

Acknowledgements. The current research described in this communication was supported by INSERM and in part by grants from Association pour la Recherche sur le Cancer, Fondation pour la Recherche Médicale, and Ligue Nationale Française Contre le Cancer. I wish to thank Professors Jean Dausset and Laurent Degos for their continuous encouragement and helpful and provocative discussions. I am also grateful to all members of my laboratory who have shared with me the pleasure as well as the difficulties of this venture.

Individual Differences Among Syngeneic Mice in Immune Response to Alloantigens and Modified Self-MHC-Antigens

P. Ivanyi

Memories

I felt close to Milan Hašek out of affection even more then of admiration. I must have been the first among the contributors to this volume to have seen Hašek, since it happened in 1950 when I began to study at the medical school of Charles University in Prague and Hašek was an assistant professor at the Institute of General Biology. Hašek was a doctor of medicine but had decided to work in research in genetics and he was a typically enthusiastic post-war communist. It so happened that these two devotions resulted in a chimeric state because it was the time to "defend and elaborate" the Lysenko-Micurin genetic dogmas.

I received my secondary education at a school in Kosice (eastern Slovakia) when, in 1949 and 1950 we were taught for the first time about the new Lysenko-Micurin genetics, the basis of which was that genes were not located in the cell nucleus, but that heredity was regulated by the environment. Changes in general cellular metabolism would induce new hereditary information and could be transmitted to the progeny. The terms Lamarckism and Darwinism were used frequently, but without precise definition. The antithetical relationship between the new science and its opposite, the reactionary old science, was presented very clearly.

Because of my strong feelings and love of dialectics, I realised that this was an intriguing situation. Either one or the other was right! And I wanted to find out who was right. Therefore, I studied the original works of Lysenko and Micurin, something I believe nobody had done, certainly not our biology teacher. Consequently, I was dubbed as Pavol-Micurin at the grammar school farewell party. However, I also visited the university library and borrowed the "reactionary" books by T. H. Morgan, *Physical Basis of Heredity* (which I never returned), the book by J. A. F. Roberts *Medical Genetics* and the book by B. Sekla (in Czech) *Heredity in Nature and Society*.

One month after matriculation (1950) to the medical faculty in Prague, I arrived at the Institute of General Biology, where Professor Sekla was standing out against the "new science". I was included in Hašek's group. This was the only way to get into the institute, and I accepted this rather than standing out as a "science dissident".

Hašek allocated to me a project to investigate how cells were formed from the yolk of an egg (the Lepesinskaja doctrine), which did not get off the ground. Then

I got another deal. Ovary transplantations in rabbits had been started with the aim of showing that progeny of a white father and a white mother with transplanted ovaries from a black donor would have white pigmentation. Moreover, as a parallel experiment, it became my duty to show that the blood groups of the foster mother, but not of the biological mother (the donor of the ovaries) would be expressed in the progeny. However, all the ovaries were rejected, and no progeny was born.

During that time I succeeded in producing alloimmune antibodies and rediscovering some interesting blood group systems in rabbit. I became interested in alloantigens and became a "rabbit man". At the same time Hašek succeeded in producing embryonal parabiosis of chicken eggs (1952) and wanted me to stop "my" rabbit work and elaborate protein serology to analyse antibody response in "his" chicken born after interspecies embryonal parabiosis. We had an hour of serious discussion, and I refused; Hašek accepted my love of alloantigens and let me be a rabbit man. "Well, if you want ...". I succeeded in my first opposition to a scientific authority and I missed the chance of cooperating and contributing in the discovery of immunological tolerance. Then Hašek left as his group became the Department of Experimental Biology and Genetics within the Academy of Science and was moved to another part of Prague.

After I finished my studies at the medical school I did not succeed in obtaining a post at the Prague research institute(s) because I was not involved in public activities, and so I began as a doctor of medicine at a district hospital in Nitra, Slovakia. Because I was an expert in rabbit alloimmunity, my contacts with Milan remained. With Dagmar, my wife, we induced immunological tolerance in newborn rabbits and drove 600 km to Prague to show Milan the adult white rabbits with black skin grafts. To help me, Hašek arranged for a respected Russian scientist who was also interested in rabbit blood groups to visit me. It boosted my popularity as he was welcomed by a festival gateway by the Nitra hospital authorities, but this was not sufficient to overcome my difficulties in getting a research job because I was still not involved in public activities. Thus Hašek made alternative arrangements for my "come back" to Prague. I know that he acted in a similar way for others. He never made an issue of the arrangements he had made, and I never had the feeling that I was in any way in his debt for such help. At the institute I had several serious discussions with him. He always wanted me to stop my work on rabbit blood groups and histocompatibility antigens. Why not mice or humans? I refused a few times over several years: an illustration that Milan was a boss who accepted arguments, with the comment: "Well, if you want ...". The compromise was that I had to take responsibility for chicken histocompatibility. Finally, when I gave up rabbit (and chicken) work and turned to "mice and men", I said him: "You are a very bad director. You should have stopped my rabbit work much earlier." My enthusiasm for alloantigens remained with me, and it was the C'-dependent lymphocytotoxicity test (on rabbit lymph node cells) which interested Jean Dausset and resulted in an invitation to work in Paris for 1 year. This succeeded only because Hašek, who was now very enthusiastic about the scientific possibilities, arranged the necessary formalities.

We had many good times together in the mid-1960s, the years of growth for the institute and of frequent evening parties. We also travelled a lot together. Once, after a long drive in my Fiat 600, we arrived, together with Miss K., in Stuttgart after midnight (we had been invited to explain immunology at a meeting of homeopaths). We had already had a few drinks on the way and Milan asked the hotel reception for some more cognac: "Cognac! Small or large glasses?" asked the receptionist. "Bring us the whole bottle" was the answer.

After the HLA workshop I drove Milan from Italy to Paris with Peter Demant on the back seat – still in my Fiat 600. In Italy I had bought two giant bottles of chianti as a fabulous present to take home. During our drive "we" finished both bottles. And so I experienced, in a very small car, all the stages which Hašek the giant went through: from excitement' and singing; stops in village squares, which all happened that night to have lovely parties; to falling asleep before our arrival at the avenue Rapp in Paris.

Once Milan arrived alone in his car at the Czech-German border. The German customs official inspected his car and discovered three 20-litre jerry cans for petrol. "You cannot take that much petrol into Germany" was the objection, "You will have to pay duty". After the official had prepared the forms, Milan said: "I won't pay, the jerry cans are empty". However, there was some petrol in *one* of the jerry cans. "You have to pay for this", said the annoyed bureaucrat. "No", said Milan, "I shall fill my tank with this". But why were the three jerry cans empty? Petrol was much cheaper for crowns in Prague than for marks in Germany, and we all had to drive as far as possible with Czech petrol. Hašek's jerry cans were empty because the road went through Plzen, the city where the only real Pilsner is served; Milan had made a stopover in a brasserie in Plzen and had no cash left for the cheap petrol.

In August 1968, on the night of 21st August, Milan came to my room at the Genetics Congress in Tokyo. I had bought a 2-litre bottle of sake as a present for friends and family. We finished the bottle that night and early morning.

And so I learned to love Milan Hašek. He was always interested in life and science. The last time I saw him was in Paris a few years ago. Or was it a few days ago?

Non-conventional *H-2* Serology

Individual Differences Among Highly Inbred Mice in Immune Responses to Alloantigens

Before I left the institute in Prague (1976), we observed an interesting phenomenon together with Dr. Milada Mickova. Owing to some irregularities in the reactivity pattern of conventional anti-*H-2* sera, Milada made separate bleedings from individual mice. Before, anti-*H-2* "sera" were serum pools of several mice of one (inbred) strain. Really, how much serum can be obtained from one mouse? Serum pools (sometimes from even 100 immunised mice) are the routine way of preparing anti-*H-2* sera. Immunologists know that such sera (serum pools) are mixtures of many antibody specificities. They are all directed against the same *H-2* molecule, but differ by their cross-reactivity pattern on third party cells. Serum pools can be rendered more specific (even anti-private) by absorptions with third party cells. Sera from individual mice are also mixtures of antibodies, but their heterogeneity might be much less than that of large serum pools. Nobody had examined to what degree anti-*H-2* sera from individual genetically identical mice differ in their specificity. In other words, how much do individual mouse sera deviate from the average of a large serum pool? By specificity of a serum, I mean its reactivity pattern on a large panel of third party target cells, possibly on a panel of all known *H-2* haplotypes. Moreover, due to extensive interspecies homology of MHC molecules, *H-2* sera can also be tested against cells from other species, e.g. human cells, for cross-reactions with HLA antigens.

The first time we examined the specificity of sera from individual mice we saw that their reactivity pattern on third party cells differs sharply. This implies a new phenomenon in MHC immunobiology: genetically identical individuals immunised with the same complex immunogen express various dominant clones of antibody-producing B cells. It was not clear what the mechanism and consequences of this type of lymphocyte diversification were.

Soon after this observation, I emigrated to Amsterdam and had to make my choice for further research project(s). I wanted to stay with alloantigens of the mouse and man. Therefore, I continued studies on MHC interspecies cross-reactions. For the analysis of cross-reaction of anti-*H-2* antibodies with HLA antigens I used mouse alloantisera. However, we analysed sera from individual mice and never serum pools. Certainly, the amount of work increased exponentially. Instead of one, many sera were analysed on large panels of mouse and human cells. We observed that Db-anti-Dd [B10.A(4R)-anti-B10.A] antibodies in the serum of one mouse cross-reacted with HLA-A11, in the serum of another mouse with HLA-B27, and a third serum cross-reacted with HLA-B5 and B12. The specificty of the individual sera also differed on the *H-2* panel of mouse cells. It was not surprising that this type of diversity existed; but it was surprising that the individual mouse sera differed that much (Ivanyi et al. 1978). It appeared as if one isolates, from one immunisation experiment a series of monoclonal antibodies (MAb) of various specificities. There was a constancy in the reactivity pattern of an individual mouse for at least several months. We still do not understand how such an high degree of diversification (amongst genetically identical individuals) in the acting B cell repertoire can be generated and whether such individual differences do have some biological consequences. We tried but could not switch or bias the B cell repertoire intentionally. Certainly, individual differences occur at "random", but at random only for the given individual. There must be some mechanism which is able to bias the repertoire of an individual mouse in one direction or other.

The phenomenon is disturbing and has also been noticed in other situations related to MHC, namely for the specificity of MHC restriction of T cells (Pala et al. 1986). Recognition of H-Y antigen by T cells is restricted by *H-2*Db (de Waal et al. 1983). However, Wettstein (1981) and Fierz et al. (1982) have shown individual variations (restriction by Kb) in the anti-H-Y response between genetically identical responders. Similarly, recognition of Moloney virus is restricted by Db (Stukart et al. 1981; Kast et al. 1988). However, occasionally individual mice show an *H-2*Kb restriction component in their Moloney virus-specific response (Stukart et al. 1981; Kast et al. 1988). In Dbm13 mutant mice, owing to gene conversion (Hemmi et al. 1988), Kb becomes the exclusive restriction element for Moloney virus (Stukart et al. 1982). The important notion is that neither the specificity of restriction (in vivo), nor the "switch" in the mutant can be seen as an all or nothing phenomenon. In other words, occasionally in individual non-mutant mice the *switch in the repertoire* can also occur. Possibly, some discrepancies among laboratories regarding the immune response of the "same" inbred strains (Juretic et al. 1985) might be due to similar situations.

Our suggestion for the explanation of variations in MHC regulation of immune responses among highly inbred mice was that the virus status – of the individual mouse or strain – was the cause of the observed variations. Variations in the virus status can be environmental or germ line dependent (evidence for the latter was presented by Herr and Gilbert, 1982).

Probably individual mice also differ in their T cell allo-repertoire. This was suggested for the allo-CTL precursor frequencies (Sherman 1980), but it is almost impossible to perform systematic work with individual mice. Possibly, there are unexpectedly great variations. Maybe they are decisive for individual variations in oncogenesis (Prehn 1975, 1983). It is also an almost general belief that HLA-regulated variations in the immune responses to self and foreign antigens are the basis of at least some HLA and disease associations. However, experts are still mistified by the occurrence of diseases with a very high association to a certain HLA antigen in only one of uniovular twins. Maybe variations in the T cell repertoire parallel variations in gene effect penetration for immune response traits.

We were not able to explain the mechanism responsible for the observed individual variations in the anti-*H-2* immune responses, but profited at the operational level by selection of strong sera with suitable specificity. The simple fact that we examined individual sera instead of serum pools opened horizons which would have otherwise remained closed. Three such situations are described below.

Anti-*H-2* Antibodies Induced by Injections of Syngeneic Cells

Anti-*H-2* antibodies are produced by injection of allogeneic cells, i.e. by immunisation with an *H-2* antigen. Our serendipity started when we observed *H-2* antibodies after injections of syngeneic cells.

BALB/c-Ldm2-loss mutant mice were immunised with BALB/c lymphocytes. The only antigen difference in this coisogenic combination is due to the absence of the Ld molecule in the responder strain. We wanted to induce anti-Ld antibodies with the aim of examining their cross-reaction with HLA on human cells. First, we had to analyse their specificity on mouse cells. This work was done with 22 individual mouse sera. The sera reacted differently, but the results were even more surprising than expected (Ivanyi et al. 1979). Some sera reacted as expected, i.e. they detected the Ld antigen. However, most sera exerted an unexpected reactivity pattern by reacting not only with Ld but also with Kk and *H-2*r. Such a reactivity pattern had not been observed before with anti-Ld antibodies. In half of the sera the anti-Kk (and anti-*H-2*r) component was the strongest. These might have been rare anti-Ld antibodies strongly cross-reactive with Kk. However, seven individual sera were negative on the stimulator (BALB/c) cells, but positive on other targets. Two of these sera reacted *only* with *H-2*k and *H-2*r cells. Moreover, these unexpected antibodies could be induced by the Ld immunogen and exerted a heterolytic activity on third party cells.

The critical experiment to be done was to examine whether donor (BALB/c, H-2d) cells absorb all activity. Our data indicated that this really was the case. By independent experiments similar results were obtained by Hansen et al. (1979). One out of the six individually tested mice produced, along with the anti-Ld antibodies, also anti-Kk antibodies and they could be also absorbed by H-2d cells. In a joint publication we concluded that we were facing cross-reactivity between K, D and L molecules (Hansen et al. 1979).

However, I did not believe that this would be the final explanation, because (a) the anti-Kk component in most of our individual sera was dominant; and (b) two sera were negative on the donor cells but positive on H-2k cells.

Before continuing with next experiments, I have to confess that the above-mentioned absorption experiments on anti-Ld sera could not be confirmed, as reported recently (Ivanyi et al. 1988). When we repeated the absorption experiments several times with various anti-Ld sera, we could not confirm that the donor (BALB/c) cells absorb all antibody activity (i.e. also the anti-Kk). We finally came to the opposite conclusion. The donor cells (BALB/c) could not absorb anti-Kk and anti-H-2r activity from the sera. We do not know why we originally obtained the ambigous result. Most probably, there are some anti-Ld sera which cross-react with Kk, and individual mouse sera differ also from this point of view. It might have also been technical, which I am more inclined to believe. The antibodies were mostly IgM and could lose activity during the course of the absorption experiment. The absorption experiments with the same sera could not be repeated because we were working with sera of individual mice.

I suspected some very non-conventional situation. The antigen difference between donor and recipient is exclusively Ld. However, some individual sera react with Kk but not with Ld. Thus, possibly, the antibodies were not induced at all by the Ld antigen. If so, if for the origin of the anti-Kk antibodies the immunisation with Ld was not decisive, what then induced the occurrence of the antibodies? In control, non-immunised mice we could not detect such antibodies. Possibly, it was the mere fact that we injected them with "the cells". If the injections are seen without the Ld antigen difference, we actually performed injections of syngeneic cells. Hence, we had to try to discover whether injections of syngeneic cells would induce H-2-specific antibodies. We injected BALB/c mice with BALB/c cells and we did actually obtain anti-Kk antibodies in the sera of about 40% of the injected mice (Ivanyi et al. 1980). Similar results were obtained with C57Bl/6 (H-2b) mice (Ivanyi et al. 1982). Hence, we observed induction of H-2-specific antibodies by injections of syngeneic cells.

Induction of H-2-specific antibodies by injection of syngeneic cells appeared as a new and interesting phenomenon. The difficulty was that the induction of such antibodies was irregular. In such a situation criticism came from various sources. Our grant application to elaborate the finding was rejected because the genetic homogeneity of all individual mice was not (and never can be) formally confirmed. Independently, Capkova et al. (1983), Gunther (1988) and Schmidt (1987) obtained similar results, and H-2-specific MAb was isolated from a mouse after injection of syngeneic cells (Cramer et al. 1988). Because the induction of antibodies was not regular, the situation was very difficult, and elaborated only by further serendipity.

Naturally Occurring *H-2*-Specific Antibodies

It was not clear how *H-2*-specific antibodies were induced by injection of syngeneic cells. A hypothetical explanation was that they were induced by MHC + X, i.e. by modified self-MHC. Modified self-MHC had been described in aged mice. Therefore, we performed syngeneic immunisation of young mice by cells from aged mice and vice versa (in C57Bl/Rij mice). Sera of individual mice were examined before and after the injections. To our surprise, about 20% of sera from the old mice contained *H-2*-specific antibodies before the injections. Again, we would have not seen this if we had examined serum pools. In individual sera the phenomenon was very clear. The antibodies in some sera reacted with a broad reactivity pattern on the panel of *H-2* congenic mouse strains. However, many sera had a specificity for only one or two *H-2* haplotypes. Exceptional sera had surprisingly high anti-*H-2* titres for "short" public *H-2* antigens. Hence, we discovered *naturally* occurring *H-2*-specific antibodies (Ivanyi et al. 1982, 1988) and analysed various aspects of their existence. They are not frequent and occur irregularly. Naturally occurring anti-A, B blood group antibodies appear as their "analogy". But the situation is not analogous at all. The "natural" anti-A, B blood group antibodies occur regularly, and develop soon after birth due to stimulation by the ubiquitous A, B blood group substances in nature. Thus, they are induced by environmental triggering. The naturally occurring anti-*H-2* antibodies are not regular at all, and the specificity of the antibodies in individual sera from genetically identical individuals is sharply different. Their occurrence is clearly age dependent (Fig. 1).

Thus, both the above-mentioned phenomena, i.e. induction of *H-2*-specific antibodies by injections of syngeneic cells, and the occurrence of natural *H-2*-specific antibodies, are irregular and occur only in a percentage of mice of some inbred strains.

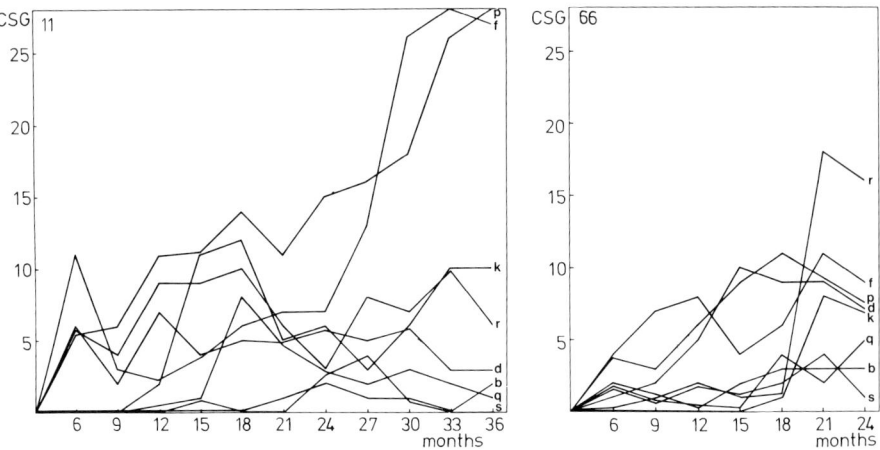

Fig. 1. Time occurrence and *H-2* specificity of antibodies in samples of serum from individual C57Bl/KaLwRij (*H-2*b) mice (no. 11 *left* and no. 66 *right*). All serum samples collected at 3-month intervals were tested against lymph node cells with haplotypes *H-2*b, d, f, k, p, q, r, s on the B10 background. Cytotoxicity scoring grade (CSG) values no higher than 5 are weak reactions under the background level. (From Cerny-Provaznik et al. 1985)

Induction of *H-2* Antibodies by Injections of Virus-Infected Cells

H-2-specific, naturally occurring antibodies and antibodies induced by injections of syngeneic cells might be due to triggering by MHC + X (X for non-MHC self or foreign antigen). If so, two different situations can be outlined. The first is that the MHC + X complex expresses *neodeterminants*. Presumably, neodeterminants expressed by MHC + X induce antibodies which react with MHC + X and cross-react with allogeneic *H-2* molecules. This is what one would except by analogy with the T cell restriction phenomenon. The antibodies would be analogous to anti-MHC + X CTL. Thus *MHC-restricted antibodies* are anti-X but recognise X (on cell membranes) only in the context of self-MHC. The criterion for such antibodies is specificity for X and negative on self-MHC without X.

A second possibility is that antibodies are induced by modified self MHC. The modified expression of self-MHC is due to the action of X on the MHC molecules. Today we believe that this is the effect of non-MHC peptide(s) in the groove of MHC molecules. In other words, there are MHC + X neodeterminants, or composite determinants, for the T cell receptor and modified expression of self-MHC for the B cell receptors. Consequently, the antibodies are not MHC-restricted anti-X antibodies, but simply anti-MHC antibodies induced by modified MHC. Such antibodies do not recognise X (neither with nor without MHC) but do recognise MHC (either with or without X).

Beyond these theoretical considerations, our great wish was to find an experiment in which MHC-specific antibodies would be induced regularly. Injections of syngeneic Sendai virus-infected cells fulfilled this wish completely (Kievits et al. 1987). In several experiments, injections of Sendai virus-infected cells induced *H-2*-specific antibodies regularly. There are still strain-dependent variations in the percentage of responding animals, but in C57Bl strains the majority of injected mice (in several independent experiments in two animal houses) produced *H-2*-specific antibodies upon injections of Sendai virus-injected syngeneic lymphocytes. The antibodies were characterised by various aspects (immunoprecipitation, capping, absorptions, extensive studies of reactivity pattern on panels of *H-2* congenic strains) and were found to be alloreactive *H-2* class 1-specific antibodies. Antibodies of individual mice differed again in *H-2* specificity. Five *H-2*-specific MAb have been isolated from mice injected with syngeneic Sendai virus-infected cells.

Comparable results were obtained in the primary and secondary immune responses (Kievits et al. 1988b). These antibodies are not antiviral and MHC restricted, they are only *H-2* specific and not virus specific at all. There was a disturbing resemblance to MHC-restricted antiviral antibodies, because most sera bound better to virus-infected cells than to normal cells (Kievits et al. 1987, 1988a). Weak sera exhibited detectable binding only on virus-infected cells and remained (falsely) negative on normal cells. However, it became clear that the antibodies also bound more strongly to cells infected by a different virus or otherwise modified to express more *H-2* antigen. Our conclusion became that we could not detect antiviral MHC-restricted antibodies (Ivanyi and Kievits 1988). The new phenomenon was that it is possible to induce *H-2* class 1-specific antibodies by virus-infected syngeneic cells.

Today we can not regularly repeat the induction of *H-2*-specific antibodies by injections of *normal* (i.e. not virus-infected) cells. Such experiments are now used as negative controls for injections of virus-infected cells. Only occasionally do some mice produce *H-2* antibodies after injection of syngeneic cells. We think that this situation supports our general conclusions, because at the time when we had "the positive results" we were approaching, in our open animal house, a period of serious viral infections which later eliminated a part of our mouse strains. We therefore established our SPF animal house. We now work with SPF mice and we cannot effectively induce *H-2* antibodies by injections of normal syngeneic lymphocytes. This is yet another reason to believe that, in the results reported previously, the antibodies were induced by MHC + X.

Whatever the explanation is, the field we have explored can, in all fairness, be designated *non-conventional H-2 serology*. In my investigations, I have never had so many problems as with non-conventional *H-2* serology. I believe that we have described some new phenomena, but I have no final explanation for their mechanism, and we do not know whether, if at all, they are functionally relevent.

The experiments on the induction of *H-2*-specific antibodies by injections of virus-infected syngeneic cells were similar to those of others in an effort to examine the existence of MHC-restricted antibodies. We arrived at the interpretation that such antibodies do not exist. It is always difficult "to prove" that something (that is more or less expected) does not exist. However, it is also difficult to define precisely what various authors understand by the therm "MHC-restriced antibodies" (Ivanyi and Kievits 1988). We could find no such antibodies. A similar conclusion has been reached by others (Tamminen and Barber 1988; Pla et al. 1988; Pestalozzi et al. 1987). Wylie et al. (1982), Froscher and Klinman (1986) claim that they represent a considerable part of the B cell repertoire. Parham (1988) said that MHC-restricted antibodies is a perplexing problem and that "devising strategies of immunization and screening for MHC restricted antibodies is difficult".

The perplexing problem for me is how it is possible that none of the *determinants* formed by the association of foreign peptides and MHC, which are perfectly recognised by the T cell receptor, is seen by antibodies? This appears to me the interesting question which can be raised on the basis of our data with non-conventional *H-2* serology.

Summary

We have described class 1 *H-2*-specific antibodies induced by injections of syngeneic virus infected cells and naturally occurring *H2* antibodies. A common denominator for these experiments is *non-conventional H-2 serology*. It remains unclear how naturally occurring *H-2*-specific antibodies are induced, and how *H-2*-specific antibodies are induced after injections of syngeneic virus-infected cells. The answer(s) to these questions might contribute to some aspccts of MHC functions, for example, in autoimmunity or resistance to foreign antigens or autologous tumours. Possibly further research, maybe using an indirect approach, will contribute to solve these problems. We could not detect self-MHC-restricted antiviral antibodies. The specificity of *H-2*-specific antibodies, which we obtained after primary or secondary immune responses to syngeneic virus-infected cells, have been anti-*H-2* and not antiviral *H-2*-restricted antibodies. We have suggested that the antibodies observed in all these situations are due to triggering by self-MHC modified by virus infection. In the course of this work differences in MHC-specific immune responses among genetically identical individuals became apparent. The amazing finding was how great such individual differences can be.

The experiments described in this contribution were performed by a number of coworkers and published in a series of papers which have not all been quoted here. The most relevant references and much of the work from other laboratories are summarized in Ivanyi (1988). The original papers, rather than this personal overview, should be quoted for the data summarized in this contribution.

Living and Working Abroad

We came to the Netherlands in 1976. Sven welcomed us with tulips when we arrived. Discussions with Vincent Eijsvoogel were decisive in shaping my research prospects. I continued to work on both the HLA and *H-2* system. The availability of the HLA-typed cell panel of Paul Engelfriet and of the *H-2* congenic and mutant strains of Kees Melief allowed me to start work a few days after arriving. Recently a utopian dream became reality: in cooperation with Hidde Ploegh and Ton Berns (Netherlands Cancer Institute) HLA-transgenic mice were created, and so I am now doing HLA research on mice. I was very lucky and happy with my Dutch PhD students Martijn, Gijs, Femia and Birgitta.

In the Netherlands my job was arranged without one single document, and immediately. What a kingdom! I have no difficulties in continuing my research work and interests along the same lines as in Prague. Certainly, the circumstances were different. In Prague I was one among few, in the Netherland I am one among many.

I had to learn to understand new aspects. Beyond the service support by my institute, I must apply for research grants for all experimental work. Thus, my projects must be approved by a "commission". All this is self-evident here, but was quite new for me. Research in Prague was supported from the budget of the institute, i.e. by the research director and his advisory team (of which I was a member). Here I had to learn that money was very valuable, not only at the supermarket but also in the research market, and each Dutch florin could be used only once! Hence, competition is much stronger here than I experienced in Prague. However, much has changed everywhere in the last 15 years, probably also in Prague.

The Netherlands is practically a bilingual country. English is used without any hesitation, and for me to talk a meeting at whatever level in English is as normal as to say *merci* when somebody opens a door for you. But here again, in Prague my English was excellent, in Amsterdam it is rather lousy.

Sascha and Jon showed us the beauties of the North Holland waterside; isn't sailing the great dream of all "landlocked" people? Erna and Jochem showed us Cobra art; our secret plans for the future became to open an art gallery. We discovered the flower auction at Schiphol ourselves and proudly showed a great many of our visitors around.

There is a definite resemblance in the history and life style of the Netherlands and Czechoslovakia. Nevertheless, the Dutch are different from the Czechs. But the Czechs are also different from others, even the Slovaks! And I was brought up bilingually as my parents spoke Hungarian. Maybe this was all more difficult for my wife Dagmar as she was born and bred in the centre of Prague.

However, diversity is what we have been selected for. That is the enigma of MHC immunogenetics. We have all those alloantigens to reflect our *individuality* and we are willing to accept this. Why should we not accept that the Dutch are different? If one understands this, it is very pleasant to live in this country: *a Realm of Tolerance*. Nevertheless, I would very much like to revisit all those places around Prague, Bratislava and Budapest which I liked so much and all those people whom I still consider to be my good friends. I hope that *Realm of Tolerance* will make this possible.

References

Capkova J, Hasek M, Kousalova M, Holan V, Boubelik M (1983) Alloreactive cytotoxic anti-H-2 antibodies in sera of the syngeneically immunized C57Bl/10ScSnPh, BALB/cJPh, and B10.A/SnPh mice. Folia Biol (Praha) 29: 200–210

Cerny-Provaznik R, Radl J, Leupers T, van Mourik P, Brondijk R, de Greeve P, Ivanyi P (1985) Anti-MHC immunity detected prior to intentional alloimmunization. I. Naturally occurring H-2-specific antibodies in C57Bl/KaLwRij (H-2b) mice. Nat Immun Cell Growth Regul 4: 138–159

Cramer M, Mierau R, Kuon W, Weiss E, Robinson PJ (1988) A monoclonal antibody induced by syngeneic ConA blasts: its reactivity pattern with mouse and human MHC class I antigens. In: Ivanyi P (ed) MHC + X complex formation and antibody induction. Springer, Berlin Heidelberg New York

De Waal LP, Melvold RW, Melief CJM (1983) Cytotoxic T lymphocyte nonresponsiveness to the male antigen H-Y in the H-2Db mutants bm13 and bm14. J Exp Med, 158: 1537–1546

Fierz W, Brenan M, Mullbacher A, Simpson E (1982) Non-H-2 and H-2 linked immune response genes control the cytotoxic T-cell response to H-Y. Immunogenetics, 15: 261–270

Froscher BG, Klinman NR (1986) Immunization with SV40-transformed cells yields mainly MHC-restricted monoclonal antibodies. J Exp Med, 164: 196–210

Gunther E (1988) Naturally occurring anti-MHC class I antibodies in the rat. In: Ivanyi P (ed) MHC + X, complex formation and antibody induction. Springer, Berlin Heidelberg New York, pp 14–17

Hansen TH, Ivanyi P, Levy RB, Sachs DH (1979) Cross-reactivity among the products of three nonallelic H-2 loci, H-2Ld, H-2Dq and H-2Kk. Transplantation, 28: 339–342

Hemmi S, Geliebter J, Zeff RA, Melvold RW, Nathenson SG (1988) Three spontaneous H-2Db mutants are generated by genetic micro-recombination (gene conversion) events. J Exp Med, 168: 2319–2335

Herr W, Gilbert W (1982) Germ line MulV reintegration in AKR/J mice. Nature, 296: 865–868

Ivanyi P (ed) (1988) MHC + X; complex formation and antibody induction. Springer, Berlin Heidelberg New York

Ivanyi P, Kievits F (1988) MHC-restricted antibodies: facts and interpretations. In: Ivanyi P (ed) MHC + X; complex formation and antibody induction. Springer, Berlin Heidelberg New York, pp 119–127

Ivanyi P, van den Berg-Loonen EM, de Greeve P (1978) Individual mice of one inbred strain produce anti-H-2 and anti-HLA antibodies of different specificities. Tissue Antigens 12: 32–38

Ivanyi P, Melief CJM, de Greeve P, van Mourik P (1979) Individual mice recognize the complex nature of H-2 antigens; unexpected reactions (anti-Kk) in anti-BALB/c-H-2d sera produced in the BALB/c-H-2db mutant. Transplant Proc, 11: 642–646

Ivanyi P, van Mourik P, Breuning MH, Melief CJM (1980) Anti-H-2 antibodies induced by syngeneic immunization. Immunogenetics 10: 319–332

Ivanyi P, van Mourik P, Breuning MH, Kruisbeek AM, Krose CJM (1982) Natural H-2 specific antibodies in sera of aged mice. Immunogenetics, 15: 95–102

Ivanyi P, Cerny-Provaznik R, van Mourik PC (1988) Naturally occurring H-2 specific antibodies. In: Ivanyi P (ed) MHC+X complex formation and antibody induction. Springer, Berlin Heidelberg New York

Juretic A, Juretic E, Nagy ZA, Klein J (1985) Cytotoxic T cell response to H-Y antigen by C6.C-H-2bm12 and B10.BR mice. Immunology, 55: 671–675

Kast WM, Boog CJP, Roep BO, Voordouw AC, Melief CJM (1988) Failure or success in the restoration of virus specific cytotoxic T lymphocyte response defects by dendritic cells. J Immunol, 140: 3186–3193

Kievits F, Rocca A, Opolski A, Limpens J, Leupers T, Kloosterman T, Boerenkamp WJ, Pla M, Ivanyi P (1987) Induction of H-2 specific antibodies is triggered by injections with syngeneic Sendai virus coated cells. Eur J Immunol, 17: 27–35

Kievits F, Boerenkamp WJ, Ivanyi P (1988a) Searching for MHC restricted antibodies: antibodies induced by injections with syngeneic cells coated with Sendai virus, trinitrophenyl, and xenogeneic beta-2-microglobulin are not restricted by the mouse MHC. In: Ivanyi P (ed) MHC+X, complex formation and antibody induction. Springer, Berlin Heidelberg New York

Kievits F, Boerenkamp WJ, Ivanyi P (1988b) Immunization with syngeneic Sendai virus-infected cells induces no MHC-restricted antibodies but antibodies specific for H-2 class I determinants. Immunogenetics, 29: 108–111

Pala P, Townsend ARM, Askonas BA (1986) Viral recognition by influenza A virus cross-reactive cytotoxic T (Tc) cells: the proportion of Tc cells that recognize nucleoprotein varies between individual mice. Eur J Immunol, 16: 193–198

Parham P (1988) A problem perplex, MHC+X. In: Ivanyi P (ed) MHC+X complex formation and antibody induction. Springer, Berlin Heidelberg New York

Pestalozzi B, Stitz L, Zinkernagel PM (1987) Monoclonal antibodies against viral determinants are not restriced to the K/D end of the major histocompatibility complex. J Exp Med, 166: 295–299

Pla M, Opolski A, Rocca A, Degos L (1988) Immunization with fibroblasts transfected with a cloned retroviral DNA induces H-2 specific antibodies in syngeneic recipients. In: Ivanyi P (ed) MHC+X, complex formation and antibody induction. Springer, Berlin Heidelberg New York

Prehn RT (1975) Non-genetic variability in susceptibility to oncogenesis. Science, 190: 1095–1096

Prehn RT, Karcher CA (1983) Splenic variations affecting sarcomagenesis among mice of an inbred strain. Int J Cancer, 31: 65–66

Schmidt W (1988) MHC specific monoclonal antibodies induced by injection of syngeneic leukemia cells. In: Ivanyi P (ed) MHC+X, complex formation and antibody induction. Springer, Berlin Heidelberg New York

Sherman LA (1980) Dissection of the B10.D2 anti-H-2Kb cytolytic T lymphocyte receptor repertoire. J Exp Med, 151: 1386–1397

Stukart MJ, Vos A, Melief CJM (1981) Cytotoxic T cell response against lymphoblasts infected with Moloney (Abelson) murine leukemia virus. Methodological aspects and H-2 requirements. Eur J Immunol, 11: 251–255

Stukart MJ, Vos A, Boes J, Melvold RW, Bailey DW, Melief CMH (1982) Crucial role of the H-2D locus in the regulation of both the D- and K-associated cytotoxic T lymphocyte response against Moloney leukemia virus demonstrated with two Db mutants. J Immunol, 128: 1360–1364

Tamminen WL, Barber BH (1988) Searching for MHC restricted monoclonal antibodies recognizing the determinants seen by anti-influenza virus cytotoxic T lymphocyte receptors. In: Ivanyi P (ed) MHC+X, complex formation and antibody induction. Springer, Berlin Heidelberg New York

Wettstein PJ (1981) H-2 effects on cell-cell interactions in the response to single non-H-2 alloantigens. IV. Variations in the proliferative response to H-Y and H-3. Immunogenetics, 14: 241–252

Wylie DE, Sherman LA, Klinman NR (1982) Participation of the major histocompatibility complex in antibody recognition of viral antigens expressed on infected cells. J Exp Med, 155: 403–414

Immunology and Cytology in Bacterial, Viral and Tumor Diseases

Immunological Analysis of Mycobacterial Disease

J. Ivanyi

Personal Reflections

One night Milan unexpectedly called at our flat in central Prague in an elated mood and asked for a cup of strong, black coffee. However, before coffee was prepared, he dozed off on the sofa. After a while, we opted to make him comfortable with a pillow and blanket and went to bed. In the middle of the night we were woken by the weight of Milan's body diagonally across us on the bed. Milan, while asleep, resisted all our efforts to move him into a parallel position in the middle of the bed. Defeated, we retreated next door and went to sleep on the floor. In the morning, amazed by the situation, Milan disappeared and soon returned with an enormous bouquet of flowers for my wife Lida.

Milan's generosity of mind was reflected by the overriding positive emphasis he had always given to other people. This was true not only of his conversations but also of his correspondence. Nevertheless, I have attempted to extract a few sections from his letters, written under difficult circumstances during 1970, which may illuminate his attitudes and feelings.

13.3. 1970

... I am writing to boost my morale for a moment, at least by reminiscence. I don't feel sad because I think that matters cannot get worse. ... Occasionally, I enjoy walking with my dog, I carry on with a few experiments and a bit of writing. We keep chasing the antisera ... it is easy to invent factors ... but we must first exclude the role of antibodies ... I am working on a book *Immunology and Medicine* (reading for "each doctor") ...

14.7. 1970

I would like to come to London, but you know our system; it is ridiculous that all members of the Institute are banned from travel to Western countries. ... I hope that at least scientific contacts will return to normal soon, but you know that such decisions are not for us to make. I was expelled from the party, and demoted from directorship; and the Council [of the Academy] was disbanded. I feel, hey, go bathing, have more time for work, and keep thinking that our system is actually extremely beneficial by saving creative potential. Instead of chasing large numbers of publications as they do in America, we get the opportunity to think over matters from an appropriate perspective. I keep thinking about the theoretical and practical problems of transplantation ...

There was a nice symposium here about Mendel, unfortunately, still not matching his stature. We are still in debt in this respect and the rest of the world should help us out ...

31.8. 1970

Do you know the story about the Roman emperor who, after conquering Jerusalem, wanted to see this one-god of the theirs. The old rabbi came and said: "Mr. Emperor, look at the sun." He looked up to get a glimpse and said: "But you cannot look there." And the rabbi replied: "Well, you see, Mr. Emperor, this is only a tiny reflection of our God." I think that, if God is angry with us, it is only when we become somewhat sad and take matters too seriously. I do like John Lord with Deep Purple and Ian Gillam singing "When You Speak to Silent Me." When thinking of the sciences and arts, I subscribe to Bertrand Russell who said (while deserting from the army in 1914) that deeds still prevail over words in politics.

25. 12. 1970

Science (and the world) is like an ameba with pseudopods in each direction but with the ability to move merely in one direction ... I heard rumours that Peter Harper gave a lecture in London claiming that he could transfer a conditioned reflex with a brain extract ... I enjoyed reading Taylor's *Biological Bomb* and the *Future of Men* (Ciba Foundation) ... After 20 years of personal efforts, I want to come to terms with racism in relationship to the genetics of man. Nature can do anything by codes and programs but talking to it is like talking to someone who is deaf and dumb.

3.11. 1975

I have a good team and a laboratory now, I also collaborate with friends outside the Institute and sometimes feel like a student who has just started. I feel excited about future plans ... We hope to go hiking and camping in the Romanian Carpathian mountains next year ...

Mycobacterial Disease

Immunological research on tuberculosis and leprosy has been attracting increasing attention during recent years. I shall discuss here the main areas of interest in which advances have been achieved or could be expected in the future. The background to a renewed emphasis on fundamental studies on the host-parasite relationship in mycobacterial diseases has been the realization that chemotherapy is unlikely to accomplish, as originally expected, the eradication of tuberculosis. The reasons for this outcome are operational since the implementation of effective, but protracted chemotherapeutic regimens requires a level of support which is not attainable in countries with generally poor health care resources. Transmission of the infection is perpetuated by late diagnosis and escalated by relapsed patients defaulting on chemotherapy. Consequently, tuberculosis and leprosy each affect at least 10 million people worldwide with associated mortality or physical disability. In recent years, the declining trend in the incidence of tuberculosis has been halted or even reverted, which is suspected of being associated with the global spread of human immunodeficiency virus (HIV) infection.

The great majority of individuals who get infected with *Mycobacterium tuberculosis* or *Mycobacterium leprae* do not develop disease. This outcome results from combined innate and aquired (immune) resistance. Protective immunity is mediated by T cells which are effective in adoptive transfer experiments, whilst passive transfer by serum does not confer protection. Hence, T cell-deficient mice show greatly increased susceptibility to mycobacterial infection. The effector mechanisms of protection have been attributed to CD4 cell-derived lymphokines which activate macrophages for the bacteriocidal activity against the intracellular mycobacteria. This concept based on the original work by Mackaness is probably correct, although attempts to obtain direct evidence of killing of mycobacteria by infected macrophages in vitro have yielded only equivocal results. The problems which had been encountered are the difficulties in maintaining functional macrophages in tissue culture and the slow growth rate of tubercle bacilli (*M. leprae* can be grown only in vivo). As far as the effector lymphokine is concerned, gamma interferon (IFN) is the main candidate involved in macrophage activation, but other humoral factors have also been implicated. In addition to the CD4 non-cognate type immunity, it was suggested recently that CD8 cells may lyse infected targets which are not equipped or have lost their bacteriocidal capacity; subsequently, the released bacteria would be taken up and killed by freshly matured and activated macrophages with unimpaired bactericidal function (Kaufmann 1988).

In view of the experimental problems discussed above, none of the parameters which would measure T cell, lymphokine or macrophage function in vitro represents an adequate immunological assay for the host protective immunity against mycobacterial pathogens. This lack of a relevant test represents probably the main limitation for exact assessment of prophylactic immunization in man and consequently the reason for the ongoing controversy about the efficacy of the bacille Calmette-Guérin (BCG) vaccine. Moreover, the interpretation of conventional skin delayed-type hypersensitivity (DTH) reactions or in vitro T cell proliferation often discounts the compelling evidence against the role of DTH reactivity in protective immunity to mycobacterial infection (Lovik and Closs 1982).

Another consequence of the non-cognate macrophage-mediated type of resistance is our complete ignorance about the molecular nature of antigens which can stimulate the protective immunity. Unlike any antibody-mediated immunity to microbial pathogens or T cell-mediated anti-virus immunity, the immunological models of study with mycobacteria are yet to be developed. The difficulties of experimental analysis are further aggravated by the fact that protection can be imparted only by a live attenuated organism such as BCG. Consequently, evaluation of any isolated antigenic constituents from mycobacteria would require a delivery within an live vector (e.g. vaccinia or Salmonella) or with a novel adjuvant which could substitute the qualities of the "live" inoculation which so far remain elusive.

The biological aspects discussed above are of major concern in view of the extensive achievements in the molecular study of mycobacterial antigens in recent years (Ivanyi et al. 1988b). Since 1981, monoclonal antibodies have been produced, and their specificities have been well defined in several laboratories. Since 1985, the lambda gt11 genomic libraries of R.A. Young have enabled the sequencing and expression of an increasing number of protein constituents. This wealth of structural information derived by advanced technologies allows one to study the topography of T cell epitopes (Lamb et al. 1987) and the immunogenicity of corresponding synthetic peptides (Cox et al. 1989). In the latter study, the immunogenicity was increased by the construction of a dimeric peptide. Furthermore, immunogenicity was conferred on previously non-immunogenic peptides by linking them as heterodimers with another immunodominant peptide.

The bacteriological diagnosis of tuberculosis has several limitations, and therefore the possibility of developing a serodiagnostic test has been of interest for several years. Monoclonal antibodies have identified several antigenic determinants which are species specific for either *M. tuberculosis* or *M. leprae*. These were evaluated in a competition assay which showed some of these epitopes to be immunodominant, i.e. a high proportion of sera from patients with multibacillary tuberculosis or leprosy containing antibodies of corresponding specificity (Ivanyi et al. 1988a). It is of particular interest that the pattern of immunodominance when comparing several specificities varies with the form of disease or infection (Jackett et al. 1988; Bothamley et al. 1988).

The virulence of mycobacteria results probably from multiple factors involved in their interaction with the infected host. Intracellular multiplication is one mandatory requirement, but toxins, commonly found in other bacteria, have not been identified. Instead, mycobacteria contain in their cell wall powerful immunomodulatory (adjuvant) substances such as muramyldipeptide and lipoarabinomannan (Moreno et al. 1988). These constituents, probably in association with other cell wall structures, can enhance or suppress immune responses and also have granulomatogenic activity. It has been speculated that mycobacteria could not have evolved potent adjuvants to boost host-protective immunity for their own destruction, but rather as decoys to subvert host resistance into pathogenic cellular reactions which cause damage to the host (Ivanyi 1986). More recently, this concept could be expanded towards certain protein constituents with structural homology between bacteria and eucaryotic cells (Young et al. 1988). These proteins belonging to a family of stress proteins (heat shock proteins) provide vital functions to cells by protecting the native conformation or by providing a transport/"chaperon" function to intracellular proteins. Hence, it was proposed that intracellular bacteria could perhaps supplant their stress proteins into metabolic pathways of their eucaryotic host cell (i.e. macrophage) to achieve a defective reaction and a pathogenic effect (Ivanyi et al. 1988b).

Immunology has a particularly important role in the pathogenesis of leprosy because immune reactions decide not only between protection or disease, but also the pattern of clinical manifestations. Thus, classification of leprosy has been based essentially on the balance between immune reactions, namely the paucibacillary tuberculoid leprosy represented by strong T cell reactions and multibacillary lepromatous leprosy by pronounced antibody formation. Since there is an abundance of T cell reactivity to mycobacteria in tuberculoid leprosy (likewise in tuberculosis), the perennial question is being asked about the nature of the "defect" which diverts protection into pathogenicity. Generally, the following mechanisms can be considered:

Change in the Specificity of the Immune Repertoire. So far, there is insufficient information comparing diseased, self-healed and BCG-vaccinated subjects. Recombinant antigens have, as yet, only enabled the study of individual T cell clones which are poorly representative of the whole repertoire. More promising evaluation might be obtained from the T cell proliferative assay of mycobacterial fractions separated by electroblotting (P. Mendez-Samperio, et al. 1989)

Defect in the Composition or Secretion of Lymphokines. Human CD4 clones have been found to differ in their secretion and susceptibility to interleukin 2 IL-2, whilst gamma-IFN secretion has been uniform (Mustafa et al. 1986).

Defective Response of Macrophages to Lymphokines. This hypothesis, however, would need to invoke the antigenic specificity which could occur at the level of antigen processing. Alternatively, macrophages could become selectively refractory for the killing of mycobacteria.

Any of the three mechanisms listed above could also be implicated in the generation of T cell anergy which is characteristic for lepromatous leprosy. T cell anergy could be the cause for the unrestrained growth of *M. leprae,* but the alternative view (D. S. Ridley, personal communication) that T cell anergy is merely a temporal consequence of excessive bacterial expansion cannot be excluded. Most patients fail to produce skin DTH reactions to an *M. leprae* extract whilst responding to tuberculin (PPD), but a certain proportion of patients is anergic to both extracts. The "split" anergy is an intriguing phenomenon when considering that several epitopes are shared between various species of mycobacteria. It was reported that CD8 cells with specificity for the phenolic glycolipid constituent of *M. leprae* could suppress the response of CD4 cells to the polyclonal mitogen concanavalin A (Bloom and Mehra 1984). Specific proteins from *M. leprae* were also implicated in a regulatory capacity by the demonstration that they suppressed the skin DTH reaction to tuberculin (Sengupta et al. 1987). However. this effect was demonstrable in patients with both lepromatous and tuberculoid leprosy and therefore in concordance with the view that the reported "suppressor" cells could not be responsible for the immunopathogenesis of lepromatous leprosy (Prasad et al. 1987).

Comparisons of the specificities of the immune repertoire between tuberculoid and lepromatous disease are difficult to perform since most of the former have low antibody levels and the latter, in reverse, give low T cell responses. Various attempts had been made to restore the immune capacity of lepromatous T cells in vitro. Since they retain a normal display of IL-2 receptors, exogenous IL-2 was used to supplement the media in antigen-stimulated lymphocyte cultures. The success rate varied between laboratories, and, on the whole, it appears that significant reversal can be achieved only in a minority of cases (Nogueira et al. 1983). Even so, the molecular mechanisms which could selectively dampen secretion or mop up IL-2 remain poorly understood. It is relevant for the study of the immune repertoire that differences may exist between cells in the peripheral blood and those at the site of pathological lesions (Rook et al. 1976). T cells trapped near to infected or antigen-containing cells become organized in granulomas. Their cellular constituents, structural relationship, CD4/CD8 ratio and bacillary count vary with the form of leprosy, and cloning of T cells from lesions could identify the important specificities (Modlin and Rea 1988).

The role of host genetic factors is reviewed by Skamene elsewhere in this volume. I shall mention only results from one recent study which revealed HLA class II association common for the incidence of pulmonary tuberculosis and for the antibody levels to a 38 protein antigen of *M. tuberculosis* (Bothamley et al. 1989). In this study on patients and controls from Indonesia, antibody titres only to one out of five tested antigens were associated with the *DR2* allele. The study also established the disease association with DR2 and DQw1 (36% and 39% attributable risk) and resistance to tuberculosis being associated with DQw3 (57% preventative fraction). The joint DR2 association of antibody levels and disease raises the possibility of a pathogenetic role of the 38K antigen. It seems conceivable that the high-responder antibody phenotype could cause the decline in the macrophage activating, i.e. protective immune function by T cells which had become engaged as helpers for the B cell response. If the assumption about the reciprocal relationship between humoral and protective immunity is correct, then the antibody specificity indicates a clue in the search for protective antigens. Alternatively, one cannot exclude the possibility that DR2 patients have more severe disease involving another molecular target for the DR2 gene and only secondarily elevated anti-38K antibody levels.

An important but relatively neglected subject is the mechanism by which an infected host may control the metabolic events which regulates the latency and recrudescence of bacterial multiplication. It is well known that infection with either *M. tuberculosis* or *M. leprae* at childhood can be followed by several years or even decades of dormancy. Reactivation of bacterial growth is thought to be the result of a sudden "breakdown" of host resistance, but there is practically no information about the underlying cellular mechanisms. Yet, this is a single critical event for the pathogenesis of most adult cases of tuberculosis and leprosy. Dormant mycobacteria cannot be demonstrated directly in host tissues, and prior experimental studies examined only the relapse of persister bacteria induced by cortisone in mice which had previously been given sub-sterilizing chemotherapy (Hart and Rees 1950). The immunosuppressive activity of cortisone indicated the role of host resistance in the maintenance of latent bacilli. However, the natural stimuli of reactivation remain unknown, and their mode of action could be distinct from the artificial high-dose cortisone treatment. The likely complexity of these mechanisms has been suggested by recent results which indicated that host immunity could paradoxically aggravate the spontaneous relapse of BCG growth following a course of incomplete chemotherapy (Cox and Ivanyi 1988). This interpretation was based on the observation that the relapse was greater in mice which were exposed to the infection for 3 weeks (i.e. immune) than in mice which received the chemotherapy immediately after BCG infection (i.e. non-immune).

In conclusion, it seems appropriate to note that the discussed mechanisms of anergy of T cell responses in multibacillary infection undoubtedly belong within the "Realm of Tolerance". There is also a striking parallel between theories of tolerance and mycobacterial anergy represented by a shift from clonal deletion to regulatory interpretations. However, neither of these mechanisms alone can fully explain the complexities of immunopathogenesis during natural evolution of human disease. As with other phenomena within the realm of immunological tolerance, the search for a uniform explanation has given way to multiple mechanisms.

References

Bloom BR, Mehra V (1984) Immunological unresponsiveness in leprosy. Immunol Rev 80: 5
Bothamley GH, Udani PM, Rudd R, Festenstein F, Ivanyi J (1988) Antibody levels in smear positive and smear negative thoracic tuberculosis of adults and children. Eur J Clin Microbiol Inf 7: 639
Bothamley GH, Beck J, Schreuder G, D'Amaro J, de Vries RRP, Kardjito T, Ivanyi J (1989) HLA-DR2 and DQw1 association with tuberculosis and antibody levels to the 38kDa antigen. J Inf Dis 159: 549–555
Cox JH, Ivanyi J (1988) The role of host factors for the chemotherapy of BCG infection in inbred strains of mice. Acta Pathol Microbiol Immunol Scand 96: 927
Cox JH, Ivanyi J, Young DB, Lamb JR, Syred AD, Francis M (1989) Orientation of epitopes influences the immunogenicity of synthetic peptide dimers. Eur J Immunol (in press)
Hart P D'arcy, Rees RJW (1950) Enhancing effect of cortisone on tuberculosis in the mouse. Lancet 2: 391
Ivanyi J (1986) Pathogenic and protective interactions in mycobacterial infections. Clin Immunol Allergy 60: 127–157
Ivanyi J, Bothamley GH, Jackett PS (1988a) Immunodiagnostic assays for tuberculosis and leprosy. Br Med Bull 44: 635–649
Ivanyi J, Sharp K, Jackett P, Bothamley G (1988b) Immunological study of the defined constituents of mycobacteria. Springer Semin Immunopathol 10: 279
Jackett P, Bothamley G, Batra HV, Mistry A, Young DB, Ivanyi J (1988) Epitope and whole antigen molecule specificities in the serology of tuberculosis. J Clin Microbiol 26: 2313
Kaufmann SHE (1988) CD8+ T lymphocytes in intracellular microbial infections. Immunol Today 9: 168–174
Lamb JR, Ivanyi J, Rees ADM, Rothbard JB, Howland K, Young RA, Young DB (1987) Mapping of T cell epitopes using recombinant antigens and synthetic peptides. EMBO J 6: 1245
Lovik M, Closs O (1982) Repeated delayed-type hypersensitivity reactions against *Mycobacterium lepraemurium* antigens at the infection site do not affect bacillary multiplication in C3H mice. Infect Immun 36: 768
Mendez-Samperio P, Lamb J, Bothamley G, Stanley P, Ellis C, Ivanyi J (1989) Molecular study of the T cell repertoire in family contacts and patients with leprosy. J Immunol (In press)
Modlin RL, Rea TH (1988) Immunopathology of leprosy granulomas. Springer Semin Immunopathol 10: 359
Moreno C, Angela M, Lamb J (1988) The inhibitory effects of mycobacterial lipoarabinomannan and polysaccharides upon polyclonal and monoclonal human T cell proliferation. Clin Exp Immunol 74: 206
Mustafa AS, Kvalheim G, Degre M, Godal T (1986) *Mycobacterium bovis* BCG-induced human T cell clones from BCG-vaccinated healthy subjects: antigen specificity and lymphokine production. Infect Immun 53: 491
Nogueira N, Kaplan G, Levy E et al. (1983) Defective gamma interferon production in leprosy: reversal with antigen and IL-2. J Exp Med 158: 2165–2170

Prasad HK, Mishra RS, Nath I (1987) Phenolic glycolipid-I of *Mycobacterium leprae* induces general suppression of in vitro concanavalin a responses unrelated to leprosy type. J Exp Med 165: 239

Rook GAW, Carswell JW, Stanford JL (1976) Preliminary evidence for the trapping of antigen-specific lymphocytes in the lymphoid tissu of "anergic" tuberculosis patients. Clin Exp Immunol 16: 129–132

Sengupta U, Sinha S, Ramu G, Lamb J, Ivanyi J (1987) Suppression of delayed hypersensitivity skin reactions to tuberculin by *M.lepare* antigens in patients with lepromatous and tuberculoid leprosy. Clin Exp Immunol 68: 58

Young DB, Lathigra R, Hendrix R, Sweetser D, Young RA (1988) Stress proteins are immune targets in leprosy and tuberculosis. Proc Natl Acad Sci USA 85: 4267–4270

Genetic Control of Susceptibility to Mycobacterial Infections

E. Skamene

Introduction

Inherited factors contributing to the susceptibility to mycobacterial infections have been postulated to exist for decades. Most of the lines of evidence supporting the role of genetics in the pathogenesis of tuberculosis and related infections during epidemics and in endemic areas of the world have been indirect. Among those were racial differences in susceptibility (Motulsky 1960), twin studies (Comstock 1978) and co-segregation of known chromosomal markers with the disease, both in families and in outbred populations (Singh et al. 1983). The more precise analysis of such genetic influence on the variability of susceptibility to mycobacterial infection in the human population has, generally, been rather disappointing for several reasons. First, as with any infectious disease, it has often been difficult to dissociate "nature" from "nurture." In other words, related family members share not only their genetic pool but also the air they breath and the food they eat. Secondly, it would be unrealistic to expect that host response to any infectious agent would solely be regulated by a single gene. The possession of a particular allele at one genetic locus may dramatically influence the course of disease in certain individuals but, at the level of whole population, many genes would be expected to be responsible for the, often spectral, disease profile which is frequently observed in mycobacterial infections (Lenzini et al. 1977). Furthermore, many interrelated processes which manifest themselves as susceptibility/resistance to being infected, susceptibility/resistance to the establishment of infection, progression or clearance of infection or susceptibility/resistance to reinfection take place within the host exposed to an infectious agent. These processes are mechanistically distinct and, therefore, should involve regulation by different genes.

The genetic basis of susceptibility and resistance to mycobacterial infections must, therefore, be viewed as a composite interplay of inherited mechanisms which manifest themselves as a programmed sequence of events. Only by separating the phenotype of host response into discrete steps may we reconstruct its genetic regulation.

Animal Models of Genetic Resistance and Susceptibility to Mycobacterial Infections

While most of the information regarding the influence of host genes on the outcome of mycobacterial infection in humans is circumstantial, animal models, where the influence of environmental factors can be controlled, provide direct evidence for this type of regulation. Over the last 50 years, three major approaches to the analysis of the role of genetics in the models of mycobacterial diseases in laboratory rodents have been employed:

1. Genetic variation in resistance/susceptibility to mycobacterial infection among randomly bred and inbred strains of animals.
2. Selective inbreeding for resistance/susceptibility to mycobacterial infection.
3. Variation in resistance/susceptibility among lines of rodents which were selectively inbred for other phenotype traits (e.g., magnitude of antibody production to antigens unrelated to mycobacteria).

The earliest formal genetic analysis of the trait of resistance and susceptibility to tuberculosis dates back to the 1930s (Lurie and Dannenberg 1965). The experimental system comprised a colony of rabbits derived from four families which were selectively inbred for resistance or susceptibility. The typing criterion used for selective inbreeding was the quantitation of primary pulmonary tubercules which developed 5 weeks after inhalation of virulent human-type *Mycobacterium tuberculosis* (H37Rv). The trait of resistance to tuberculosis was shown to be dominant, multiple and additive over susceptibility by Mendelian analysis experiments (Lurie et al. 1952). The studies on phenotypic expression of this trait revealed that the genetically resistant lines of rabbits were innately endowed with a superior capacity to sequester and inactivate the mycobacterial pathogens within their alveolar macrophages and that they were, furthermore, superior in generating an immune response. Although the gene(s) regulating resistance to tuberculosis in rabbits was not identified, the experimental results have withstood the test of time and they are now being confirmed, extended, and explained in experimental models of tuberculosis in inbred strains of mice.

The genetic regulation of macrophage function has also been postulated to explain the phenomenon of innate resistance to mycobacterial infection (and to other infections with intracellular pathogens) which was documented in "Biozzi mice" that were selectively bred for high (HL) or low (LL) antibody responsiveness to sheep erythrocytes (Gheorghiu et al. 1985). A hypothesis offered to explain the HL and LL phenotypes was derived from the observation that LL-type macrophages exhibited superior metabolic activity (resulting in poor antigen retention) which translated into the expression of stronger bacteriostatic function against intracellularly ingested pathogens (Plant and Glynn 1982).

Genetic restriction of macrophage function thus appeared to be the common denominator in various models of inherited resistance/susceptibility to mycobacterial infection and it signaled the importance of nonspecific phase of resistance in these systems of host defense. As it turns out, the control of macrophage priming for activation into bactericidal cell is also the functional expression of the *Bcg* gene which regulates the innate resistance of mice to mycobacterial infection and which appears to be the first single gene demonstrated to exert an unequivocal influence on the course of host response to mycobacteria.

Population Genetics of the *Bcg* Gene

Strain variation in resistance to mycobacterial infection among mice has been noted since the mid-1940s. Reports by Donovick et al. (1949), Gray (1960), and Sever and Youmans (1957) showed that the survival time of various mouse strains after intravenous infection with *M. tuberculosis* varied considerably. Lynch et al. (1965) performed a Mendelian segregation analysis of the trait of resistance to *M. tuberculosis* in the progenitors of C57BL/6J (susceptible) and Swiss (resistant) mice and demonstrated that it was controlled by a single dominant gene which, with all probability, was identical to the *Bcg* gene which is the major topic of this review.

Using the *Mycobacterium bovis* bacille Calmette-Guérin (BCG) strain Montreal as the typing pathogen, our group (Forget et al. 1981) demonstrated a clear discontinuous variation in the response of inbred mouse strains to intravenous infection with a small dose (10^4 colony forming units, CFU) of this agent. Approximately one half of all inbred mouse strains tested typed as resistant, i.e., they did not allow any bacterial proliferation to occur in the spleens, livers, or lungs. There was a logarithmic growth of mycobacteria in the organs of the other half of inbred (susceptible) strains, the difference between the two groups often being significant as early as 24 h after infection (Fig. 1). Such segregation into resistant and susceptible strains, without any evidence of strains with an intermediate susceptibility, suggested that the trait might be under single gene control (Forget et al. 1981).

This hypothesis was confirmed by the Mendelian analysis of numerous crosses between resistant and susceptible progenitors. A bimodal distribution of resistant and susceptible animals was observed among the backcross progeny (Gros et al.

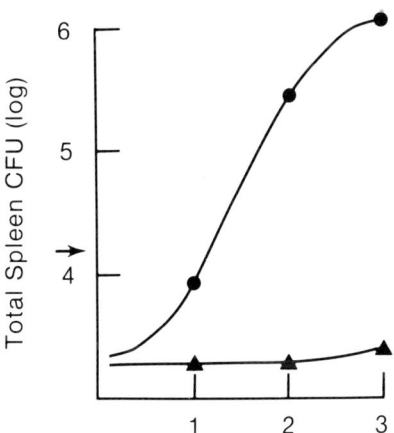

Fig. 1. Genetic variation in the control of BCG proliferation in vivo. *Arrow,* dose of BCG injected; *circles,* susceptible strain; *triangles,* resistant strain. (From Skamene, Forget 1988)

1981) and the trait has continued to breed true for up to 25 generations. Innate resistance to BCG infection (measured as the ability to restrict mycobacterial multiplication in the reticuloendothelial organs within the first 2–3 weeks after intravenous infection with a small BCG dose) was thus found to be under the control of a single, dominant, autosomal gene named the *Bcg* gene. The location of the *Bcg* gene on the chromosomal map of the mouse genome was achieved by typing recombinant inbred (RI) strains of the BXH, BXD, and BXA genes derived from the C57BL/6J (B) susceptible progenitor and the C3H/HeJ (H), DBA/2J (D), and A/J (A) resistant progenitors, respectively. The strain distribution pattern of resistant *(Bcg^r)* and susceptible *(Bcg^s)* alleles was found to be very similar to the strain distribution pattern of two isoenzyme loci, *Idh-1* (isocitrate dehydrogenase) and *Pep-3* (dipeptidase 3), located on the centromeric part of chromosome 1. The gene order was established by recombination frequencies to be *Idh-1–Bcg–Pep-3*.

Molecular Genetics of the *Bcg* Gene

In the absence of a precise knowledge of the structure of the *Bcg* gene or of its product, the strategy towards elucidating the molecular genetics of this locus has been to identify a linkage group overlapping the *Bcg* gene by restriction fragment length polymorphism (RFLP) analysis. The aim of the ongoing investigation has been to generate and position a large group of polymorphic markers in the portion of mouse chromosome 1 carrying the *Bcg* gene. RFLPs which are identified in that region of the chromosome are positioned with respect to *Bcg* by segregation analysis in RI strains and analysis of individual segregating progeny of known *Bcg* phenotype. This approach, taken in our laboratory and by others, has led to the identification of a large linkage group surrounding the *Bcg* gene (Fig. 2). Finer mapping and evaluation of the physical distance of the RFLPs to the *Bcg* gene is now being done by techniques such as pulse field gel electrophoresis. Cloning of genomic sequences overlapping the gene could then be envisioned by utilizing chromosome walking or chromosome jumping in appropriate genomic DNA libraries. In order to generate a large number of RFLPs, the chromosome-specific

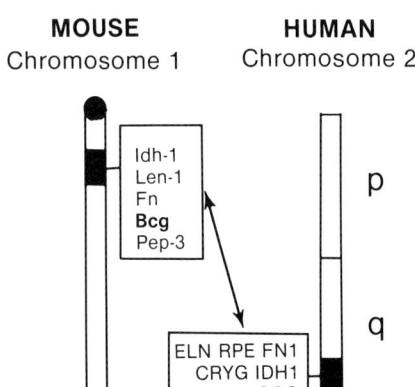

Fig. 2. Conservation of murine and human linkage groups (*Len-1* is a gamma crystallin gene, homologous to CRYG). (From Skamene, Forget 1988)

libraries obtained from somatic cell hybrids carrying the portions of mouse chromosome 1 on a primate background are being used. The linkage group involving the *Bcg* gene, as identified to date, reveals a striking homology with a conserved linkage group present on the long arm of human chromosome 2. It is thus conceivable that the human analogue of the murine *Bcg* gene exists in that part of genome. It is of interest that a similar sequence homology is also found in the bovine model. The hypothesis of the existence of a human equivalent of the *Bcg* gene is, at present, being examined by the search for co-segregation of these RFLP markers with the pattern of resistance and susceptibility to tuberculosis in families living in the tuberculosis-endemic areas of the world.

Phenotypic Expression of the *Bcg* Gene

The identification of the *Bcg* gene and of the in vivo trait of resistance to infection which is under its control allowed the construction of mouse lines which are *Bcg* congenic, i.e., genetically identical except for the small chromosomal segment containing the *Bcg* linkage group (Potter et al. 1983). The functional studies analyzing the cellular mechanism controlled by this gene could, therefore, be performed in a system where the interference from the remainder of the genome was practically nonexistent.

The first interesting finding made by the analysis of this model was that, in addition to regulating innate resistance to mycobacterial infection, this genetic locus also controls early host response to *Salmonella typhimurium* and *Leishmania donovani*. This fact was described prior to the *Bcg* gene work by British investigators (Plant and Glynn 1979; Bradley et al. 1979). This was one of the most tangible pieces of evidence attesting to the value of gene mapping for our understanding of genetic mechanisms of resistance and susceptibility: a single gene controlling innate resistance to a group of immunologically distinct and taxonomically unrelated pathogens was identified. The property which is shared by these microorganisms is the possession of a lipopolysaccharide-like surface sequence called integrins which allow for efficient macrophage-parasite interaction. Given the fact that all three pathogens restricted by the *Bcg* gene are intracellular parasites, it seemed plausible that the gene controls some facet of macrophage function (Skamene et al. 1982).

The observation that the initial events of host response, demonstrable as the difference between the susceptible and resistant phenotype as early as 24 h after infection, are being regulated by the *Bcg* gene further emphasized the notion that the acquired immune response was *not* the primary mechanism of this genetic control (Gros et al. 1983). This was further supported by the demonstration that the depletion of T cell, B cell, and natural killer (NK) cell populations from the resistant animals had not altered their response and, furthermore, that they remained resistant even after 900 R of total body irradiation. Radiation chimera experiments documented that the cell population expressing the resistant phenotype originated from bone marrow. The only manipulation which transformed the genetically resistant mouse strain into a phenotypically susceptible one was long-term treatment with silica (Gros et al. 1983). Thus, by exclusion, the mature macro-

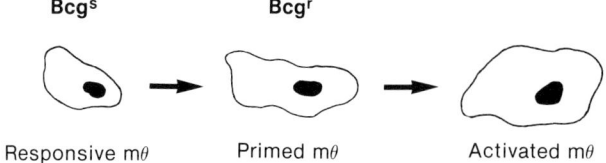

Fig. 3. Proposed mechanism of *Bcg* gene control at the cellular level. (From Skamene, Forget 1988)

phage remained the only candidate for the cell population expressing the *Bcg* gene.

The next series of experiments, initiated in order to understand what particular facet of macrophage function is regulated by the *Bcg* gene, led to the conclusion that it influenced the process of T cell-independent macrophage activation. It was shown that Bcg^r macrophages, isolated from the peritoneal cavity or from the spleens of normal, uninfected donors were superior to Bcg^s macrophages in their ability to interfere with the intracellular growth of BCG (Stach et al. 1984). The Bcg^r macrophages showed a quantitatively enhanced ability to become activated by a variety of specific and nonspecific stimuli. This was demonstrated by the up-regulation of Ia antigen expression following the in vitro exposure to lymphokines or after the phagocytosis of mycobacteria (Zwilling et al. 1985). As a consequence, the Bcg^r macrophages were observed to possess superior accessory functions in supporting both the antigen-induced and the mitogen-induced T cell proliferation when compared to Bcg^s macrophages (Denis et al. 1988a). Other markers of macrophage activation such as enhanced activity of the respiratory burst, down-regulation of 5' nucleotidase activity in the macrophage plasma membrane, and an enhanced bactericidal activity against a large spectrum of bacterial targets were induced either at a higher level, in a shorter period of time, or with a lower concentration of the appropriate stimulus in the genetically resistant Bcg^r macrophages in comparison with their genetically susceptible Bcg^s congenic macrophages.

Macrophage activation is a stepwise chain of events in which cells at different stages of maturation and/or differentiation become receptive to primary and activating signals to acquire cytostatic or cytotoxic effector responses (Meltzer and Nacy 1985). In its simplified form the cascade involves the stimulation of responsive macrophages into the primed state by molecules such as exogenous or endogenous interleukins (e.g., gamma interferon). Primed macrophages are then able to respond to a variety of membrane stimuli, among them lipopolysaccharides, integrins, and other components of microbial cell walls, to become activated for microbicidal function. According to this concept and based on our results and those of others, the Bcg^r and Bcg^s macrophage phenotypes represent two stages in a series of progressive activation steps (Fig. 3).

The Bcg^r macrophage is genetically programmed to be at a more advanced level in the activation sequence; it seems to have, phenomenologically, many characteristics of a *primed* cell. The phagocytosis of BCG or the interaction with other activating stimuli leads to membrane perturbation and to a range of pleiotropic effects which are characteristic of activated macrophages: up-regulation of Ia, down-regulation of 5' nucleotidase, increased oxidative burst, enhanced nonspecific bacteriostatic and bactericidal activity. It should be emphasized that these processes only represent *markers* of the activated state of the macrophage. It is not implied that any one of these particular markers is actually *the* expression of the resistant phenotype at a molecular level. It appears that the Bcg^r macrophage can respond, by activation, to the phagocytic mycobacterial stimulus very early in the course of infection without the need for priming by the specifically sensitized T cells. To unravel the molecular basis of the immunologically nonspecific priming of Bcg^r macrophages (e.g., effective membrane processing and transduction of priming signal) is the current experimental challenge.

The Bcg^s macrophage, on the other hand, is quantitatively lower in the cascade of macrophage activation, it appears to be in a responsive but not yet a primed state. The phagocytosis of mycobacteria does not lead to the completion of activating sequence – the state of priming has not yet been achieved (Denis et al. 1988 a, b, c).

It should be pointed out that the Bcg^s macrophage does, however, have the capacity to develop into a fully activated cell when exposed to a higher concentration or to longer exposure to such priming stimuli as, for example, T cell-derived lymphokines in the course of acquired immunity. The genetically susceptible Bcg^s host is able to control the mycobacterial load in the immune phase of response through the process of T cell-dependent macrophage activation (Pelletier et al. 1982). However, when the T cell arm of immunity is carefully analyzed and corrected for equal antigenic load, the genetically susceptible Bcg^s mice are again inferior to their Bcg^r counterparts. This is undoubtedly due to the differences in antigen presentation caused by the differential Ia expression on the two macrophage populations (Buschman and Skamene 1988). Thus the Bcg gene has a profound effect on the host response to mycobacteria, regulating not only the nonspecific antimicrobial function of the macrophage in the innate phase of resistance but, indirectly, also restricting the magnitude and the type of specific immune response during the course of natural infection and after vaccination (Buschman et al. 1988).

Conclusion

The genetic system described in this paper is undoubtedly just one of many directing the complex process of host response to mycobacterial infection. It is presented here as an example of the usefulness of the genetic analysis as a tool to probe the mechanisms of resistance and susceptibility to mycobacterial infections. The murine model has a potential importance in understanding the response of the human host to tuberculosis both at a genetic level (search for the inherited markers of susceptibility) and at a functional level (search for the macrophage dysfunction as a basis of susceptibility to the disease). Further elucidation of the physiological and biochemical determinants of the genetic resistance and susceptibility should form the basis of genetic epidemiology of tuberculosis with a subsequent quest for more targeted strategies for vaccination and treatment of those who are genetically susceptible to the disease.

Acknowledgement. Original work in this paper was supported by MRC grants 6756 and 6431 and PHS grant AI 18693.

References

Bradley DJ, Taylor BA, Blackwell JM, Evans EP, Freeman J (1979) Regulation of Leishmania populations within the host. III. Mapping of the locus controlling susceptibility to visceral leishmaniasis in the mouse. Clin Exp Immunol 37: 7-14

Buschman E, Skamene E (1988) Immunologic consequences of innate resistance and susceptibility to BCG. Immunol Letters 19: 199-210

Buschman E, Apt AS, Nickonenko BV, Moroz AM, Averbakh MH, Skamene E (1988) Genetic aspects of innate resistance and acquired immunity to Mycobacteria in inbred mice. In: Miescher PA (ed) Immunology of mycobacterial infections. Springer, Berlin Heidelberg New York, pp 319-336 (Springer seminars in immunopathology series, vol 10)

Comstock GW (1978) Tuberculosis in twins: a reanalysis of the Prophit survey. Am Rev Respir Dis 117: 621-624

Denis M, Forget A, Pelletier M, Jodoin A, Skamene E (1988a) Pleiotropic effects of the *Bcg* gene. I. Antigen-presentation in genetically - susceptible and resistant congenic mouse strains. J Immunol 140: 2395-2400

Denis M, Forget A, Pelletier M, Skamene E (1988b) Pleiotropic effects of the *Bcg* gene. III. Respiratory burst in *Bcg*-congenic macrophages. Clin Exp Immunol 73: 370-375

Denis M, Buschman E, Forget A, Pelletier M, Skamene E (1988c) Pleiotropic effects of the *Bcg* gene: genetic restriction of responses to mitogens and allogeneic targets. J Immunol 141: 3988-3993

Donovick R, McKee CM, Jambar WP, Rake G (1949) Use of the mouse in standardized test for anti-tuberculous activity of compounds of natural or synthetic origin: choice of mouse strains. Am Rev Tuberc 60: 109-120

Forget A, Skamene E, Gros P, Miailhe AC, Turcotte R (1981) Strain differences in the response to infection with small dispersed doses of Mycobacterium bovis BCG among inbred mice. Infect Immun 32: 42-48

Gheorghiu M, Mouton D, Lecoeur H, Lagranderie M, Meuel JC, Biozzi G (1985) Resistance of high and low antibody responder lines of mice to the growth of avirulent (BCG) and virulent (H37Rv) strains of mycobacteria. Clin Exp Immunol 59: 177-184

Gray DF (1960) Variations in natural resistance to tuberculosis. J Hyg (Lond) 58: 215-227

Gros P, Skamene E, Forget A (1981) Genetic control of natural resistance to Mycobacterium bovis (BCG) in mice. J Immunol 127: 2417-2423

Gros P, Skamene E, Forget A (1983) Cellular mechanisms of genetically controlled host resistance to *Mycobacterium bovis* (BCG). J Immunol 131: 1966-1972

Lenzini L, Rottoli P, Rottoli L (1977) The spectrum of human tuberculosis. Clin Exp Immunol 27: 230-237

Lurie MB, Dannenberg AMJr (1965) Macrophage function in infectious disease with inbred rabbits. Bacteriol Rev 29: 466-476

Lurie MB, Zappasodi P, Dannenberg AMJr, Weiss GH (1952) On the mechanism of genetic resistance to tuberculosis and its mode of inheritance. Am J Hum Genet 4: 302-314

Lynch CJ, Pierce-Chase CH, Dubos R (1965) A genetic study of susceptibility to experimental tuberculosis in mice infected with mammalian tubercle bacilli. J Exp Med 121: 1051-1070

Meltzer MS, Nacy CA (1985) Macrophage cytotoxicity against tumor cell and microbial targets: genetic control of the activation network. Prog Leuk Biol 3: 595-604

Motulsky AG (1960) Metabolic polymorphisms and the role of infectious disease in human evolution. Hum Biol 32: 28-62

Pelletier M, Forget A, Bourassa D, Gros P, Skamene E (1982) Immunopathology of BCG infection in genetically-resistant and susceptible mouse strains. J Immunol 129: 2179–2185

Plant J, Glynn AA (1979) Locating Salmonella resistance gene on mouse chromosome 1. Clin Exp Immunol 37: 1–6

Plant J, Glynn AA (1982) Genetic control of resistance to Salmonella typhimurium infection in high and low antibody responder mice. Clin Exp Immunol 50: 283

Potter M, O'Brien A, Skamene E, Gros P, Forget A, Kongshavn PAL, Wax JS (1983) A BALB/c congenic strain of mice that carries a genetic locus (Ity^r) controlling resistance to intracellular parasites. Infect Immun 40: 1234–1235

Sever JL, Youmans GP (1957) The enumeration of non-pathogenic viable tubercule bacilli from the organs of mice. Am Rev Tuberc 75: 280–294

Singh SPN, Mehra NK, Dingbey HB, Pande JN, Vaidya MC (1983) HLA-A, -B, -C, and -DR antigen profile in pulmonary tuberculosis in North India. Tissue Antigens 21: 380–384

Skamene E, Forget A (1988) Genetic basis of host resistance and susceptibility to intracellular pathogens. Adv Exp Med Biol 239: 23–38

Skamene E, Gros P, Forget A, Kongshavn PAL, St Charles C, Taylor BA (1982) Genetic regulation of resistance to intracellular pathogens. Nature 297: 506–510

Stach JL, Gros P, Forget A, Skamene E (1984) Phenotypic expression of genetically-controlled natural resistance to *Mycobacterium bovis* (BCG). J Immunol 132: 888–892

Zwilling BS, Johnson S, Vespa L, Kwasniewski M (1985) BCG infection induces continuous I-A expression in BCG resistant mice. Prog Leuk Biol 3: 299–304

From Serology of the Chicken MHC to Polymorphism of Malaria Antigen Genes

J. S. McBride

Memories

Koleč, the detached laboratories and experimental animal farm of the Institute for Experimental Biology and Genetics is some 10 miles northwest of Prague. A green graduate in 1968, I spent the very first year of my research apprenticeship there. My task was to produce sera for typing of chicken blood group antigens, which turned out to be the B locus. I recall chasing the birds around their outside runs to be bled, immunised and bled again, through the changing seasons and fortunes of that historic year. I acquired an allergy to the uncooperative dirty beasts but, in compensation, also a lasting appreciation of serology as a tool of genetic analysis.

Who could ever forget the people and the social life in Koleč? The chief, Karel Hála, with his expectation of twice the impossible as the minimal achievement level from all his staff; Ivan K., ever ready to debate any topic including the work; Patrick W.J., the Sleeping American and our teacher of colloquialisms; the technicians and the farm staff always willing to help. There were the congenial afterwork stopovers in the village pub, and there were the memorable parties attended by everyone including Milan Hašek. It was Milan's famous zest for life which dominated at the parties, but I remember most vividly the generous and courageous man who gave me encouragement and practival support at the start of a journey to Scotland and, eventually, to immunoparasitology.

Malaria Antigens and Their Polymorphisms

Malaria is a major infectious disease of man with the incidence estimated to be as high as 489 million new cases annually (Stürchler 1989). There are four species of human malaria parasites, of which *Plasmodium falciparum* is the principal pathogen, responsible for about a half of all cases and for practically all of 1–2 million of malaria-related fatalities. Since the malaria problem has been steadily deteriorating due to the emergence and global spread of multidrug-resistant parasites, research towards the development of malaria vaccines has assumed increasing importance (Miller et al. 1986).

The clinical manifestations of malaria are all associated with proliferation of the erythrocytic stages of the parasite, and thus any prospective vaccine will have to effectively control the blood phase of the infection. In endemic areas, individuals naturally exposed to *P. falciparum* suffer many reinfections and clinical attacks before any degree of protection is acquired (Greenwood et al. 1984), while experimentally induced immunity to the blood forms has a significant isolate-specific component (James et al. 1932; Boyd et al. 1936; Cadigan and Chaicumpa 1965). This pattern of immunity argues for the existence within the parasite species of antigenically diverse strains. Stimulated by this hypothesis, we have demonstrated serological polymorphism of several *P. falciparum* antigens, including candidates for vaccine against the blood forms (McBride et al. 1982, 1985; Clark et al 1985; Fenton et al. 1989). I select some of our recent results illustrating the polymorphic nature of one of these molecules.

GP43-53K is a major glycoprotein expressed on the surface of the merozoite, the invasive extracellular stage of the parasite which is responsible for dissemination of the infection among erythrocytes. Consistent with the surface location and accessibility of the antigen to antibody, inhibition by GP43-53K antibodies of infection of red cell has been found in vitro (Clark et al. 1989). The molecule is immunogenic in people who frequently produce specific antibodies in response to *P. falciparum* infection. These observations identify the antigen as a possible vaccine candidate whose promise, however, may be compromised by the fact that the molecule is polymorphic in *P. falciparum* populations.

We have biochemical, serological and genetic evidence consistent with allelic polymorphism of the GP43-53K antigen. The analysis has been simplified by two factors, the availability of homogenous (cloned) lines of the parasite and the fact that the blood forms expressing the antigen are haploid (Walliker et al. 1987).

Comparison by two-dimensional polyacrylamide gel electrophoresis (2D-PAGE) identified several variants with different isoelectric points and ranging in M_r from 43K to 53K among strains (with any one strain expressing only one of these variants (Fenton et al 1989). More importantly, the 2D-PAGE variants also differ serologically, as demonstrated by monoclonal antibodies.

Monoclonal antibodies (McAbs) reactive with the 43-53K molecule have been raised against parasites expressing different variants, and were tested by titration in immunofluorescence assays (IFA) for ability to react with a panel of 20 selected standard strains of *P. falciparum*. Significantly, out of nine McAbs tested only one reacted equally well with all strains, identifying a common epitope. The other McAbs clearly detected antigenic differences, some reacting with certain isolates at up to 1:100000 dilutions while failing to recognise the antigen of other isolates even when used neat.

To determine the distributions of the restricted epitopes, the McAbs were used to type over 200 *P. falciparum* isolates from several endemic regions. The results are illustrated by representative examples listed in Table 1, and are summarised as follows. (a) All isolates expressed the common epitope as well as one or more of the restricted sites, indicating that the antigen is expressed by all strains of the parasite species. (b) The restricted epitopes were found in several different combinations which are assumed to represent serotypic variants of the GP43-53K. The variants are phenotypically stable characters of parasites maintained in culture. They are also stable after meiosis and transmision through the insect vector, and behave as allelic forms in a genetic cross of *P. falciparum* (Walliker et al. 1987, and unpublished data). (c) While the full extent of the antigen's polymorphism re-

Table 1. Serological variants of GP43-53K antigen of *P. falciparum* defined by monoclonal antibodies in immunofluorescence typing[a]

Isolate	Origin	Epitopes recognised by anti-GP43-53K monoclonals									Serogroup
		16.4	13.4	4-4F	8-5D	12.3	12.5	12.7	8G10/48	8F6/49	
T9/23	Thailand	++	-	-	-	+++	+++	+++	+	-	A
FCH-C2	Tanzania	++	-	-	-	+++	+++	+++	+++	-	A
GF6	Gambia	+++	-	-	-	+++	+++	+++	±	-	A
TM28	Thailand	++	-	±	±	+++	+++	+++	-	-	A
CH12/12	Thailand	++	-	+++	+++	+++	+++	+++	±	-	A
TM15	Thailand	+++	-	+++	+++	+++	++	+++	-	-	A
TM54R	Thailand	+++	-	+++	+++	+++	+++	+++	-	-	A
PA17	Uganda	+++	-	+++	+++	+++	+++	+++	+	-	A
033	Ghana	+++	-	+++	+++	+++	+++	+++	±	-	A
GF90	Gambia	+++	+++	+++	+++	+++	+++	+++	-	-	A
GF23	Gambia	+++	+++	+++	+++	+++	+++	+++	+	-	A
W	Nigeria	+++	-	+++	+++	+++	+++	+++	-	-	A
FCB-1	Colombia	+++	-	+++	+++	+++	+++	+++	-	-	A
T9/94	Thailand	+++	-	+++	+++	+++	+++	+++	-	-	A
3D7[b]	not known	+++	++	+++	+++	+++	+++	+++	-	-	A
NT112	Thailand	++	-	-	-	-	-	+	+++	-	B
PR7	Thailand	+++	-	-	-	-	-	-	+++	-	B
PR9	Thailand	++	-	-	-	-	-	±	+++	-	B
K9	Thailand	++	-	-	-	-	-	±	+++	-	B
GF91	Gambia	++	-	-	-	-	-	-	+++	+++	B
GF7	Gambia	+++	-	-	-	-	-	-	+++	+++	B
GF36	Gambia	++	-	-	-	-	-	-	+++	+++	B
053	Cameroun	++	-	-	-	-	-	-	+++	+++	B
056	Ethiopia	++	-	-	-	-	-	-	+++	+++	B
JP	East Africa	+++	-	-	-	-	-	-	+++	+++	B
H1	Honduras	++	-	-	-	-	-	-	+++	+++	B
K1[b]	Thailand	+++	-	-	-	-	-	+	+++	+++	B
FCQ27[b]	Papua New Guinea	++	-	-	-	-	-	±	+++	+++	B
MAD20	Papua New Guinea	++	-	-	-	-	-	-	+++	+++	B

[a] The GP43-53K is synthesised only by the schizont, the mature asexual haploid stage of the malaria parasite which inhabits erythrocytes (Clark et al. 1989). Approximately 2000 blood schizonts from each isolate were screened for reactivity with each antibody and the results were scored as follows: +++ and ++ for strong or medium positive reactions confined to schizonts; + and ± for weak positive reactions which were neither limited to schizonts nor always reproducible in repeated tests, and which are believed to reflect cross-reactions of some antibodies with other molecule(s) than GP43-53K; - negative reactions.

[b] See Fig. 1 for partial amino acid sequences of GP43-53K variants of the marked isolates.

mains to be determined, five of the most frequent variants are represented worldwide and account for over 90% of all parasites tested. Most of the currently recognised variants could be assigned to one or the other of only two distinct major serogroups designated A and B.

The complete sequence of a cDNA clone encoding one variant of the antigen has been published (Smythe et al. 1988), providing starting information for our studies aimed at the elucidation of the genetic basis of the serological findings.

First, we used a series of oligonucleotides representing different parts of the published sequence in hybridisation analyses of genomic DNA from parasites expressing variants from one or the other major serogroups of the antigen. Probes derived from the central regions of the gene of the FCQ27 strain hybridised only to DNAs of strains placed in the same serogroup as FCQ27 (Table 1, group B), but not to DNAs of strains from the other serogroup. This indicated that the group-specific antigenic epitopes are encoded by a variable region of the structural gene. In contrast, probes derived from the 5' and 3' ends of the gene hybridised to genomic DNAs of all tested strains.

This information served in the choice of primers for the polymerase chain reaction (PCR) used to amplify, and subsequently sequence, the GP43-53K gene of parasites selected according to the serotype of their expressed product (Table 1). The parasites included the 3D7 strain from group A, and strains K1 and FCQ27 from group B. Two stretches of PCR-amplified genomic sequences from FCQ27 were identical to the published cDNA sequence, thus confirming the accuracy of PCR and the subsequent procedures.

Although to date we have only partial sequences for the other two strains, their comparison to each other and to FCQ27 has been informative (Fig. 1). At the N-terminus, the first 43 amino acids are identical. After this conserved part, the rest of the known sequences diverge very significantly between group A strain (3D7) and group B strains (K1 and FCQ27). The divergent regions include characteristic blocks of tandemly repeated sequences (Smythe et al. 1988) found to be different in each of the three alleles compared here. The 3D7 repeat consists of 12 identical copies of the AGGS block, preceded by one copy of ASGS which is also found once in the other two alleles. Repeats of K1 and FCQ27 have no homology with the 3D7 sequence, and also differ from each other, though less dramatically. The K1 repeat contains five identical copies of a 12-amino-acid sequence which is clearly homologous to a unique sequence in the FCQ27 strain (containing two amino acid changes). Similarly, the two copies of the 32-amino-acid-reapeat of FCQ27 are homologous to a sequence present once in K1 (one residue difference). The data show a good correlation between the degrees of the sequence and the serological divergence, leading to the conclusion that polymorphism of the GP43-53K antigen is largely determined by its structural gene. We wish to continue work on several aspects of this molecule, including the question of its evolution in the sexually breeding populations of the parasite.

Advice and suggestions from the eminent ex-members of the Prague Institute will be welcome and much appreciated.

Acknowledgements. I thank Dr. J.T.Clark and Mrs. J.Robinson for making available their sequence data, and to Dr. R.Ridley and Professor J.G.Scaife for accom-

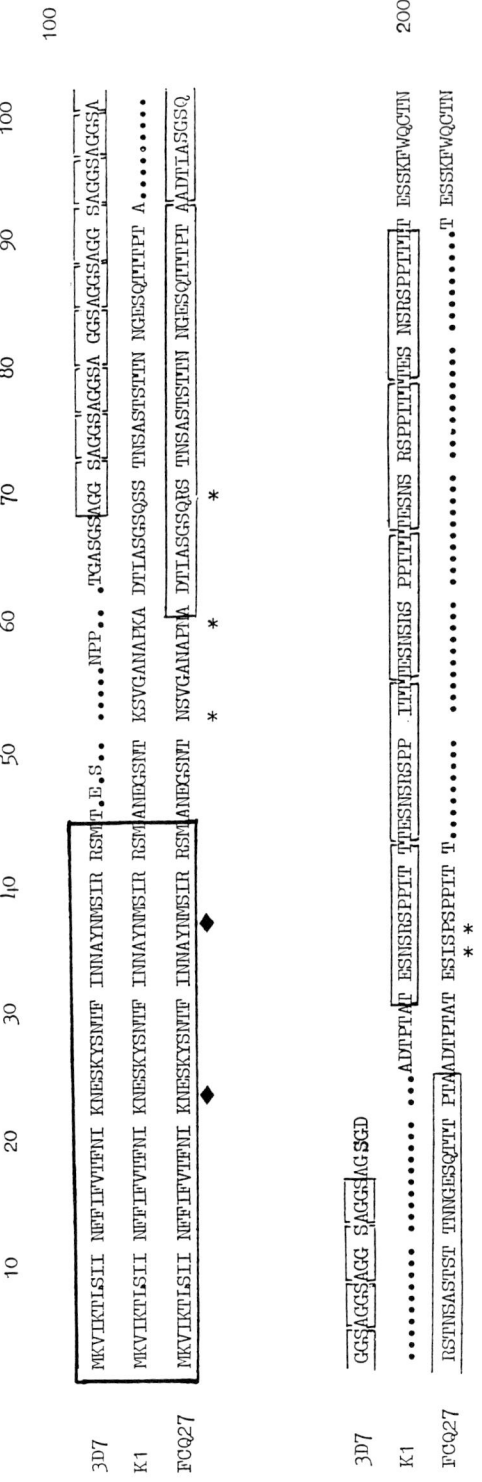

Fig. 1. Comparison of deduced amino acid sequences from the N-terminal part of GP43-53K antigen variants of the 3D7 (origin unknown), K1 (Thailand) and FCQ27 (Papua New Guinea) strains of *P. falciparum*. The sequences correspond to cDNA clone of the FCQ27 allele (Symthe et al. 1988), or to cloned genomic sequences of the other alleles. Amino acids are indicated by single letter code. The available sequences of 3D7 and K1 end at residues 106 and 168 respectively, and are aligned for best fit with the first 152 residues of FCQ27 (total length 264 amino acids). To maximise the number of identities, gaps, indicated by *dots*, were introduced into the sequences. Conserved first 43 amino acids are boxed in *thick lines* and potential N-glycosylation sites are indicated by *lozenges*. Also *boxed* are characteristic tandem repeats which vary among the alleles (12 copies of the AGGS sequence in 3D7; five copies of a TESNSRSPPITT repeat in K1; two copies of 32 residues in FCQ27). *Asterisks* mark positions of additional differences between the related K1 and FCQ27 alleles. See Table 1 for serological profiles of GP43-53K variants expressed by the three parasite isolates

modation and continuous advice on our attempts at DNA work. I also thank Dr. A. Saul and Dr. R. Reese for monoclonal antibodies, and Professor D. Walliker, Dr. S. Thaithong, Dr. C. Wongsrinachalai and D. Conway for parasite isolates. Supported by the Wellcome Trust and the UNDP/World Bank/WHO Special Programme for Research and Training in Tropical Diseases.

References

Boyd MF, Stratman-Thomas WK, Kitchen SF (1936) On acquired immunity to *Plasmodium falciparum*. Am J Trop Med 16: 139–145

Cadigan FC, Chaicumpa V Jr (1969) *Plasmodium falciparum* in the white-handed gibbon: protection afforded by previous infection with homologous and heterologous strains obtained in Thailand. Military Med 134: 1135–1139

Clark JT, Donachie S, Anand R, Wilson CF, Heidrich HG, McBride JS (1989) 46–53 Kilodalton glycoprotein from the surface of *Plasmodium falciparum* merozoites. Mol Biochem Parasitol 32: 15–24

Fenton B, Clark JT, Wilson CF, McBride JS, Walliker D (1989) Polymorphism of a 35–48kDa *Plasmodium falciparum* merozoite surface antigen. Mol Biochem Parasitol 34: 79–86

Greenwood BM, Bradley AK, Greenwood AM, Byass P, Jammeh H, Marsh K, Tulloch S, Oldfield FSJ, Hayes R (1987) Mortality and morbidity from malaria among children in a rural area of The Gambia, West Africa. Trans Soc Trop Med Hyg 81: 478–486

James SP, Nicol WD, Shute PG (1932) A study of induced malignant tertian malaria. Proc R Soc Med 25: 1153–1181

McBride JS, Walliker D, Morgan D (1982) Antigenic diversity in the human malaria parasite *Plasmodium falciparum*. Science 217: 254–257

McBride JS, Newbold CI, Anand R (1985) Polymorphism of a high molecular weight schizont antigen of the human malaria parasite *Plasmodium falciparum*. J Exp Med 161: 160–180

Miller LH, Howard RJ, Carter R, Good MF, Nussenzweig V, Nussenzweig RS (1986) Research towards malaria vaccines. Science 234: 1349–1356

Smythe JA, Coppel RL, Brown GV, Ramasamy R, Kemp DJ, Anders RF (1988) Identification of two integral membrane proteins of *Plasmodium falciparum*. Proc Nat Acad Sci USA, 85: 5195–5199

Stürchler D (1989) How much malaria is there worldwide? Parasitol Today 5: 39–40

Walliker D, Quakyi IA, Wellems TE, McCutchan TF, Szarfman A, London WT, Corcoran LM, Burkot TR, Carter R (1987) Genetic analysis of the human malaria parasite *Plasmodium falciparum*. Science 236: 1661–1666

Virus-Induced Neutropenia

T. A. Rakusan

Introduction: 1968–1988

In January 1969, 2 months after our arrival to the United States, I started as a postdoctoral fellow in the laboratory of Albert S. Kaplan and his wife, Tamar Ben Porat, at the Albert Einstein Medical Center in Philadelphia, PA. They were both classical virologists interested in the effects of virus infection (in particular, pseudorabies virus, a pig herpesvirus) on protein and nucleic acid synthesis in the infected mammalian cells. I spent almost 3 years in their laboratory, and during that time we described the so-called immediate early viral messenger RNA (mRNA) (Rakusanova et al. 1971), showed that early after virus infection cell-specific mRNA is displaced from polysomes by virus-specific mRNA (Ben Porat et al. 1971); and characterized cellular RNA synthesized in the infected cells (Rakusanova et al. 1972).

In the fall of 1972, I joined the laboratory of Paul H. Black at Massachusetts General Hospital. At that time he was interested in the mechanism(s) of virus-induced carcinogenesis using an in vitro model of hamster cells transformed by SV40 (a simian papova virus, small DNA virus). We described three clones of SV40-transformed hamster cells which differed in their ability to release SV40 spontaneously and in the response to induction treatments such as ultraviolet or gamma irradiation, or mitomycin C. Cells of one clone released SV40 spontaneously, the second clone produced SV40 only after induction treatment and the third clone failed to release infectious SV40 even after induction. We showed that the cells of all three clones contained a similarly low number of SV40 genomes per cell, that SV40 DNA was integrated into cellular DNA (Kaplan et al. 1975), that an early consequence of induction treatment was an excision of SV40 DNA from its integrated position on the cellular genome (Rakusanova et al. 1976), and that excision and replication of SV40 DNA occurred after induction in the cells of all three clones, even in those which did not release infectious virus after induction (Rakusanova et al. 1978, 1979).

In 1978 I decided to complete may medical training in the United States and spent the next 6 years in pediatric residency programs and obtained a pediatric infectious disease fellowship. In 1984 I joined the faculty in the Department of Pediatrics at the University of Texas Medical Branch in Galveston. Since then I have been largely involved in clinical work (Teele et al. 1981; Schuster et al. 1984; Chonmaitree et al. 1984; Congeni et al. 1985; Christie et al. 1986; Hajare et al. 1989).

Virus-Induced Neutropenia

My interest in the subject of virus-induced neutropenia (absolute neutrophil count < 1500/mm³ – mild, < 1000/³ – moderate, < 500/mm³ – severe neutropenia) originated in a clinical observation made while caring for a child with a symptomatic congenital cytomegalovirus (CMV) infection.

Neutropenia Accompanying Congenital CMV Infection

Infection with CMV, a human herpesvirus, is widespread; most adults worldwide have been infected sometime in their lives. CMV infections in healthy individuals are usually asymptomatic, few patients present with a clinical picture of infectious mononucleosis. Severe or fatal infections occur in immunocompromised hosts, such as organ transplant recipients, and in congenitally infected infants. Congenital CMV infection is frequent, it occurs in 0.5%–2.5% of all live-born infants in the United States. However, more than 95% of such congenitally infected infants are asymptomatic, and the majority of these remain well. About 5% of infants with congenital CMV infection are symptomatic at birth, presenting with findings such as microcephaly or hydrocephalus, hepatosplenomegaly, pneumonia, thrombocytopenia, or disseminated intravascular coagulation. Some of the severely affected infants die, the survivors have a high incidence of sequelae in later life (Hanshaw 1982).

Our patient had several of the above symptoms and, in addition, had severe neutropenia (Table 1). When it was noticed that several well-known textbooks fail to list neutropenia among symptoms of congenital CMV infection, I reviewed hospital charts of other congenitally infected infants identified in the course of another study and compared their white blood cell counts with control, uninfected infants. It became apparent that the congenitally infected infants, even asymptomatic ones, were more likely to have unexplaines neutropenia than the uninfected newborns, that neutropenia usually occurred after the 1 week of life , and, in the few infants we studied, it did not appear to be clinically significant (Tables 1–3) (Rakusan et al. 1984).

Table 1. Neutropenia and thrombocytopenia in an infant with a symptomatic congenital CMV infection

Age (days)	White blood cell count (cells/mm³)	Polymorphonuclear Leukocyte count[a] (cells/mm³)	Platelet count (per mm³)
1	8200	2296	28000
3	9100	3000	23000
5	6700	1100	57000
7	8300	720	35000
8	8000	880	76000
16	11600	1760	446000
20	9500	480	301000
139	12200	*1300*	393000

Abnormal values are underlined.
[a] Mature neutrophils and bands.

Table 2. Incidence of neutropenia and thrombocytopenia in infants with congenital CMV infection

Patient	Age observed		Thrombocytopenia <150000 platelets/mm³
	Neutropenia		
	Polymorphonuclear <1500	leukocytes per mm³ <1000	
1	None		Day 3
2	Day 26	Day 1, 11	Day 4
3	Days 7-29	Day 36	None
4	Days 6, 14, 16, 24, 25, 36	Days 7, 19, 27, 29, 33	None

Table 3. Incidence of neutropenia and thrombocytopenia in control infants

Patient	Age observed			Etiology
	Neutropenia		Thrombocytopenia <150000 platelets/mm³	
	Polymorphonuclear per mm³ <1500	leukocytes <1000		
1	None		None	
2	None		None	
3	None		Days 18-24	Severe NEC*
4	None		None	
5		Days 1, 2	Days 2-9	Sepsis
6	None		None	
7	None		None	
8	None		None	
9	None		None	
10			Days 7-20	Severe NEC
11	None		None	Sepsis
12	None		Days 2-12	Sepsis
			Days 25, 27, 30	Sepsis

* NEC, necrotizing enterocolitis.

Inhibition of Hempoietic Colony Formation by Human CMV In Vitro

CMV was previously noted to cause neutropenia in symptomatically infected immunocompromised patients (Suwansirikul et al. 1977) and in newborn infants infected by blood transfusions (Yeager et al. 1981). The mechanism of CMV-associated neutropenia is unknown. An old observation of CMV inclusion within megakaryocytes detected on histological examination of bone marrow from a congenitally infected child suggested that a direct infection of hemopoietic presursor cells by CMV could be an explanation (Chesney et al. 1978). We therefore decided to investigate the effect of infection of human hemopoietic cells with CMV in vitro.

Normal human bone marrow (BM) or cord blood (CB) was used as a source of hemopoietic cells. Mononuclear cells (MNC) were isolated, infected with CMV or mock infected and cultured in a semisolid medium in the presence of fetal calf

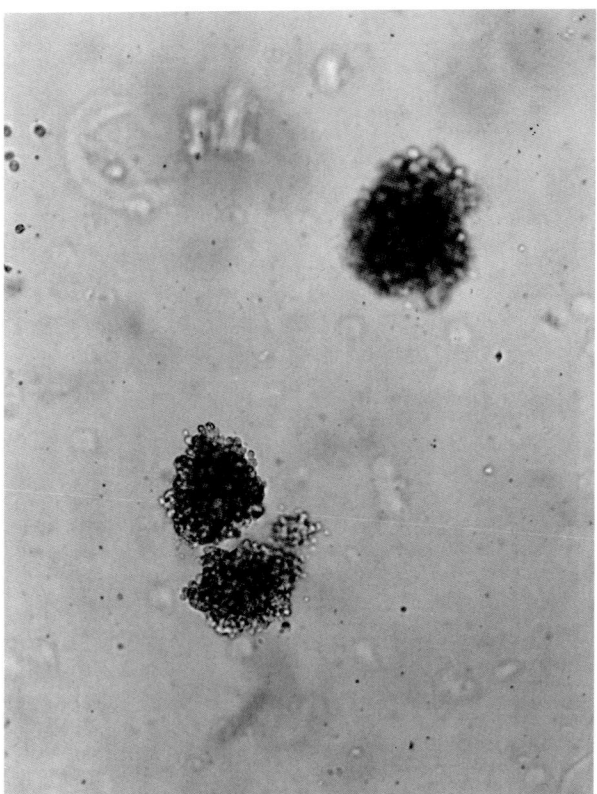

Fig. 1. Three GM colonies and one cluster

serum and either placental or lymphocyte-conditioned media. Granulocytic/macrophage colonies (GM) (≥ 39 cells) and clusters (3–38 cells) were enumerated after a 7-day incubation (Fig. 1). Erythroid colonies (BFU-E) formed in the presence of erythropoietin and burst-promoting activity were counted after a 14 day incubation. Several different recent clinical isolates of CMV (CMV C1 – CMV C65) were used in these experiments in addition to a laboratory strain, AD 169 (Rakusan et al. 1989).

As indicated in Tables 4 and 5, CMV inhibited the GM colony and BFU-E formation by BM and CB MNC in vitro. Recent clinical isolates were more efficient inhibitors than AD169, even though multiplicity of infection of AD169 exceeded that of clinical isolates by 10–1000-fold. The capacity of individual clinical isolates to suppress GM colony and BFU-E formation varied between the individual virus stocks and between the experiments. We identified a unique isolate of CMV, CMV-C1, which consistently inhibited GM colony formation both by BM and CB MNC, even after 10–15 passages in vitro. Plaque-purified CMV-C1 stocks (purified three times) were prepared, and all the plaque isolates tested retained the inhibitory properties.

Since interferon (IFN) has been shown to inhibit hemopoietic colony formation in vitro (Klimpel et al. 1982), we determined IFN production by MNC simul-

Table 4. Effect of CMV infection in vitro on GM colony formation by BM and CB MNC

Experiment	Source of MNC	Virus[a]	GM colonies on day 7[b]	Inhibition (%)	Interferon on day 2[c]
1	BM	MI control	114± 3	–	ND
		AD169	94±20 NS[d]	18	ND
		CMV C1	5± 2	96	ND
		CMV C24	61± 7	47	ND
		CMV C65	43± 1	62	ND
2	BM	MI control	41± 7	–	12
		AD169	18± 5	56	140
		CMV C24	12± 3	71	98
		CMV C24	24± 3 NS	42	98
3	BM	MI control	63± 3	–	12
		AD169	43± 2	32	140
		AD169	49±14	22	49
		CMV C24	48±16	24	70
4	CB	MI control	49±22	–	<5.5
		AD169	40±10 NS	19	<5.5
		CMV-C1	0	100	<5.5
5	CB	MI control	21± 6	–	<18
		CMV C21	24± 1 NS	0	31
		CMV C24	13± 3 NS	39	65
		CMV C25	17± 4 NS	20	46
6	CB	MI control	39±10	–	ND
		AD169-cocultuse	12± 2	69	ND

[a] BM and CB MNCs were mock infected or infected with stocks of virus for 1 h at 37 °C before a colony assay in experiment 6, the CB MNCs were co-cultivated with HCMV-infected or mock-infected fibroblasts for 3 days.
[b] Number of GM colonies per 10^5 cells (BM experiments) or 3×10^5 cells (CB experiments). Data are means+SD.
[c] Data are interferon units per 10^5 cells.
[d] $P > 0.05$, Student's t test, compared with controls.
GM, granulocyte/macrophage; BM, bone marrow; CB, cord blood; MNCs, mononuclear cells; ND, not done, MI, mock infected; NS, not significant.

Table 5. Effect of CMV infection in vitro on BFU-E formation by BM MNC

Experiment	Virus[a]	BFU-E[b] day 15	Inhibition (%)
1	MI control	115±10.7	–
	AD169, moi[c]=9	23± 7.0	80
	AD169, moi[c]=0.9	66±14.9	43
	CMV-C1	0	100
2	MI control	49± 4.1	–
	AD169	26±11.9	46
	CMV-C2	26± 3.5	46

[a] MNC were infected or mock infected (MI) for 1 h at 37 °C.
[b] Burst forming units, erythrocytin; number/10^5 cells, data are means±SD.
[c] moi, multiplicity of infection, plaque-forming units per cell.

taneously with GM colony formation. Similar quantities of IFN were released by MNC infected with a laboratory strain as by MNC exposed to recent clinical isolates (Table 4). Levels of IFN detected did not correlate well with the observed inhibition of GM colony formation. CB MNC infected with CMV eleborated a somewhat lower concentration of IFN than BM MNC. CMV failed to replicate over a 3-7-day period in BM and CB MNC incubated under our conditions.

We have thus demonstrated that infection of human BM or CB MNC with CMV in vitro inhibits formation of hemopoietic colonies in semisolid medium. The suppression of hemopoietic cell proliferation could be at least partially responsible for neutropenia and thrombocytopenia that may occur in the course of acute and congenital CMV infections.

Resent clinical isolates of CMV were found to interact more effectively with CB and BM MNC than the laboratory strain AD169, which is in agreement with previous reports (Einhorn 1984; Schrier et al. 1986). In addition, we observed large difference in the effect of CMV on GM colony formation between individual clinical isolates of CMV. Why some isolates exert no inhibitory effect on hemopoietic cells while another (CMV-C1) is consistently and profoundly inhibitory is not clear at present. BM MNC appear to be more sensitive to the inhibition by CMV than are CB MNC though the nature of this difference is unknown. It is of interest that mitogen-induced proliferation of CB MNC is also less readily suppressed by CMV than proliferation of adult peripheral blood MNC (Rakusan et al. 1987).

We have not addressed directly the question of the mechanism(s) underlying the observed inhibition of hemopoietic colony proliferation by CMV. Three major possibilities are:

1. Hemopoietic stem/precursor cells are the targets of CMV infection with resulting impairment of their proliferation and function. Since the inhibition of colony formation observed in cultures of MNC infected with clinical isolates of CMV occurs under conditions of low multiplicity of infection which is sufficient to infect only a small proportion of the cells, this explanation seems unlikely.
2. CMV infects accessory cells with subsequently diminished production of colony stimulating factor(s). We cannot exclude this possibility; however, the assays of colony formation are carried out in the presence of either placental or lymphocyte-conditioned media, which supply the colony stimulating factor(s), thus the presumed diminished production within the system should be inconsequential.
3. The third, most likely, alternative is that CMV-infected accessory cells such as monocytes release inhibitory substance(s). IFNs, which are produced by CMV-infected MNC and which are capable of inhibiting hemopoietic colony formation (Klimpel et al. 1982), were considered to be potential inhibitory factors in our system. However, we have not found a consistent, reproducible relationship between the amount of IFN produced in MNC cultures and the degree of inhibition of GM colony formation. A possibility remains that it is not the overall quantitiy of IFNs, but rather a level of IFN-γ which accounts for GM colony inhibition in our experiments. Rodgers et al. (1985) have reported the presence

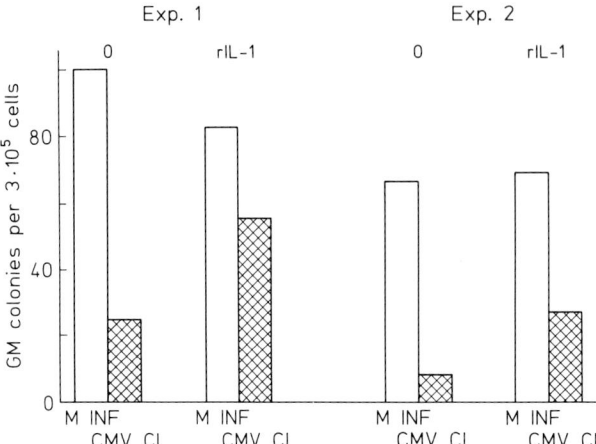

Fig. 2. Effect of rIL-1 on CMV-induced inhibition of GM colony formation. *0*, nor rIL-1 added; *rIL-1*, rIL-1 (50 units) added to the cultures after infection/mock infection; *M INF*, mock infected; *CMV C1*, infected with the clinical isolate CMV-C1

of an inhibitor of interleukin-1 in cultures of monocytes infected with a laboratory strain of CMV. The role of a similar inhibitor in our system has not been determined.

However, our preliminary results indicate that the CMV-induced inhibition of GM colony formation in vitro can be partially reversed by the addition of recombinant interleukin-1 (rIL-1) to the cultures (Fig. 2).

The similarities between the effect of CMV on lymphocyte function described by others (Einhorn 1984; Schrier et al. 1986) and the effect of CMV on hemopoietic colony formation described in the present report, i.e., greater activity of recent clinical isolates when compared with a laboratory strain, individual variation between different clinical isolates, apparent independence of the inhibition of the amount of IFN produced by the infected MNC, and an apparently low proportion of MNC which became infected with CMV, are of interest. Monocytes are thought to mediate CMV-induced inhibition of lymphocyte functions (Kapasi and Rice 1986). Their role, if any, in the inhibition of hemopoietic colony formation remains to be assessed.

Acknowledgement. The work was supported in part by BRSG 2 SO7 RR 05427-24 awarded by the Biomedical Research Support Grant Program, Division of Research Resources, National Institutes of Health and by Cancer Center Grant (CA 17701) awarded to Tamara A. Rakusan.

References

Ben Porat T, Rakusanova T, Kaplan AS (1971) Early functions of the genome of herpesvirus. II. Inhibition of the formation of cell specific polysomes. Virology 46: 890–899

Chesney JP, Taher A, Gilbert EMF, Shahidi NT (1978) Intranuclear inclusions in megakaryocytes in congenital cytomegalovirus infection. J Pediatr 92: 957–958

Chonmaitree T, Congeni BL, Munoz J, Rakusan TA, Powell KR, Box QT (1984) Twice daily ceftriaxone therapy for serious bacterial infections in children. J Antimicrob Chemother 13: 511–516

Christie JD, Rakusan TA, Martinez MA, Lucia HL, Rajamanan S, Edwards SB, Hayden CK (1986) Hydranencephaly caused by congenital infection with herpes simplex virus. Pediatr Infect Dis 5: 473–478

Congeni BL, Chonmaitree T, Rakusan T, Box QT (1985) Once daily ceftriaxone therapy of serious bacterial infections in children. Antimicrob Agents Chemother 27: 181–183

Einhorn L, Ost A (1984) Cytomegalovirus infection of human blood cells. J Infect Dis 149: 207–214

Hajare S, Gibson FB, Rakusan TA, Strunk CL, Kalia A (1989) Laryngeal coccidioidomycosis causing airway obstruction. Pediatr Infect Dis 8: 54–56

Hanshaw JB, (1982) Cytomegalovirus. In: Remington JS, Klein JO (eds) Infectious diseases of the fetus and newborn infant. Saunders, Philadelphia, pp 104–142

Kapasi K, Rice GPA (1986) Role of the monocyte in cytomegalovirus – mediated immunosuppression in vitro. J Infect Dis 154: 881–884

Kaplan JC, Wilbert SM, Collins JJ, Rakusanova T, Zamansky GB, Black PH (1975) Isolation of SV40 transformed inbred hamster cell lines heterogeneous for virus induction by chemicals or radiation. Virology 68: 200–214

Klimpel GR, Fleishman WR Jr, Klimpel KD (1982) Gamma interferon (IFN γ) and α/β suppress murine myeloid colony formation (CFU-C). Magnitude of suppression is dependent upon level of colony stimulating factor (CSF). J Immunol 129: 76–80

Rakusan TA, Patten ED, Richardson CJ, Pollard RB (1984) Neutropenia associated with congenital cytomegalovirus infection. Clin Res 32: 894A

Rakusan TA, Rowlands K, Juneja HS (1987) Inhibition of lymphocyte proliferation and hemopoietic colony formation by human cytomegalovirus in vitro (abstr R21.50). In: Abstracts of the VIIth International Congress of Virology, Edmonton, Alberta, 1987. National Research Council, Ottawa

Rakusan TA, Juneja HS, Fleischmann WR Jr (1989) Inhibition of hemopoietic colony formation by human cytomegalovirus in vitro. J Infect Dis 159: 127–130

Rakusanova T, Ben Porat T, Himeno M, Kaplan AS (1971) Early functions of the genome of herpesvirus. I. Characterization of the RNA synthesized in cycloheximide treated, infected cells. Virology 46: 877–889

Rakusanova T, Ben Porat T, Kaplan AS (1972) Effect of herpesvirus infection on the synthesis of cell specific RNA. Virology 49: 537–548

Rakusanova T, Kaplan JC, Smales WP, Black PH (1976) Excision of viral DNA from host cell DNA after induction of SV40 transformed hamster cells. J Virl 19: 279–285

Rakusanova T, Smales WP, Kaplan JC, Black PH (1978) Replication of simian virus 40 in SV40-transformed hamster kidney cells induced by mitomycin C or Co60-irradiation. Virology 88: 300–313

Rakusanova T, Smales WP, Kaplan JC, Black PH (1979) Effect of mitomycin C and Co60-irradiation on the replication of SV40 in cell lines of varying permissivity for PS40 replication. J Gen Virol 43: 235–239

Rodgers BC, Scott DM, Mundin J, Sissions JGP (1985) Monocyte-derived inhibitor of interleukin 1 induced by human cytomegalovirus. J Virol 55: 527–532

Schrier RD, Rice GPA, Oldston MBA (1986) Suppression of natural killer cell activity and T cell proliferation by fresh isolates of human cytomegaloviruses. J Infect Dis 153: 1084–1091

Schuster JD, Rakusan TA, Chonmaitree T, Box QT (1984) Tuberculous osteitis of the skull mimicking histiocytosis X. J Pediatr 105: 269–271

Suwansirikul S, Rao N, Dowling JN, Ho M (1977) Clinical manifestations of primary and secondary cytomegalovirus infections after renal transplantation. Arch Intern Med 137: 1026–1029

Teele DW, Dashefsky B, Rakusan T, Klein JO (1981) Meningitis after lumbar puncture in children with bacteremia. N Engl J Med 305: 1079–1081

Yeager AS, Grummet CF, Hafleigh EB, Arvin AM, Bradley JS, Prober CG (1981) Prevention of transfusion acquired cytomegalovirus infections in newborn infants. J Pediatr 98: 281–287

Tumor Immunotherapy

P. Koldovsky

In 1951, when I started to study medicine at the Karlova Universita (Charles University) in Prague, I was interested in working at the Institute of General Biology. An older, politically powerful student manipulated me into the department of "aspirants." These aspirants were so called because they hoped to become Candidate of Science (corresponding to a PhD). The department was headed by a young man fresh from medical school - Milan Hašek. His wife Vera, Marta Vojtiskova, and Jan Grozdanovic also belonged to the group. The technicians were Ludek Martinek and Eva Linkova. One year later Tomas Hraba came, and the following year Jan Hort joined the group.

Around 1953 the group became the Department of Experimental Biology and Genetics within the Institute of Microbiology at the Czechoslovac Academy of Science and it moved to another part of Prague - to Dejvice. A few years later this department became an institute of the same name. This institute became known worldwide for its excellent work in immunology; nevertheless, its name emphasizes genetics and not immunology. The reason is the history of the institute. The group, which I joined when it was still at Albertov, was not working in immunology. The main topic of interest was Micurin's and Lysenko's genetics. The principles were quite simple - heredity is determined by the environment, and the most important factor is metabolism. Micurin came to conclusion that genetic changes are best induced when the genetic background is made unstable. In Czech we used the term *rozviklana dedicnost* ("wobble heredity") and I always had the impression of a loose tooth. Micurin also said that the best period to induce genetic instability was in a young organism and that the best way was to change the metabolism.

The other big stars of Soviet biology were the mother-daughter team Olga Borisovna and Olga Pantelejemovna Lepesinskaja. They were studying the origin of cells from noncellular material. Olga Borisovna described it as being from egg yolk droplets and Olga Pantelejemovna Lepesinskaja from protein crystals of egg white.

Before entering medical school I had read the biology textbook by Belehradek and the wonderful book by Sekla *Heredity in Nature and Society*. The reasons for my attraction to our group's program were twofold. First of all, Hašek told me that we should study claims by Soviet biologists objectively and prove or disprove them. It was probably a party order which Hašek was ready to fulfil in a critical way. Secondly, Hašek's approach was logical. The work was done on chicken embryos – certainly a very young organism. Vera Haskova introduced coal particles into the egg white and some time later boiled the eggs when it could be seen that the embryos really had digested the egg white. So exchanging the egg whites of embryonated eggs of different strains changes the metabolism at a very early stage (so-called plastic stage – to use Micurin terminology) of development. My first duty was to help Marta Vojtiskova to exchange the egg whites. The egg white has two phases – a more fluid one immediately under the shell and a more gelatinous one around the yolk. It was easy to exchange the fluid part, and we hatched many chickens from such eggs. However, after many complete exchanges of the egg white, only four chickens hatched. I still remember the wild party celebrating the first of these chickens. Ferdinandov had written that the fluid part, being directly under the shell, was the origin of skin and feathers, and so, if it were exchanged, it would cause a change in color. Our recipients were White Leghorn embryos, and the donors were Black Minor or Rhode Island Red embryos; we never saw a color change! One of Hašek's students outside Prague was exchanging chicken and duck egg whites and produced a chicken with webbed feet. Hašek forced him to add that in birds such changes can also occur spontaneously.

The fourth member of the group – Jan Grozdanovic – was in charge of repeating Lepesinskaja's experiments; he worked on both projects – the origin of cells from egg yolk and egg white. He did not consider the exchange of egg white by syringe to be physiological and wanted a slower exchange. So he made openings in the egg shells of two eggs and joined them with a paraffin bridge. Hašek was sure that the exchange of blood would cause an even greater metabolic change than just the exchange of egg white. He made the openings above a vessel and inserted tissue from a third embryo in between. The resulting vascularization caused both extracorporal blood systems to join, and the method of embryonal parabiosis was born.

Already at that time Milan recognized immunology as a powerful tool and demonstrated that chicken parabiotic pairs do not produce antibodies against each other. In 1953 Hašek wrote a monograph (in Czech) about these experiments – *Vegetative Hybridization in Animals*. The title emphasizes the relation to Micurin's vegetative hybridization in plants. And so *immunological tolerance* was discovered a few months before the experiments of Billingham, Brent, and Medawar were published. Later Peter Medawar wrote to his friend Milan that he was sorry that Hašek was not sharing the Nobel Prize for tolerance.

I have mentioned the early stages of our beloved institute in Prague not only to explain the title of the institute, but mainly to demonstrate what a critical and innovative person like Milan could achieve from such a chaotic start. The discovery of immunological tolerance resulted in the whole group starting to work on problems of transplantation immunity. I did my share – for example, polyvalent tolerance in outbred rats, skin grafting in cattle differing in one blood group only – but I wanted a "problem" of my own. Hraba suggested that I should work on tumor immunity, and Hašek not only agreed, but gave me all possible support. The first inbred mice were a gift from Avrion Mitchison, and with Radslav Kinsky we started to breed them. Later, when more mice were needed, Hašek organized not only excellent breeding facilities within the institute, but also used his political power so that we could buy mice from one of the last private enterprises in Prague. Right at the beginning of my experiments with mice I was interested in the therapeutic potentials of immunology so I did some combination experiments with radiotherapy and surgery in animal models. The only clinical experience at that time was work done with Jakoubkova and Pavol Ivanyi on choriocarcinoma. After many years of experimental work, I am now working in a clinic – to prove to critical and supportive clinicians alike that immunology can be a useful additional tool in cancer treatment.

The dream of tumor immunotherapy is over 100 years old and very simple. Immunotherapy would be a gentle method of cancer treatment: no blood, no pain, the tumor would just disappear. The patient would be immunized or receive antiserum. Some scientists wanted even more – to prevent cancer by vaccination. Both dreams are becoming a little bit more of a reality nowadays. There is a lot of speculation as to what the influence of immunization against hepatitis virus will be on the incidence of cancer. The dream of a powerful antiserum led to the production of monoclonal antibodies. These antibodies can be used for direct therapy or in combination with anticancer drugs. Moreover, the idiotype of these antibodies could represent the inner image of the tumor antigen, and they could thus be used for immunization. However, what is true of viral infection does not apply to the tumor. The tumor was, and is, often compared to an infection, and the production of dog antisera against human tumors was based on this assumption (Héricourt and Richet 1895). However, the tumor represents many problems from the immunotherapeutic point of view. First of all, nobody has succeeded in proving beyond reasonable doubt the existence of a tumor-specific transplantation-type antigen in any human tumor. Moreover, the tumor originates from autologous tissue, and a certain degree of nonreactivity or tolerance is to be expected. Finally, the tumor is composed of many cell clones, and each can carry a different tumor-associated antigen (TAA). These TAA can be various differential antigens or embryo-antigens. The expression of these antigens on the cell membrane need not be stable, as they can undergo antigenic modulation induced by antibodies. Antigenic modulation was the reason for the therapeutic failure in the treatment of T cell leukemia with monoclonal antibodies against the corresponding differential antigen (Ritz and Schlossman 1982).

Nevertheless, many clinical observations support the idea that a patient is able to react immunologically against his or her own tumor. The idea is not so strange, because anybody can react against many autologous tissues; tumor is an autologous tissue and can carry organ-specific antigen(s) of the tissue of origin (Koldovsky and Weinstein 1973). Therefore, some tumor immunologists try to improve a tumor patient's immune reactivity by nonspecific stimulation of the immune system. It all started with bacille Calmette-Guérin (BCG) many years ago. Today there are many compounds known as "biological response modifiers." They range from ill-defined tissue extracts to recombinant interleukins. A very encouraging fact is that so far the clinical results with nonspecific stimulation are better than specific cancer therapy with monoclonal antibodies or vaccination. It seems that in recent years a bridge has been formed between specific and nonspecific cancer immunotherapy. It has been discovered that, in vitro, nonspecifically stimulated lymphocytes can kill tumor cells selectively (but not exclusively). Such activated lymphocytes are able to kill tumor cells which are resistant to natural killer (NK) cells. After initial experiments with phytohemagglutinin (PHA)-stimulated lymphocytes, recombinant interleukin-2 (rIL-2) is used today, and the cells are called "lymphokine activated killer (LAK) cells" (Grimm and Wilson 1985). In 1987 we organized a meeting in Düsseldorf which was devoted to cancer therapy with lymphocytes (Koldovsky et al. 1989), an area in which there is quite a large amount of clinical experience.

It is important to note that therapy which is not directed at the cancer, but supports the immune reactivity of the patient, produces objective improvements. One must bear in mind that until now these clinical trials have been performed on terminally ill patients with very advanced cancer, in whom other therapy methods had already failed. Better results can be expected in patients with less advanced cancer. The ideal situation would be patients immediately after operation when they are clinically free of tumor. Many of these patients carry microscopic tumors, and from animal experiments it is known that immunotherapy is able to destroy only a limited number of tumor cells. At present I do not know of any clinician who would give the green light for such trials. There must first be evidence that the therapy with lymphocytes can be improved and that they can specifically find even small tumors and kill them with no hidden dangers for the patient.

I am now working at the ear-nose-throat (ENT) clinic in Düsseldorf, and there are several aspects of tumors of the head and neck region which make them attractive for therapy with lymphocytes. First of all, there is a need for additional therapy - in some cases the tumor cannot be removed completely but the operation must still be performed for palliative reasons. The possibilities of radiation and chemotherapy have almost been exhausted, and immunotherapy can be a good additional treatment. Furthermore, the tumors are almost always accessible, so the lymphocytes can be injected directly into the tumor, which is far better than any other application, and the effect of the therapy can be followed objectively. However, personal experience in animal models, a few clinical observations, and some experiments in vitro give me enough warning against an overenthusiastic use of such a therapy. I have two objections against therapy with LAK cells: (a) nobody knows how safe the therapy is, and patients with advanced tumors might react differently from patients with a limited tumor burden; (b) the LAK cells are not tumor specific, and it would be extremely difficult to produce enough LAK cells to eliminate a larger tumor. There is always the danger that immunotherapy would cause a reverse effect, i.e., enhance tumor growth. In vitro experiments with LAK cells and ovarian carcinoma have shown that LAK cells can, in some cases, enhance tumor growth (Peri et al. 1986). These in vitro experiments could not be explained on the basis of immunological enhancement. Enhancement is a specific phenomenon, and LAK cells operate nonspecifically. Either the LAK cells in these experiments were producing a growth factor, or the immune cells were stimulating tumor growth, as described in some of Prehn's experiments (Prehn 1977; Bubenik and Koldovsky 1964).

For these reasons I feel it is necessary to develop additional methods which would allow the immunobiological properties of the lymphocytes to be used for therapy to be tested. These tests should not only exclude the danger of tumor growth acceleration as far as possible, but they should also demonstrate the actual capability of the lymphocytes to kill tumor cells in vitro as well their capability to substantially inhibit tumor growth. Experiments in tissue culture systems with primary tumors are very difficult. Only a few tumors such as glioma, ovarian carcinoma, or melanoma have good plating efficiency. Practically all the tumors of the head and neck region have very low plating efficiency, and most of them do not start to grow at all. Therefore, we have developed an in vivo system in nude mice which allows us to test the activity of the lymphocytes from each individual against its own tumor. This approach is an adaptation of a subrenal capsule assay (SRCA) used for testing chemotherapeutic drugs (Bogden et al. 1979; Kau et al. 1989; C. Kürten, R. Kau, H. Kumazawa, P. Koldovsky, to be published). In the subrenal capsule space of a mouse, the tumor will start to grow practically in all cases. In order to test chemotherapeutic drugs, a period of 6 days is sufficient, and normal mice can be used. We need a longer period of time for our purposes, and we therefore use nude mice. There is great variation in the primary inoculum from the tumor biopsy, and therefore we have to know how much this variability influences tumor growth. We use various amounts of solid tumor and a permanent tumor line, HT-29 (colon carcinoma). The growth curves are shown in Figs. 1 and 2, and it can be seen that there were some differences only at the beginning of growth, but towards the end of the experiment the size of the initial inoculum did not play any substantial role. Using the tumor line HT-29, we have shown that

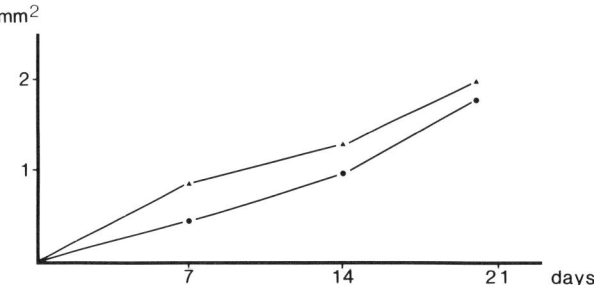

Fig. 1. Growth of laryngeal carcinoma starting from two sizes of inoculum: *triangles,* 9 mm^3; *circles,* 18 mm^3

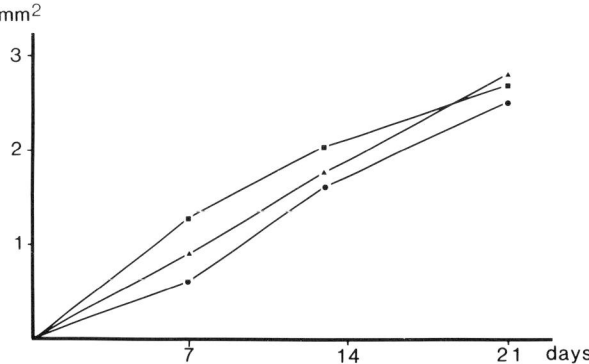

Fig. 2. Growth of HT-29 tumor starting from various numbers of cells: *circles,* 10^5; *triangles,* 2×10^5; *squares,* 4×10^5

Table 1. Growth of HT-29 with and without nonspecifically stimulated allogenic lymphocytes

	Lymphocytes	0
Nonstimulated	0.14 + 0.08	0.12 + 0.05
PHA	0.08 + 0.03	0.15 + 0.1
IL-2	0.08 + 0.04	0.15 + 0.06

Table 2. Influence of specifically stimulated allogenic lymphocytes on the growth of HT-29 cells

	Lymphocytes	0
IL-2	0.12	0.18 + 0.06
IL-2 + HT-29		0.21 + 0.09

LAK cells, not being major histocompatibility complex (MHC) restricted, can inhibit the growth of tumor under the renal capsule. In other words, this experiment shows that human lymphocytes are able to function in the subrenal capsule space (Table 1).

The capability of human lymphocytes to inhibit growth of human tumors in nude mice has already been demonstrated for subcutaneously growing tumors (Coates and Crawford 1977). For this experiment the tumor cells were first incubated with the lymphocytes and than injected subcutaneously. It would be more relevant to prove that lymphocytes are able to inhibit growth of an already established tumor. The SRCA is a well-defined anatomical localization, the tumor is visible under the capsule and so the lymphocytes can be injected either into the already growing tumor or in its immediate vicinity. We usually allow the tumor to grow for 7-10 days; during this time the lymphocytes are stimulated in vitro so that they will be ready for injection. In the HT-29 model we have also shown that antitumoral activity can be increased by cocultivation of the lymphocytes with the HT-29 cells (Table 2).

To evaluate the actual activity of the autologous lymphocytes on the patient's tumor, we use the following protocol. Tumor material obtained during surgery is implanted in both kidneys of five to seven mice. Figure 3 shows a melanoma growing under the renal capsule. Patient lymphocytes from heparinized peripheral blood are isolated on lymphocyte separation medium (LSM, Flow Laboratories), cultivated in RPMI medium with fetal calf serum and rIL-2 (Boehringer). The LAK cells are than injected in the vicinity of the tumor growing in the left kidney, and the right kidney tumor is injected with control material. LAK cells are able to inhibit the growth of the tumor, but as they are not specific, they are not able to localize selectively in the tumor after i.v. application. Most of them are trapped in the lung and produce undesired side effects. Vose (1984) suggested stimulating the lymphocytes in vitro with autologous tumor to increase their tumor specificity or selectivity. We tested this possibility using the SRCA and were able to show that lymphocytes stimulated with autologous tumor material and rIL-2 produce a better inhibitory effect than LAK cells alone (Tables 3, 4).

Another possibility to increase or induce specificity of the lymphocytes is antibody-dependent cell cytotoxicity (ADCC) (Table 5). For these experiments we

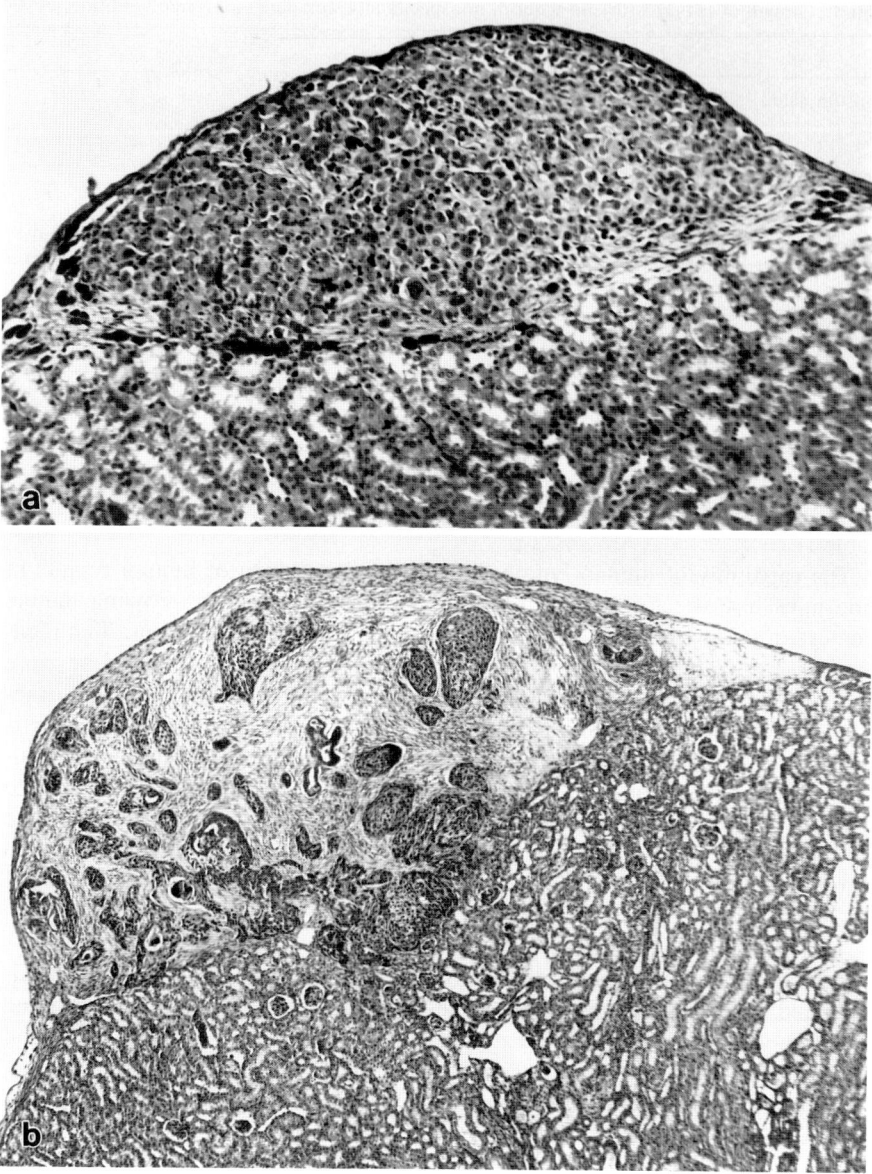

Fig. 3. a Melanoma. b Laryngeal carcinoma

used the melanoma line M21 established by Dr. Morton (UCLA, Los Angeles, California). All cells of this line carry a membrane antigen – GD3 – and Dr. Reisfeld (Scripps Clinic and Research Institute, San Diego, California) provided us with monoclonal antibodies against this antigen. We incubated LAK cells obtained from healthy donors with these antibodies, washed off the excess antibodies, and injected the lymphocytes coated with anti-GD3 antibodies in the vi-

Table 3. Influence of autologous activated lymphocytes on tumor growth

Stimulation	Experiment (mm)	Control (mm)
IL-2	0.14 ± 0.07	0.24 ± 0.1
IL-2 + autologous tumor	0.09 ± 0.05 (4/6)	0.27 ± 0.07

Table 4. Influence of autologous in vitro activated lymphocytes on the growth of the tumor xenograft in kidney capsule assay

No.	Mice grafted (n)	Lymphocytes injected (left side) (n)	Tumor detected at the end of experiment	
			Left	Right
1	5	2×10^6	4	5
2	5	5×10^6	3	5
3	4	5×10^6	4	4
4	6	4×10^6	4	6
5	5	10×10^6	2	5
6	5	6×10^6	3	5
7	6	2×20^6	5	6
8	4	10×10^6	1	4
	40		26	40

Table 5. Models for studying ADCC

Tumor	TAA	Antibodies
NPC (xenotransplant, EBNA)	Lydma, Ma, EBNA (all cells)	Rabbit anti-EBV subcomponents (Wolf)
M21 Melanoma line	GD3 (all cells)	MAb (mice) (Reisfeld)
Biopsy (fresh tumor material)	Epithelial associated antigens	Commercial MAb (mice)

cinity of M21 growing in the kidney capsule. The antibody-coated LAK cells produced a far better inhibitory effect than LAK cells alone (Table 6).

The tumors of the head and neck region do not express GD3 antigen, and therefore we have to use a different strategy. Frozen sections were prepared from the tumor material obtained by surgery and tested by immunoperoxidase reaction with a battery of monoclonal antibodies. Antibodies reacting with more than 50% of the tumor cells were then used in a similar fashion to that described for the melanoma model. The patient's lymphocytes were stimulated with rIL-2 and coated with the respective antibodies. These lymphocytes were then injected in the vicinity of the tumor from the same patient growing under the renal capsule. As seen in Table 7, in all cases the antibody improved the antitumor effect of LAK cells. In-

Table 6. The influence of allogenic LAK cells with and without MAb

Tumor	Experiment (LAK+AB)		Control (LAK)	
	(n)	Growth (mm)	(n)	Growth (mm)
NPC	6/6	0.14±0.08	6/6	0.12±0.05
M21	2/5	0.07±0.03	5/5	0.21±0.09

Table 7. The influence of autologous LAK cells with and without MAb

50% Tumor cells positive with MAb	LAK Tumors/total (n)	LAK+MAb Tumors/total (n)
EMA	4/5	1/5
Cytokeratin	5/5	2/5
Vimentin	3/5	1/5
D 11	4/5	2/5
D 8	4/5	3/5

terestingly, even antibodies against nonmembrane antigens produced this effect. It is known that ADCC can operate with the help of such antigens. It is also possible that such antigens are present in the tumor tissue (outside the cells – from the dead tumor cells), and that this is sufficient for the LAK cells with the antibodies to be attracted into the vicinity of tumor cells. The nude mouse system seems to be suitable for such studies, but has two disadvantages. First, the nude mouse is not immunologically nonreactive, and thus an antihuman reaction could improve the tumor inhibition caused by the patient's lymphocytes. However, this is not likely as the tumor growing in the right kidney is also exposed to the immune system of the same mouse and serves as a control. Secondly, of more significance could be the fact that human lymphocytes cannot function properly in the nude mouse. For this reasons and also because we wanted to know more about the lymphocyte-tumor cell interaction, we started a series of in vitro experiments. Preliminary results are as follows.

The lymphocytes were incubated in suspension with target cells for various periods of time. The tubes were kept in an upright position, and the cells were left to settle for 1, 2, 4, and 8 h. Then the supernatant was carefully removed, and fibrinogen (20 µl, 1 mg/ml) was added to the sediment which was gently resuspended; then trombin (10 µl, 1 mg/ml) was added, and the solution was allowed to clot for 10 min at 37 °C. The clot was fixed with glutaraldehyde and processed for electron

Fig. 4a, b. Interaction of LAK cells with tumor cells. a Phagocytosis. *1*, First contact – LAK cell on the left; *2*, adaptation of surfaces of both cells (LAK on the left); *3*, the tumor cell is engulfed, the nucleus of LAK is elongated; *4*, completely destroyed tumor cells inside the LAK cell. b Cytolysis. *1*, Attachment of LAK cell to tumor cell; *2*, cytoplasmic bridge, vacuoles within the tumor cell; *3*, three damaged tumor cells, LAK in the middle; *4*, destroyed tumor cells surrounded by LAK cells

Tumor Immunotherapy

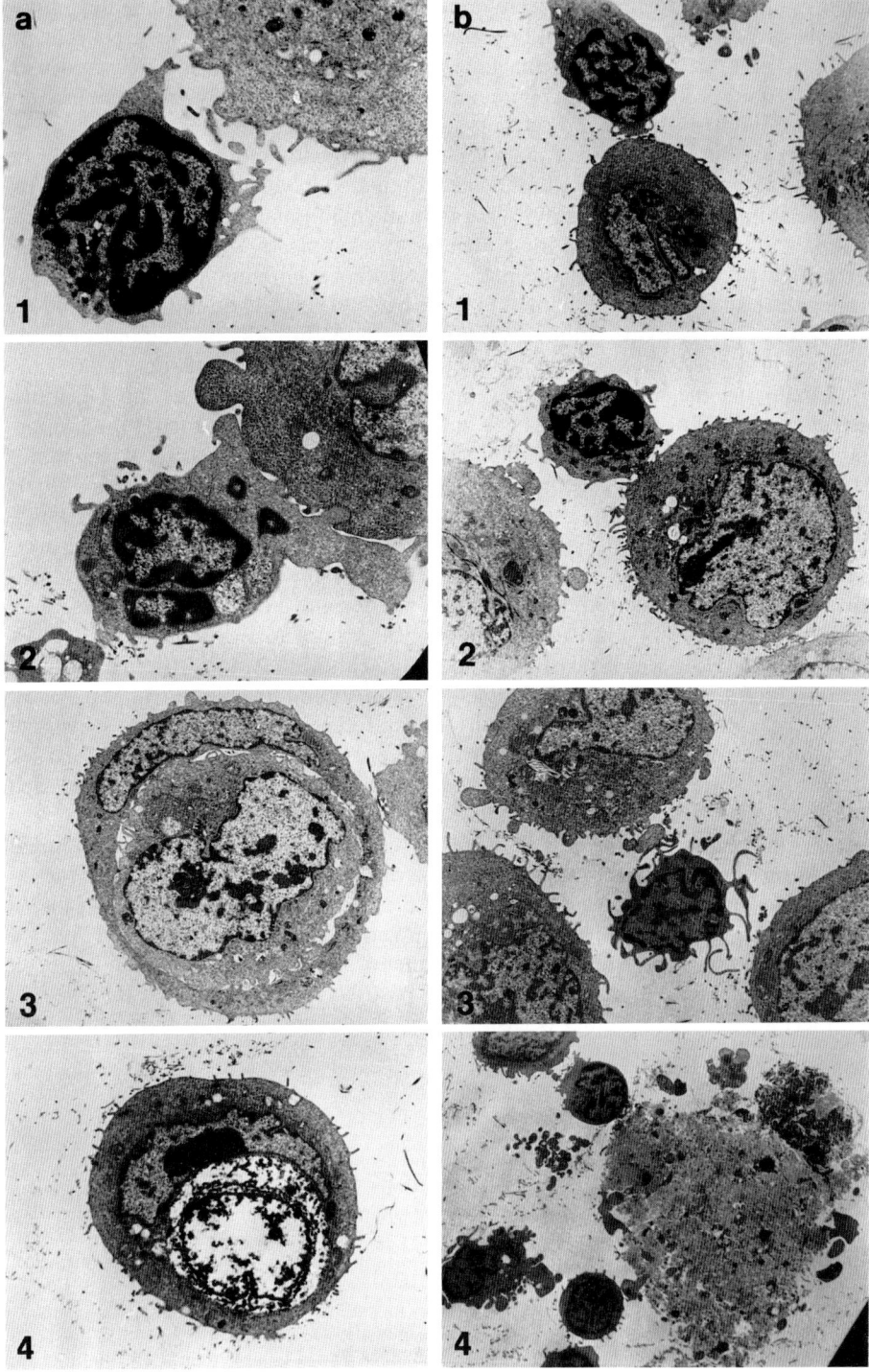

microscopy. The effector cells were either LAK cells, in vitro stimulated cytotoxic T cells, or LAK cells coated with monoclonal antibodies against the target cells. In the case of LAK cells alone, phagocytosis or a cytotoxic reaction occurred with equal frequency. In ADCC experiments only the cytoxic (cytolytic) reactions were observed. Figure 4 shows the various steps of both reactions.

Looking into the future, I do not believe, as mentioned above, that it will be possible to produce enough lymphocytes stimulated in vitro to destroy even the tumor remaining after the surgery. What immune manipulation can achieve is to restore the immune capacity of the patient – for example, by injecting specific helper cell clones, which will than enable the patient's immune system to fight the cancer effectively. Only the patient him- or herself is able continuously to produce enough lymphocytes to eliminate the cancer and find all the micrometastases. Rare clinical observations of spontaneous remissions support this possibility.

Finally, let me return to Milan Hašek. If Milan had been just an ingenious scientist, none of us would have been at the meeting held in Ommen. More important than his scientific talent was his capacity to create a wonderful working atmosphere, to bring people together, to inspire them, and to encourage team work. There are now more than 25 scientists from Hašek's institute working successfully abroad. The institute in Prague lost many scientists, but it is still producing respectable work. I know of no other director who has been able to create such an institute. It must be emphasized that Milan did not become a director of an existing institute; there was not even an immunological school in Czechoslovakia. Hašek created both. How was it possible? I spent 17 years with Milan, 10 years in Philadelphia, and the last 10 years in Düsseldorf, so I should be able to compare. But it is still very difficult for me to identify the differences between Milan's institute and the other laboratories where I have worked. One big difference is that Hašek taught us not to compete but to collaborate. We communicated freely with each other, we discussed all our problems, and were willing to share even our crazy ideas. One reason for this was that Hašek removed any worries about obtaining money for research. There was no need to write grant applications, prepare for extramural visits, or hide the results before a paper was accepted. We also had a kind of family life, spending a lot of time together after working hours. When we were together in the Netherlands, I felt some of the old atmosphere and I regret that it is impossible to make trips into the past. Nevertheless, I hope that we will all meet again on some other occasion.

References

Bogden AE, Haskell PM, Le Page DJ, Kelton DE, Cobb WR, Ester HK (1979) Growth of human tumor xenografts implanted under the renal capsule of normal immunocompetent mice. Exp Cell Biol 47: 281–293

Bubenik J, Koldovsky P (1964) The mechanismus of anti-tumor immunity studied by means of transfer of immunity. Folia Biol (Praha) 10: 427–441

Coates AS, Crawford M (1977) Growth of human melanoma in nude mice: suppression by T-lymphocytes from the tumor donor. J Natl Cancer Inst 59: 1325–1329

Grimm EA, Wilson DJ (1985) The human lymphokine activated killer system. Cell Immunol 94: 568–578

Héricourt J, Richet C (1895) Remarques à propos de la note de M. Boureau sur la sérothérapie des néoplasma. C R Seances Acad Sci 21: 273–281

Kau R, Kürten C, Kumazawa H, Koldovsky P (1989) Antibody dependent cellular cytotoxicity against tumors of the head and neck region measured by subrenal capsule assay. Arch Otorhinolaryngol (in press)

Koldovsky P, Weinstein J (1973) Expression of non-tumor-specific antigens in human tumor cells. Natl Cancer Inst Monogr 37: 33–35

Koldovsky P, Koldovsky U, Beck L, Vosteen KH (eds) (1989) Lymphocytes in cancer therapy. Springer, Berlin Heidelberg New York

Peri G, Zanaboni F, Rossini S, Mangioni C, Landoni F, Epis A, Mantovani A (1986) Evaluation of the interaction of mononuclear phagocytes with ovarian carcinoma cells in a colony assay. Br J Cancer 53: 47–52

Prehn RT (1977) Immunostimulation of the lymphdependent phase of neoplastic growth. J Natl Cancer Inst 59: 1043

Ritz J, Schlossman SF (1982) Utilisation of monoclonal antibodies in the treatment of leukemia and lymphoma. Blood 59: 1–11

Vose BM (1984) Activation of lymphocytes antitumor responses in man. Cancer Immunol Immunother 17: 73–75

Radiation-Enhanced Oncogene Expression

V. Klement

Milan Hašek – In Memoriam

"Doctor Hašek will see you now" said the secretary and looked at me over her glasses. The door was open, and in the air there was a pleasant fragrance of aromatic tobacco. In the center of a rather modest office was standing a tall, athletic man in a dark business suit, white shirt and a tie, lighting a pipe. An unusual-looking pipe, with a brier bowl and an aluminum stem. Through the smoke I saw the man's face with distinctly cut features, an angular jaw, a tanned and relaxed face. He was smiling.

"What can I do for you?"

I introduced myself and explained that I was a radiation oncologist interested in learning more about tumor biology and that I would like to apply for the vacant position at the Institute.

"What do you read?" he asked.

"Paterson's Cancer, Haddow's Chemical and Genetic Mechanisms of Carcinogenesis, Homburger's and Fishman's Pathophysiology of Cancer."

"Sit down." He continued with more questions pertinent to the literature quoted. "That's fine." To the secretary: "Let us call Jan Svoboda."

Jan Svoboda appeared, young, almost boyish looking, also tanned, relaxed, and smiling, holding the same brier and aluminum pipe.

"Here is your man" said Hašek. "Why don't we arrange the exam for him sometime in the fall."

In the fall of the year 1961 I entered the Institute. For 6 years I had the good fortune of working closely with Milan Hašek. I remember him as a man of a great personal charm; a strong man in both the physical and intellectual sense; a natural leader who makes things and other people move and who can do it with social grace and without losing the friendship and admiration of his colleagues; a man who seemed always to be relaxed yet endowed with an excellent capacity for methodical planning, analysis, and intuitive scientific thinking.

I complained to him once, in my 2nd year of training, that I did not have enough data for publication. He said: "It is like the four seasons. You cannot rush things, but you can be sure the time for harvest always comes." The next year I had enough data to write five papers.

For all this, for your encouragement, for giving me a chance at the beginning of my professional career, I thank you, Milan.

Radiation-Enhanced Oncogene Expression

The genes which are relevant to a malignant cell phenotype are known as oncogenes (for review see Bishop 1985). Historically, oncogenes were first recognized to be a part of a genome of transforming retroviruses. A transfer of an exogenous, acutely transforming viral oncogene and its insertion into the genome of a non-malignant cell through retrovirus infection leads to transformation (Bishop 1985), while the loss of the inserted exogenous oncogene from such a cell leads to a reversion of the transformed state (Yang et al. 1979). In spontaneous oncogenic transformation where insertion of exogenous genetic material does not take place, certain genes, which under normal conditions participate in cell growth and differentiation, might induce a malignant phenotype when their function is altered as a result of various genetic mechanisms such as chromosomal translocation, insertional or deletion mutation, gene rearrangement, and gene amplification (Brodeur et al. 1984, Seeger et al. 1985; Benedict et al. 1983; Cavenee et al. 1983; Dryja et al. 1984; Ali et al. 1987). Some of these functionally altered cellular regulatory genes (proto-oncogenes) have been shown to have a prognostic significance and indicate a poor prognosis for the patient when they are present in the tumor cells in an amplified state (Brodeur et al. 1984; Seeger et al. 1985; Slamon et al. 1987).

Ionizing radiation is an effective modality for local and regional cancer therapy, where the effect is thought to be associated strictly with the lethal effect of radiation on the target cell. Ionizing radiation, however, is also known to be a potent mutagen and, when administered in sublethal doses, it can be expected to modify the expression of genes, including proto-oncogenes, which determine the malignant cell phenotype. Such modification might be permanent or temporary and it might hypothetically include inactivation of already activated proto-oncogenes, activation of additional proto-oncogenes, or activation of tumor suppressor genes.

As there was little information on this subject in the literature, we have studied the effect of gamma radiation on human breast cancer cells and we have obtained evidence that the expression of certain oncogenes is enhanced in the cell population previously exposed to radiation.

Human breast cancer cell line SK-BR-3 was obtained from the American Type Culture Collection (catalog no. HTB-30) in the 28th in vitro passage and propagated in our laboratory. This cell line was derived from a pleural effusion of a patient with metastatic breast carcinoma. The cells have epithelial morphology and in the areas of heavy growth they tend to detach and grow in suspension. They contain four to eight copies of HER-2/*neu* oncogene (King et al. 1985; Kraus et al. 1987). This oncogene was the main object of our studies. It is located on the band q21 of chromosome 17, its product is a 185000-dalton transmembrane protein which belongs to the family of oncogenes resembling the epidermal growth factor receptor. Women who develop a breast cancer which contains an amplified HER-2/*neu* oncogene have a poor prognosis (Slamon et al. 1987).

When the SK-BR-3 cells were received, we determined their basic biological characteristics. The plating efficiency was low: of the order of 5%–10%. The doubling time was 53 h. Radiation sensitivity of SK-BR-3 cells was determined by exposing cells in suspension to a single dose of gamma radiation from a ^{60}Co source. Radiation survival response is shown in Fig. 1. A dose of 7.5 Gy, which left ap-

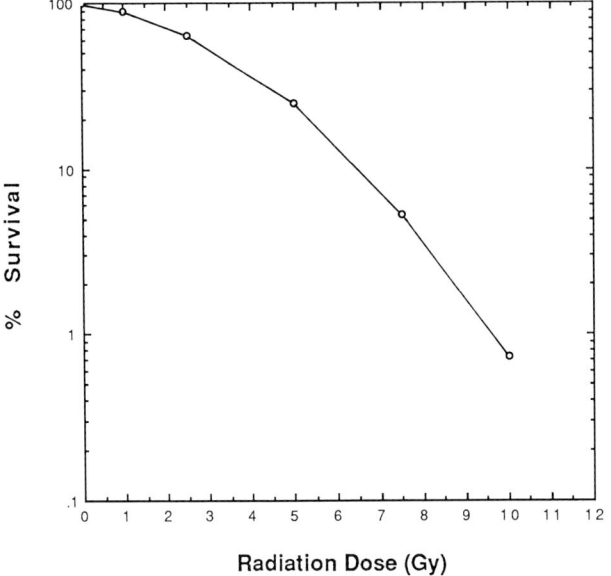

Fig. 1. SK-BR-3 cells in the 32nd in vitro passage were trypsinized and resuspended in McCoy's 5a medium with 15% fetal bovine serum (FBS). The cell suspensions of various densities, namely 10^2, 10^3, 10^4, and 10^5 cells/ml, were prepared in 50-ml Falcon plastic tubes. The tubes were irradiated in gamma cell 200, AECL (output 3.83 Gy/min) at room temperature. After irradiation various cell numbers were plated in 60-mm Petri dishes to give the expected number of colonies of the order of 10^1-10^2 per plate. Lethally irradiated (50 Gy) SK-BR-3 cells were added as a feeder layer in sufficient numbers to make the total number of cells in each plate 10^5. There were duplicate dishes for each radiation dose. Thirteen days after plating the dishes were fixed and stained with Giemsa. The colonies were counted, and the survival fraction was calculated with correlation to the plating efficiency of nonirradiated control

proximately 5% surviving cells, was chosen as a single radiation dose for the experiments below.

The plan of the experiment was to isolate cellular poly(A)-containing RNA, prepare a corresponding cDNA probe, and hybridize the probe with the DNA of HER-2/*neu* and other oncogenes. The same experiments were to be performed with irradiated and nonirradiated cells and the results compared.

Whole cell RNA was prepared from following three types of cell cultures:

1. Control SK-BR-3 cells, nonirradiated (34th in vitro passage).
2. Short-term postradiation cultures (SK-BR-3 cells of 33rd and 36th passages were harvested by trypsinization, exposed to 7.5 Gy gamma radiation and plated again. The cultures were maintained for 96 h, and then whole cell RNA was prepared).
3. Long-term postradiation cultures (SK-BR-3 cells of 31st passage were irradiated as above at a dose of 7.5 Gy, plated again, and maintained in vitro for 41 days with fluid change and subpassage as required. At the level of the 34th in vitro passage, the same as in the control, the cells were harvested for whole cell RNA preparation).

Poly(A)-RNA was prepared from each whole cell RNA preparation above by chromatography on oligo (dT)-cellulose columns (Maniatis et al. 1982). The radiolabeled cDNA was prepared from poly(A)-RNA using ^{32}p-labeled d-CTP and d-ATP. The procedure for first-strand cDNA synthesis was followed (Maniatis et al. 1982). The labeled cDNA was hybridized to oncogene DNAs on Hybond membranes as described below.

The following oncogene clones were used for hybridization with cDNA probes: v-*src*, v-*ros*, v-*abl*, v-*fos*, v-*mos*, v-*raf*, v-*myb*, v-*fes*, v-*ras* (K and H), v-*erb* A and B, v-*jun*, HER-2/*neu*, c-*myc*, N-*myc*. HER-2/*neu* plasmid was obtained from National Institutes of Health (NIH) repository of human DNA probes and libraries. The v-*jun* clone was kindly provided by Dr. Peter Vogt. Other clones, either in plasmid form or isolated fragments, were graciously provided by Dr. Roy-Burman. Plasmid DNAs were purified by CsCl density gradients. The plasmid purity was evaluted on agarose minigels. The contaminating RNA was removed by RNase treatment. The oncogene fragments were recovered by treatment of the plasmid DNA by appropriate restriction nucleases, and the fragments were separated by large-scale agarose gel electrophoresis using low-melting agarose. The cut-out segments containing the desired inserts were melted and the fragments purified by phenol-chloroform extraction.

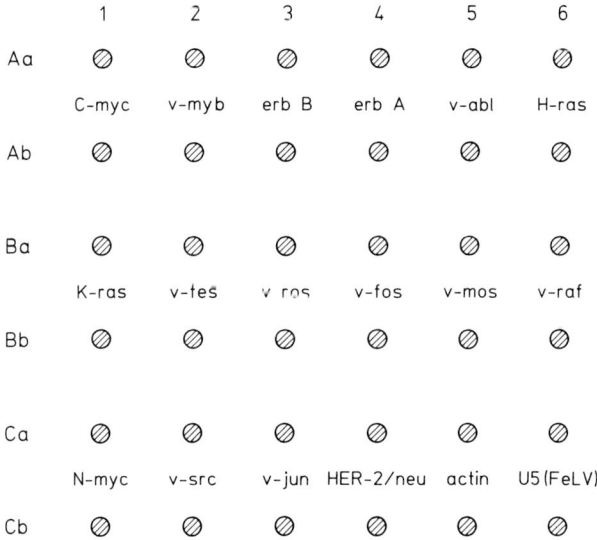

Fig. 2. Blot pattern of oncogenes hybridized with cDNA probe prepared from poly(A)-RNA of SK-BR-3 cells, both controls and irradiated; *a*, 15 pmol; *b*, 150 pmol. Equimolar concentrations (15 pmol and 150 pmol) of each cloned fragment were spotted in a total of 4 mcl volume per spot. Three membranes of the same pattern were spotted, processed in denaturing solution (0.5 M NaOH, 1.5 M Tris), followed by neutralization solution (0.5 M Tris pH 7.5, 1.5 M NaCl), and dried in a vacuum oven at 80°C for 2 h. The membranes were then prehybridized in SSPE and Denhard solution with salmon sperm DNA and 0.1% sodium dodecyl sulfate (SDS) (Maniatis et al. 1982). Each membrane was hybridized to one of three cDNA probes (^{32}P, 7×10^7 cpm) prepared on poly(A)-RNA from the following cells: control, untreated SK-BR-3 cells; SK-BR-3 cells 96 h postradiation; SK-BR-3 cells 41 days postradiation

Purified oncogenes were then dissolved to equimolar concentrations and spotted on Hybond membranes in a patern as shown in Fig. 2. Three membranes with an identical spot pattern were prepared. Each of them was hybridized against one out of three ^{32}P radioactive cDNA probes (Maniatis et al. 1982). These probes were prepared on three types of poly(A)-RNA as described above:

1. From normal, nonirradiated SK-BR-3 cells
2. From SK-BR-3 cells exposed to 7.5-Gy gamma radiation 96 h prior to poly(A)-RNA preparation
3. From SK-BR-3 cells exposed to 7.5-Gy gamma radiation 41 days prior to poly(A)-RNA preparation

After hybridization autoradiograms were obtained (Maniatis et al. 1982). Autoradiography detected poly(A)-RNA of HER-2/neu, N-*myc*, and v-*ras* (H) genes in nonirradiated SK-BR-3 cells, as well as the poly(A)-RNA of cytoplasmic actin gene which was used as a positive control. The poly(A)-RNA of other genes, spe-

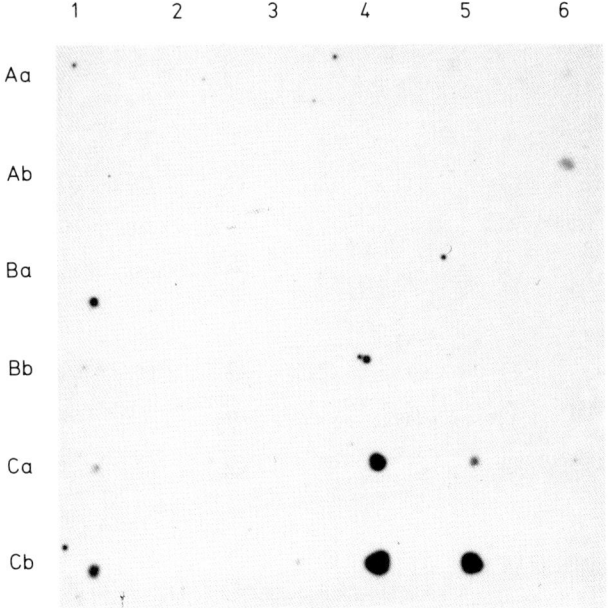

Fig. 3. Autoradiograph of a hybridization experiment using oncogenes in a blot pattern as shown in Fig. 2 and cDNA probe prepared from poly(A)-RNA of control, nonirradiated SK-BR-3 cells. This experiment showed detectable level of mRNA for H-*ras*, N-*myc*, HER-2/neu and cytoplasmic actin-related sequences in SK-BR-3 cells. Other dots are artifacts

Fig. 4. Microdensitometric traces of dot blots from hybridization of ^{32}P (d-CTP and d-ATP)-labeled cDNA probes for SK-BR-3 poly(A)-RNA to oncogene and normal cell gene clones. *1*, Control SK-BR-3 cells; *2*, SK-BR-3 cells 96 h postradiation; *3*, SK-BR-3 cells 41 days postradiation. *a*, actin, 15 pmol, 12-h autoradiography exposure, two screens; *b*, HER-2/neu, 15 pmol, 2-h exposure, two screens; *c*, N-*myc*, 15 pmol, 12-h exposure, two screens; *d*, N-*myc*, 150 pmol, 12-h exposure, one screen; *e*, v-*ras* (H), 150 pmol, 12-h exposure, two screens; *f*, v-*ras* (K), 150 pmol, 12-h exposure, two screens

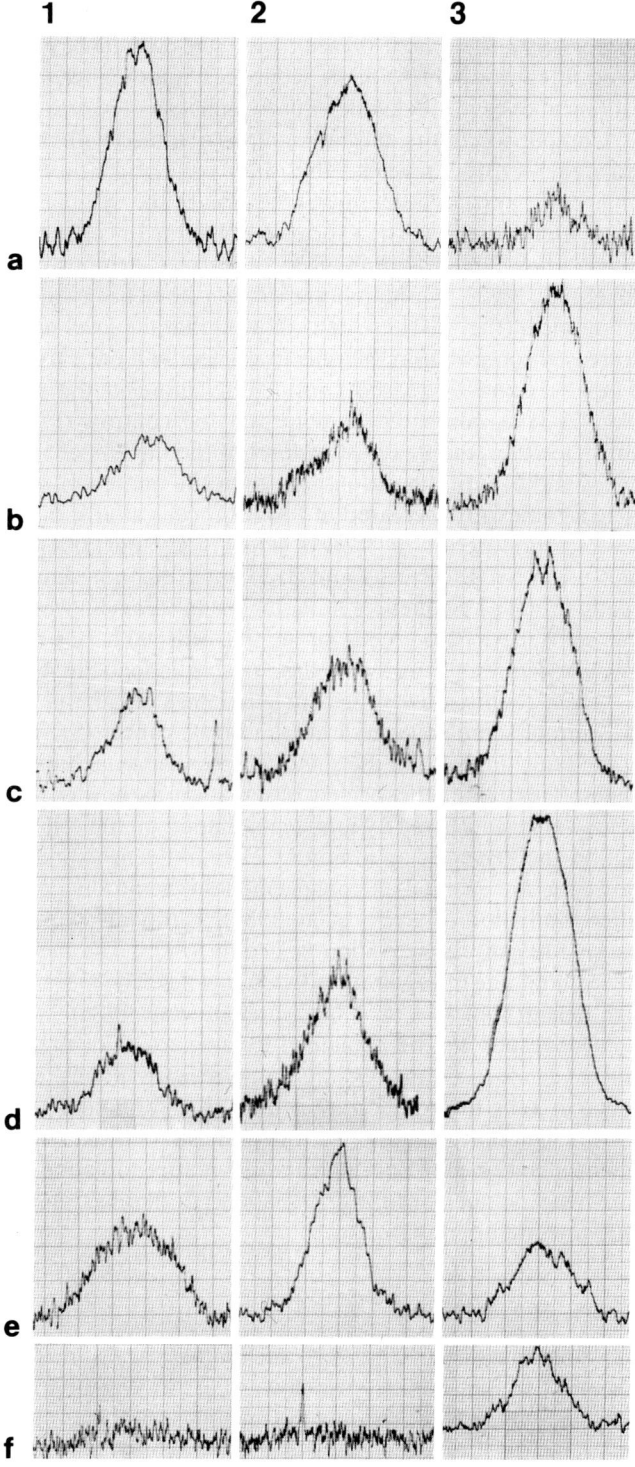

cifically c-*myc*, v-*myb*, v-*erb* A, v-*erb* B, v-*abl*, v-*ras* (K), v-*fes*, v-*ros*, v-*fos*, v-*mos*, v-*raf*, v-*src*, and v-*jun*, if present, were not detectable by our method. Equally undetectable were poly(A)-RNA sequences homologous to the U5 of the long terminal repeat of feline leukemic virus, which was used as a negative control (Fig. 3).

Comparison of the autoradiographs obtained with the probe for control and irradiated SK-BR-3 revealed that after irradiation the expression of some genes changed. It appeared that the expression of the cytoplasmic actin gene was diminished after radiation. The expression of some oncogenes, such as HER-2/*neu* and N-*myc*, however, was enhanced. This was demonstrated in an objective and quantitative way by obtaining microdensitometric readings of individual hybridization blots (Fig. 4). These data showed that the level of cytoplasmic actin mRNA decreased somewhat in the cells irradiated 96 h prior to poly(A)-RNA preparation (Fig. 4A-2) and decreased considerably more in the cells 41 days postradiation (Fig. 4A-3) as compared to nonirradiated controls (Fig. 4A-1). In the same cultures, however, the steady state level of the mRNA of two proto-oncogenes HER-2/*neu* and N-*myc* showed just the opposite trend, i.e., both of these mRNA levels were significantly increased in SK-BR-3 cells after radiation, especially in the late postradiation period of 41 days (Fig. 4B, C, and D). Oncogene v-*ras* (H) was expressed in SK-BR-3 cells and irradiation did not change the expression significantly (Fig. 4E). Sequences homologous to v-*ras* (K) were not initially expressed in the control SK-BR-3 cells or in the cells 96 h postradiation; however, a low mRNA level was detected 41 days postradiation (Fig. 4F).

These results showed that sublethal dose of gamma radiation enhanced the expression of some genes in a human breast cancer (SK-BR-3) cell population and, at the same time and in the same cell population, inhibited the expression of other genes. This is an unexpected observation as it was generally believed that the acute damage inflicted by ionizing radiation on the cell DNA had a random distribution and generally an inhibitory effect on gene expression. One previous report, however, documented an enhancement in the production of a specific cell product after irradiation (Shapiro et al. 1984). Ultraviolet light has also been shown to cause a selective inactivation of certain genes. The mechanism in this case is the differential rate of repair of individual genes. The more active genes have more active repair (Mellon et al. 1986; Madhani et al. 1986).

Our results can be explained by a selection of pre-existing cell variants with different oncogene expression. Some recently published data on increased resistance of cells to radiation after their transformation by the *ras* oncogene (Sklar 1988) might indeed support this hypothesis. Our data, however, which show oncogene enhancement to occur within 96 h after radiation and with only 5% of cells surviving, do not favor the explanation of cell selection. Experiments to clarify this question are in progress.

Living and Working Abroad

My colleague at the University of Southern California returned from the World Congress in Biochemistry which was held in Prague in July 1988. He came to me and said: "Prague is probably the most beautiful city I have ever seen. How could you have left it to come to live in Los Angeles?"

How could I? I did not answer his question. If he had been able to read my thoughts, he would have found that I really never left altogether. My heart is still there. Memories go back 20 years. Having completed my fellowship at the National Institutes of Health, my wife and I were ready to return to Prague. The events of 1968 decided otherwise. Our destiny led us on our new journey to the West. Our home was to become California. Our journey across the American continent became one of the most memorable events of our lives. The land and the people are beautiful and they welcomed us with open arms.

My professional life and experience in the United States has been very rewarding. The time spent at the National Institutes of Health working with Janet Hartley and under the direction of Robert Huebner was a valuable learning experience, a happy time of meeting new people and starting new friendships. A very special place will always be reserved for the late Wallace P. Rowe for whom I have the highest admiration as a teacher, scientist, and friend. In our new home in California I received great support from my colleagues Robert McAllister and Murray Gardner who both helped me set up the laboratory and offered advice and cooperation. In recent years my heavy involvement in the clinical field has brought new challenges and rewards. Research support here is irregular, varies from excellent to nonexistent, a situation much less predictable than in Prague. The life is intense, the work hard, competition keen, and potential rewards great.

In our daily lives, what we might occasionally miss from European culture and tradition is hopefully balanced by the incredible beauty of this state with desert plains, orange groves, snow-capped mountains, and Pacific Ocean beaches. For all this, we are very grateful and offer our thanks. But it is at Christmas when we always think of Prague.

Acknowledgement: I wish to express my sincere thanks to Dr. Pradip Roy-Burman for allowing me to conduct the research described in this paper in his laboratory while I was on sabbatical leave and for his support and encouragement. I am grateful to Dr. Satish Parimoo and Ms. Barbara Bachman for their guidance, advice, and help with the project and to Dr. David Klein for performing the autoradiographic microdensitometry.

References

Ali IU, Lidereau R, Theillet C, Callahan R (1987) Reduction to homozygosity of genes on chromosome 11 in human breast neoplasia. Science 238: 185-188

Benedict WF, Murphee AL, Banerjee A, Spina CA, Sparkes MC, Sparkes RS (1983) Patient with 13 chromosome deletion: evidence that the retinoblastoma gene is a recessive cancer gene. Science 219: 973-975

Bishop JM (1985) Viral oncogenes. Cell 42: 23-38

Brodeur GM, Seeger RC, Schwab M, Varmus HE, Bishop JM (1984) Amplification of N-myc in untreated human neuroblastomas correlates with advanced disease stage. Science 224: 1121-1124

Cavenee WK, Dryja TP, Phillips RA, Benedict WF, Godbout R, Gallie BL, Murphee AL, Strong CL, White RL (1983) Expression of recessive alleles by chromosomal mechanisms in retinoblastoma. Nature 305: 305-784

Dryja TP, Cavenee W, White R, Rapaport JM, Peterson R, Albert DM, Bruns GAP (1984) Homozygosity of chromosome 13 in retinoblastoma. N Engl J Med 310: 550-553

King CR, Kraus MH, Aaronson SA (1985) Amplification of a novel v-erb B-related gene in a human mammary carcinoma. Science 229: 974–976

Kraus MH, Popescu NC, Amsbaugh SC, King CR (1987) Overexpression of the EGF receptor-related proto-oncogene erb B-2 in human mammary tumor cell lines by different molecular mechanism. EMBO J 6: 605–610

Madhani HD, Bohr VA, Hanawalt PC (1986) Differential DNA repair in transcriptionally active and inactive proto-oncogenes: c-abl and c-mos. Cell 45: 417–423

Maniatis T, Fritsch EF, Sambrook J (1982) Molecular cloning. A laboratory manual. Cold Spring Harbor Laboratory, Cold Spring Habor

Mellon I, Bohr VA, Smith CA, Hanawalt PC (1986) Preferential DNA Repair of an active gene in human cells. Proc Natl Acad Sci USA 83: 8878–8882

Seeger RC, Brodeur GM, Sather H, Dalton A, Siegel SE, Wong KY, Hammond D (1985) Association of multiple copies of the N-myc oncogene with rapid progression of neuroblastomas. N Engl J Med 313: 1111–1116

Shapiro DL, Finkelstein JN, Rubin P, Penney DP, Siemann DW (1984) Radiation induced secretion of surfactant from cell cultures of type II pneumocytes: an in vitro model of radiation toxicity. Int J Radiat Oncol Biol Phys 10: 375–378

Sklar MD (1988) The ras oncogenes increase the intrinsic resistance of NIH 3T3 cells to ionizing radiation. Science 239: 645–647

Slamon DJ, Clark GM, Wong SG, Levin WJ, Ullrich A, McGuire WL (1987) Human breast cancer: correlation of relapse and survival with amplification of the HER-2/neu oncogene. Science 235: 177–182

Yang YHJ, Rhim JS, Rasheed S, Klement V, Roy-Burman P (1979) Reversion of Kirsten sarcoma virus transformed human cells: elimination of the sarcoma virus nucleotide sequences. J Gen Virol 43: 447–451

Oncogenes: A Pathologist's View

L. R. Donner

In the summer of 1958 I bought a book by Professor Hašek entitled *Vegetative Hybridization in Animals* at the bookstore of the Czech Academy of Sciences in Wenceslaus Square. Retrospectively, the book was a witness of the bizarre intellectual climate in our country in the 1950s. In the fall of 1962, as a medical student, I met Professor Hašek in person for the first time and became interested in doing research at his institute. Following graduation from the School of Medicine, I jointed the institute and came to know Professor Hašek better, particularly in the late 1960s and early 1970s. I remember him fondly as a man of great intellect, intellectual curiosity, and scientific creativity.

In 1975 I left the country and jointed the Division of Biochemical Virology, Baylor College of Medicine in Houston. Those were truly exciting times for me, times of great expectation. Drs. Kit and Dubbs had previously isolated a human HeLa cell line which was deficient in thymidine kinase. Upon infection of the cell line with ultraviolet-irradiated herpes simplex virus type 2 (HSV-2), some of the cells acquired a portion of the viral genome, including a gene for viral thymidine kinase. In those times the notion that HSV-2 was a culprit in human cervical carcinomas was widely entertained, and the experimental system available appeared attractive. Locations of viral genomes in malignantly or biochemically transformed cells were, at best, poorly known. In order to elucidate the question of HSV-2 thymidine kinase gene residence in the biochemically transformed human HeLa cells, I prepared, cloned, and cytogenetically analyzed several somatic cell hybrids between the biochemically transformed cells and murine cells. Expression of the viral thymidine kinase convincingly correlated with the presence of a single HeLa chromosomal marker in the somatic cell hybrids. It became certain that a portion of the viral genome was capable of integrating into the DNA of the infected cells; however, we were unable to determine whether or not the integration was site specific. Later studies by other investigators using somatic cell hybrids between biochemically transformed human cells and rodent cells, and particularly transfection studies, showed that the integration of the viral DNA into cellular DNA was apparently random and not site specific.

After 1 year in Houston I moved to Bethesda, Maryland, to join the Laboratory of Viral Carcinogenesis that was headed by Dr. George Todaro. At that time I became interested in feline sarcoma viruses. Thanks to the pioneering work of Erickson and his collaborators, it was already known that tyrosine-specific protein kinase coded by Rous sarcoma virus was an indispensable tool for malignant transformation of infected cells. His work was greatly facilitated by the availability of several biologically well-characterized avian sarcoma virus mutants. However, there were no feline sarcoma virus mutants in existence at that time. Therefore, my task was to isolate and characterize such mutants. After having spent some time playing with methycellulose gels, 5-bromodeoxyruidine, and fluorescent light without success, I came to realize that a difference in the degree of attachment between the normal and feline sarcoma virus-transformed cells to the substrate could be useful for my purpose.

Although normal uninfected cells adhered tightly to the plastic, the transformed cells, which were round, were adhering poorly, with a tendency to float off. I cultured several T 150 flasks of Snyder-Theilen feline sarcoma virus-transformed mink cells. In order to ensure that all cellular revertants I hoped to isolate would be of independent origin, the cellular population in each flask was originated from a separate small cellular inoculum. By frequently shaking off the cells and inspecting the flasks, I succeeded in isolating several cellular revertants. Luckily, several of the revertants retained feline sarcoma virus DNA. Further analysis showed that the feline sarcoma virus DNA present in the transformed cells and the revertants were of the same size. Also, these revertants expressed viral P85 glycoprotein which was, in most cases, of the same molecular weight as the protein expressed in the transformed cells. Although there was no difference in sugar moieties between P85 extracted from the transformed cells and the revertants, the protein expressed in the revertants was markedly hypophosphorylated. It became obvious that there were two mechanisms of reversion in this system: (a) a loss of feline sarcoma viral DNA; or (b) mutation of the viral oncogene responsible for malignant transformation. Further analysis of the revertants (and from them, rescued transformation-defective mutants of feline sarcoma) was performed by Dr. Mariano Barbacid who showed that the mutants lacked tyrosine protein kinase activity. These findings were subsequently confirmed, and it is now established that the fes oncogene and the identical *fps* oncogene belong to the tyrosine-specific protein kinase family of oncogenes.

Thus, tumor virology led to the discovery of oncogenes. Dr. George van de Woude started DNA cloning of murine sarcoma viruses in the same building where I worked. My boss Dr. Charles Sherr had cloned the *fes* oncogene from both the Snyder-Theilen and Gardner-Arnstein strains of sarcoma virus. There was another feline sarcoma virus strain in our laboratory that had previously received scant attention. This strain was originally isolated from a cat with multiple spontaneous fibrosarcomas by a Pennsylvanian veterinarian, Dr. Susan McDonough. Despite this promising debut, she successfully resisted being lured into tumor virology research, preferring instead, veterinary practice.

Personally, my interest in the strain increased after my analysis of Hirt's extract of the virus-infected cells revealed that the DNA of this strain was unusually long. Luckily, the viral DNA was not cleaved by commonly used restriction endonuclease *EcoRI*. However, after *EcoRI* digestion, the only nonproducer cell line we had in our laboratory yielded a viral DNA-containing fragment which was too large to attempt molecular cloning. It was necessary to isolate a nonproducer in which the viral DNA would be integrated in a more favorable site. Also, there were problems with the different strains of helper viruses needed to rescue feline sarcoma virus from the nonproducer cells, but I finally found that a strain of amphotropic murine leukemia virus gave a suitable leukemia virus to sarcoma virus ratio.

I isolated several nonproducer cell lines, and one of them contained a single, approximately 10-kb long *EcoRI* fragment that contained feline sarcoma virus DNA, a size suitable for DNA cloning using lambda phage. After having screened 150 000 plaques, two lambda phages were identified that carried integrated feline sarcoma virus insert. The cloned feline sarcoma virus DNA, which was unusually long (8.2 kb), was studied further. Restriction endonuclease cleavage patterns and heteroduplex analysis confirmed that this strain of feline sarcoma virus contained a new oncogene. This oncogene, which is now called *fms,* is located at the terminal portion of the long arm of human chromosome 5 and codes for the receptor for a macrophage growth factor CSF-1. Currently *fms* is one of the most actively studied oncogenes. Patients with 5q-syndrome, in which the gene is deleted, suffer from refractory anemia, have immature myeloid cells in their bone marrow, and 10%–20% of them develop acute myeloid leukemia.

Tumor virology appeared to be losing its once pre-eminent position, and I started to want to move closer to medicine. During my stay at the National Cancer Institute, two sons were born to us, and I wanted more time to spend with my family. Therefore, I entered a residency training program in pathology at the George Washington University Medical Center in Washington, DC, where Dr. Steve Silverberg, and excellent pathologist, teacher, and author of a widely used textbook, *Principles and Practice of Surgical Pathology,* had recently joined the faculty. After a few months, my desire for research had re-emerged. I approached Dr. Jose Costa, head of surgical pathology at the Laboratory of Pathology, National Cancer Institute, in Bethesda. His proposal was to study immunoreactivity for smooth muscle myosin in a variety of human mesenchymal tumors. I did so, using large files of human sarcomas which were at my disposal.

One year later Dr. Costa accepted a position in Switzerland, and I joined Dr. Timothy Triche, a noted pediatric tumor pathologist. With him I studied expression of several cell surface antigens in cell lines derived from small round cell tumors of childhood. Using flow cytometry and a panel of several monoclonal antibodies, I found that, using this approach, it was possible to distinguish neuroblastomas and lymphomas from remaining small, round cell tumors (Ewing sarcomas, peripheral neuroepitheliomas, and rhabdomyosarcomas). Immunoreactivity of cryostat sections of primary small round cell tumors of childhood with a panel monoclonal antibodies was consistent with cell culture study data. Theoretically interesting was finding that the basic structure of HLA-ABC is expressed in peripheral neuroepitheliomas but not neuroblastomas. Similarly, beta-2 microglobulin was expressed in peripheral neuroepitheliomas but not in neuroblastomas. Because differential diagnosis between neuroblastomas and peripheral neuroepitheliomas presents one of the most difficult diagnostic challenges to the pathologist, diagnostic utility of the finding is evident. Neuroblastomas do not express HLA-ABC and beta-2 microglobulin and show immunoreactivity with monoclonal antibodies HSAN1.2, A2B5, PI153/3, and BA-1, and malignant lymphomas express HLA-ABC, beta-2 microglobulin, leukocyte common antigen, and show no immunoreactivity with HSAN1.2. Peripheral neuroepitheliomas, Ewing sarcomas, and rhabdomyosarcomas express HLA-ABC and beta-2 microglobulin and do not express leukocyte common antigen and show no immunoreactivity with HSAN1.2.

In 1985 I successfully passed the American Board of Pathology examination and returned to Houston to become a fellow in the Department of Pathology, M. D. Anderson Hospital and Tumor Institute. The variety of tumor material available there led me to the idea of studying oncogene expressions in tumors of soft tissue and bone. Even now, it is difficult to predict the future impact of molecular biology on the practice of anatomical pathology. Rearrangement of immunoglobulin and T cell receptor genes, while of great theoretical significance, is of limited diagnostic utility and is used mainly for cases of diagnostically difficult lymphoid proliferations. So far the only oncogene of diagnostic significance is N-*myc*. Amplification of this oncogene in neuroblastomas implies dismal prognosis for the majority of patients (Brodeur et al. 1984). Moreover, because this oncogene is not amplified in any other small round cell tumors of childhood, the presence of this oncogene in amplified form can be useful for differential diagnosis of difficult cases. However, small round cell tumors of childhood are rather infrequent in the general population, and the patients are mostly confined to specialized children's hospitals. Amplification of N-*myc* in classic small cell carcinoma of lung was reported to be associated with a poor response to chemotherapy, rapid tumor growth, and short survival. However, fewer than 100 tumors were analyzed, a number insufficient for appropriate statistical conclusions.

A related oncogene, L-*myc,* is amplified in some small cell carcinomas of the lung, but the clinical significance of these findings is uncertain. C-*myc* is amplified in a large cell variant of small cell sarcoma of the lung, and the amplification appears to be associated with shorter doubling time, increased cloning efficiency, and low or absent L-dopa decarboxylase. Also, N-*myc* is amplified in some retinoblastomas, but the clinical significance of this finding is uncertain. *Neu* oncogene, which was originally isolated from chemically induced neuroblastomas and which is known to be closely related to the epidermal growth factor receptor gene, has gained considerable attention recently. This oncogene was reported to be amplified in 30% of the duct carcinomas of breast, and the amplification was a significant independent predictor of overall survival and time to relapse. According to the authors, *neu* amplification in duct carcinoma of the breast is as important a prognostic factor as the lymph node status (Slamon et al. 1987). An independent study showed that the *neu* oncogene was amplified in a subset of duct carcinomas of breast and that amplification was more common in advanced stage tumors with positive lymph nodes. The *neu* gene amplification was present in 21% of tumors that recurred within 3 years and in 6% of nonrecurrent tumors. It is obvious that this finding requires independent verification. If the findings are confirmed, it will be necessary to set up a laboratory of molecular biology in many large hospitals. Study of other oncogenes and related genes coding for cell growth factors (c-*myc,* c-*myb,* p53, *ras,* c-*fms,* epidermal growth factor receptor gene, *bcl*) added significantly to our understanding of the neoplastic process but currently has little, if any, application in anatomical pathology.

My question was: could oncogenes be of practical value for differential diagnosis of tumors of soft tissue and bone? Because I was aware of how labile RNA molecules can be, I approached this project with trepidation and I have discovered, to my relief, that the status of preservation of RNA in minced tumors directly frozen in Revco was satisfactory. Total cellular RNA was extracted by a modified quanidinium isothiocyanate/cesium chloride method. Poly(A)$^+$ RNA was selected by affinity chromatography over oligo (dT) cellulose. This RNA was size fractured by electrophoresis in 1.1% agarose gels containing formaldehyde, transferred to a nylon membrane, and hybridized to ^{32}P-labeled DNA probes. The nylon membranes were then autoradiographed at $-70\,°C$ with intensifying screens, and the signal intensity was analyzed by spectrophotometer. We studied expression of c-*myc*, N-*myc*, c-*myb*, c-*fos*, p53, c-Ki-*ras*, c-*sis*, TGF-α, and epidermal growth factor receptor gene in a total of 44 tumors. Our effort to study additional oncogenes was aborted by the fact that the yields of RNA were often low and that after several hybridizations, no RNA was left on the filters. We found that:

1. In the majority of tumors, c-*myc* was expressed or overexpressed.
2. N-*myc* was aberrantly expressed in one of two neurofibrosarcomas and one of six malignant fibrous histiocytomas and was not expressed in other tumors. It is known that poorly differentiated neurofibrosarcomas can mimic malignant fibrous histiocytomas; thus, there exists the possibility that the single positive malignant fibrous histiocytoma was in fact a neurofibrosarcoma. Also, a single malignant analyzed melanoma aberrantly expressed this oncogene. It is of interest that both neurofibrosarcoma and malignant melanoma are tumors of neural crest origin.
3. c-*sis*, c-Ki-*ras*, c-*fos*, TGF-α gene, and p53 were expressed at the normal level in the majority of the tumors and epidermal growth factor receptor gene in a third of tumors.
4. c-*myb* was not expressed in any tumors and c-*fos* was not expressed in malignant fibrous histiocytomas.
5. The following aberrant transcripts were found: 1.2-kb c-Ki-*ras* mRNA in chondrosarcoma and malignant fibrous histiocytoma, 7.0-kb and 7.5-kb c-Ki-*ras* mRNA in neurofibrosarcoma, 1.0-kb TGF-α mRNA in chordoma, 7.5-kb and 9.5-kb TGF-α mRNA in neurofibrosarcoma and malignant fibrous histiocytoma.
6. All three tumors that expressed aberrant transcripts of N-*myc* (neurofibrosarcoma, malignant fibrous histiocytoma, and melanoma) also expressed aberrant transcripts of TGF-α gene. Because both genes reside in the short arm of chromosome 2, one could speculate that the aberrant transcripts were secondary to aberrations involving this chromosomal region.
7. In all three giant cell tumors of bone studied, c-*sis* was uniquely overexpressed.
8. Except for the unique overexpression of c-*sis* in giant cell tumors of bone, no other benign tumors (uterine leiomyoma, neurilemmoma, ganglioneuroma, desmoid fibromatosis) overexpressed or aberrantly expressed any of the oncogenes. However, c-*myc*, c-*fos*, p53, c-Ki-*ras*, c-*sis*, TGF-α gene, and epidermal growth factor receptor gene were expressed in one or more of the benign tumors.

The findings demonstrated that oncogenes and genes coding for growth hormones are also expressed in benign mesenchymal tumors and that expression of certain oncogenes (c-*sis* in giant cell tumors of bone, N-*myc* in tumors of neural crest derivation, and absence of expression of c-*fos* in malignant fibrous histiocytomas) can be useful for differential diagnosis. Expression of additional oncogenes needs to be studied, and analysis of a larger number of tumors in necessary to determine whether or not expression of certain oncogenes carries prognostic implications.

I have been doing full-time research in the United States for a total of 5 years and I must admit that my level of personal satisfaction has been lower and my degree of personal frustration higher than I experienced during my early years in Prague. Retrospectively, I have started to understand that, with few exceptions, our colleagues who went to work abroad prior to 1968 did not defect. Although research possibilities in this country are clearly superior to the ones we once had, I have been unable to find the same level of fairness and friendliness that we once enjoyed at our Institute in Prague in the 1960s.

Fortunately, the atmosphere in the departments of pathology differs markedly from the atmosphere in many of the research centers here. I earnestly hope and pray that it is going to remain this way.

References

Brodeur GM, Seeger RC, Schwab M, Varmus HE, Bishop JM (1984) Amplification of N-myc in untreated human neuroblastomas correlates with advanced disease stage. Science 224: 1121–1124

Slamon DJ, Clark GM, Wong SG, Levin WJ, Ulbrich A, McGuire WL (1987) Human breast cancer: correlation of relapse and survival with amplification of the HER-2/neu oncogene. Science 235: 177–182

Natural Killer Cells:
Odyssey from Laboratory Artifact to Clinical Reality

E. Lotzová

Professor Milan Hašek – The Way I Remember Him

The unfailing features I have encountered at all immunology-oriented scientific gatherings worldwide, once my Czech background has become known, were the queries, reminiscences, and affectionate stories about Professor Milan Hašek. Virtually every immunologist knew and respected him for his contributions to modern immunology. Professor Hašek was truly international. Besides being a talented scientist, he had an exceptional gift to make friends all over the world. These friendships included not only members of the scientific and medical community, but also artists and athletes as well as ordinary people. He was versatile in his interests, with a flamboyant personality, and an audacity to face harsh times boldly.

I knew Professor Hašek as a teacher when I was a student at the Charles University in Prague, and later on as a colleague during my stay at the Czechoslovak Academy of Sciences. I found him a dedicated educator, and a generous and encouraging colleague. He was a great proponent of international scientific interaction which, as he wisely recognized, was important for progress, facilitation of knowledge, and scientific accomplishments. During his leadership, the Institute of Experimental Biology and Genetics at the Czechoslovak Academy of Sciences truly flourished. I was very sad to learn about Professor Hašek's premature death and I believe that with his departure science has lost one of its great minds.

Annotation

Even though for the first few years of my stay in the United States my research was concerned with the immunogenetics of bone marrow transplantation (the area to which I believe I have made a substantial contribution), most of my scientific career has been associated with studies on natural immune anticancer mechanisms. Thus, in this article I will review briefly the history and the immunobiology of natural killer (NK) cells and will list some of the contributions which my laboratory has made to this important field.

NK Cell Beginning

The human large granular lymphocytes (LGL), the morphological prototype of NK cells, were identified more than 40 years ago (Maximow and Bloom 1947). However, an odyssey preceded appreciation of the biological and functional entity of NK cells. Three decades passed until, during the studies on specific cell-mediated antitumor immunity of cancer patients, two unexpected observations were revealed: first, the lymphocytes of cancer patients (if reactive) exhibited cytotoxic responses not only against autologous tumors (or tumors of the same histological type), but also against cancer cells of divergent histology; secondly, lymphocytes of healthy donors, included as controls in these studies, manifested equal or higher reactivity than those of cancer patients against a variety of tumor cells (Kay and Sinkovics 1974; Kay et al. 1977; Rosenberg et al. 1974; Lotzová and McCredie 1978). These observations were quite perplexing and were initially dismissed as an in vitro artifact. However, the efforts attempting to resolve this "technical difficulty" failed, the "nonspecific cytotoxicity" was observed more frequently, and this unusual observation was extended to experimentel animal models. Finally, this phenomenon was accepted as a true biological activity and designated NK cell-mediated cytotoxicity and/or spontaneous lymphocyte-mediated cytotoxicity (for review see Lotzová and Herberman 1986a).

It was clear from the beginning that the lymphoid cells involved in natural cytotoxicity, termed NK cells, differed from conventional cytotoxic T lymphocytes. The most obvious differences were exemplified by the rapid and uninduced cytotoxic function of NK cells, unrestricted by major histocompatibility complex (MHC) antigens; NK cell presence in congenitally athymic mice; and a lack of expression of typical T cell surface markers (Lotzová and Herberman 1986a). In spite of these differences, the question of NK cell relationship to T cells persisted for another decade. Nevertheless, it has now been clearly established that NK cells are divergent from T cells and other currently known cytotoxic effector cells.

Table 1. Current definition of NK cells and their differences from MHC-unrestricted T cells

Most human NK cells are $CD3^-$, $CD16^+$, $NKH1^+$, LGL.

NK cells do not rearrange (α, β, γ, or δ) TCR genes and do not synthesize functional TCR mRNA.

NK cells antitumor activity is mediated independently of expression of class I or II MHC molecules on target cells.

MHC-unrestricted T lymphocytes, when activated, acquire the ability to kill tumor cells, including NK-sensitive targets.

These T lymphocytes, in contrast to NK cells, express CD3 structure and either α, β or γ, δ TCR heterodimers.

Because of the obvious cell surface differences, MHC-unrestricted $CD3^+$ lymphocytes should not be classified as NK cells.

These cells should be designated as T lymphocytes with "NK-like" or "MHC-unrestricted" cytotoxicity.

TCR, T cell receptor.

The most current definition of NK cells is illustrated in Table 1. This table also depicts the differences between NK cells and MHC-unrestricted cytotoxic T lymphocytes.

Are NK Cells Involved in Antitumor Activity in Vivo?

As is usual, any new observation brings about a certain degree of resistance and misbelief. Thus, the odyssey of NK cells continued. Their in vitro antitumor activity was acknowledged, but their in vivo function was doubted. This triggered numerous studies in experimental animal models addressing the question of the role of NK cells in tumor resistance in vivo. Results of these investigations uncovered that NK cell antitumor activity was not restricted to the in vitro system, but was also manifested in vivo. The latter conclusion was based primarily on the observations demonstrating that selectively NK cell-depleted animals manifested higher susceptibility to tumors (Lotzová and Herberman 1986b), whereas the animals with augmented NK cell cytotoxicity were more resistant to tumor growth and dissemination (for review see Lotzová and Herberman 1986a, b).

One example of such an association between tumor growth and NK cell cytotoxicity is shown in a representative experiment performed in our laboratory and depicted in Fig. 1. We demonstrated that induction of NK cell activity in the peritoneal cavity of mice (the compartment with no NK activity) by 2-amino-5-iodo-6-phenyl-4-pyrimidinone (AIPP) resulted in prevention of growth of ascitic mammary adenocarcinoma, ACA-755. On the contrary, depletion of NK cell cytotoxicity of AIPP-stimulated mice with NK 1.1 antiserum was associated with aggressive tumor growth and mortality of most of the animals. The treatment of mice with normal mouse serum or Thy-1.2 antibody (directed against T cells) did

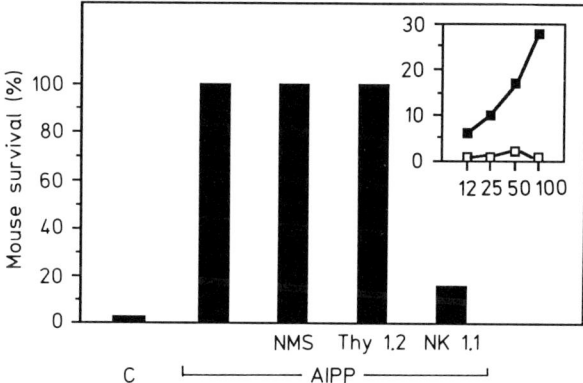

Fig. 1. Correlation between NK cell cytotoxicity and tumor resistance. B6D2F$_1$ mice were untreated *(C)* or injected with AIPP 3 days prior to cytotoxicity assay or administration of 10^3 ACA-755. AIPP-treated mice were depleted of T (Thy-1.2) or NK cells (NK 1.1) prior to tumor challenge. Normal mouse serum *(NMS)* was used as a control. *Inset* indicates peritoneal NK cytotoxicity of AIPP-treated *(solid squares)* or untreated *(open squares)* mice tested against ACA-755 in a 4-h ^{51}Cr release assay (Lotzová et al. 1986). *X axis* effector: target (E:T) ratio; *y axis,* percentage cytotoxicity

Table 2. Regional NK augmentation of ovarian cancer patients results in tumor reduction

Patient	Lytic activity		Tumor reduction (%)
	Pretreatment	Posttreatment	
1	2	62	100
2	<1	126	100
3	<1	139	87
4	<1	200	67
5	<1	59	75
6	<1	40	58

Cytotoxicity of ascitic fluid-associated lymphocytes from ovarian cancer patients treated with VMTE (for details see Lotzová 1986a) was tested against K-562 in a 3-h ^{51}Cr release assay (Lotzová et al. 1987a). The lytic activity is expressed in lytic units/10^7 lymphocytes; one lytic unit represents the number of lymphocytes required for lysis of 20% target cells (Lotzová 1986a)

not affect tumor growth. These and similar studies demonstrated the role of NK cells in in vivo defense against tumors (Lotzová and Herberman 1986b; Lotzová et al. 1986).

The involvement of NK cells in defense against human cancer is naturally more difficult to analyze. However, a functional defect in NK cells has been shown to correlate with an increased incidence of some neoplasia (Roder et al. 1986; Hoffman and Ferrarini 1983). Studies in our laboratory have revealed a close correlation between NK cell cytotoxicity of patients with epithelial ovarian carcinoma and cancer expansion. Specifically, we observed that regional (peritoneal) augmentation of NK lytic activity by virus modified tumor cell extracts (VMTE, for further information see Lotzová 1986a; Lotzová et al. 1987a) resulted in a significant reduction or total disappearance of malignant ascitic cells (Table 2). In some patients this treatment also resulted in a reduction of solid tumor masses and prolongation of life. These data indicate that NK cells may represent one of the immune effector cell components involved in the destruction of human ovarian cancer cells. During these studies we also discovered a new antiovarian cancer-directed cytotoxic factor with therapeutic promise, which is currently being patented. It is important to mention that these and similar observations from our laboratory have paved new avenues in the treatment of patients with ovarian cancer.

Other Functions of NK Cells

Another functional activity of NK cells became known practically concurrently with the demonstration of the role of NK cells in defense against cancer. In fact, prior to the discovery of NK cells, our group as well as other research groups were concerned with the characterization of effector cells responsible for the rejection of allogeneic and parental bone marrow (BM) transplants. Our previous studies had showed that the characteristics of BM effector cells deviated from T cells involved in rejection of solid tissue grafts (Lotzová 1983). BM effector cells resembled NK cells in that they exerted rapid reactivity without any previous sensitiza-

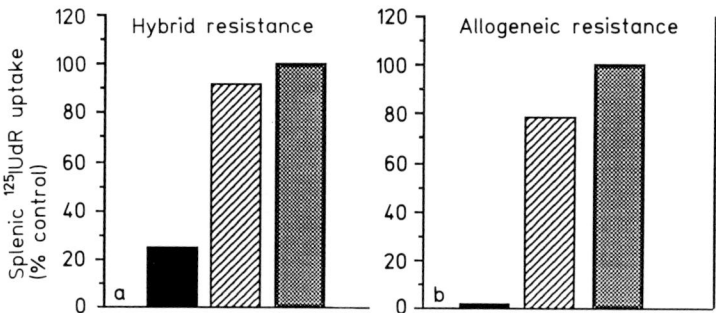

Fig. 2a, b. Abrogation of hybrid and allogeneic resistance by NK 1.1 antiserum. Lethally irradiated B6D2F$_1$ (**a**) and B6 (**b**) mice were untreated *(solid columns)* or injected with NK 1.1 antiserum *(hatched columns)* prior to transplantation with 10^6 parental B6 or allogeneic BALB/c BM cells, respectively. Syngeneic B6 and BALB/c mice *(screened columns)* were used as controls. Growth of BM cells was measured by the ^{125}IUdR uptake technique (Lotzová 1083)

tion and thymic or MHC restriction, despite the lethal dose of irradiation (Lotzová 1983; Lotzová and Savary 1977). We compared several other features of these effector cells with NK cells and found compatibility in a number of other characteristics (Lotzová 1983; Lotzová and Savary 1977; Lotzová and Gutterman 1979). A few years later, when specific NK cell antiserum (NK 1.1) became available (Pollack 1982), we demonstrated, for the first time, the direct involvement of NK cells in rejection of parental and allogeneic BM transplants (Fig. 2) (Lotzová et al. 1983). Thus, the role of NK cells was established in another biological phenomenon.

Relatively recently, the investigations into antimicrobial defense showed that depletion of NK cells by asialo GM1 or NK 1.1 antibodies resulted in a higher susceptibility of mice to a variety of viruses, including murine cytomegalovirus, vaccinia virus, Coxsackie B virus, encephalomyocarditis virus, and influenza virus (for review see Welsh 1986; Lotzová and Ades 1988). Similarly to these studies in mice, patients with complete absence of NK cells, but with other immune functions intact, were shown to develop severe viral infections (Lotzová and Ades 1988). This observation indicated that an NK cell defect contributes to the pathology of human viral infections and pointed to the role of NK cells in defense against infectious diseases.

Additional evidence for the functional activities of NK cells was generated from studies on hematopoiesis and lymphopoiesis. These investigations have shown that NK cells are involved in down- or up-regulation of the growth of hematopoietic progenitors and in differentiation and proliferation of B and T lymphocytes (for review see Lotzová 1986b). Finally, NK cells have been shown to produce a multitude of cytokines such as interleukin-1, 2, 4, and 5; interferons (IFNs); as well as tumor necrosis factor (Scala et al. 1986; Kasahara et al. 1983). It is conceivable to postulate that, via release of these biologically active molecules, NK cell may maintain the autocrine regulation as well as the regulation of various members of lymphoid and hematopoietic compartments.

NK Cell Down-Regulation by Suppressor Cells

Our laboratory was the first to describe the down-regulation of the cytotoxic function of NK cells by suppressor cells (Savary and Lotzová 1978; Lotzová 1980). After we had reported this phenomenon, a number of other laboratories made similar observations (for review see Lotzová and Savary 1986). Suppressor cells were detected in infant and old mice; in mice with low NK activity; and in animals manipulated by bacille Calmette-Guérin, *Corynebacterium parvum* (CP), pyran copolymer, adriamycin, β-estradiol, carrageenan, hydrocortisone, and irradiation. It is important to note that NK cell down-regulation by suppressor cells is not a phenomenon unique to animal models, but was also observed in humans (for review see Lotzová and Savary 1986).

In the next paragraph, I will describe briefly our original observations revealing the presence of NK cell-related suppressor cells in CP-treated mice. These studies were originally aimed at the augmentation of NK cell antitumor potential in vivo. As expected, the administration of CP to mice, resulted in initial augmentation of NK cell activity. However, this effect was later followed by a deep and relatively long-lasting depression of NK cell cytotoxicity (Fig. 3). Moreover, the ability of splenocytes from CP-treated mice to suppress NK activity of normal mouse splenocytes indicated the presence of suppressor cells. Characterization studies showed that suppressive activity was associated with T cells, since the removal of this cell population by Thy-1.2 antibody resulted in the abrogation of suppressive effect (Fig. 4). These investigations established the role of T cells in the down-regulation of NK cell cytotoxic function (Lotzová 1980; Savary and Lotzová 1987). Several investigators, using various experimental models, subsequently described the involvement of both T cells and macrophages in suppression of NK cell activity (for review see Lotzová and Savary 1986).

Augmentation of NK Cell Activity

As it can be suppressed, NK cell cytotoxic function can also be augmented. A number of synthetic and biological molecules have been shown to have NK cell-augmenting activity (Lotzová and Herberman 1986a). The most effective of these molecules are IFNs and interleukin-2 (IL-2). Interestingly, the majority of agents with NK cell-activating properties also display IFN- or IL-2-inducing activity. IL-2 is substantially more effective than IFNs in inducing NK cell antitumor activity both in vivo and in vitro (Lotzová and Savary 1984; Lotzová et al. 1987b). In addition to NK cell-activating properties, IL-2 has been shown to display NK cell growth-promoting potential (Lotzová et al. 1987b; Trinchieri et al. 1984; Lotzová 1987a; Lotze et al. 1981).

The Lymphokine-Activated Killing Phenomenon and NK Cells

Lymphokine-activated killing (LAK) was described as early as 1981 (Lotze et al. 1981) and was subsequently and prematurely attributed to a unique population of cytotoxic lymphocytes (LAK), divergent from NK cells (Grimm et al. 1983). One

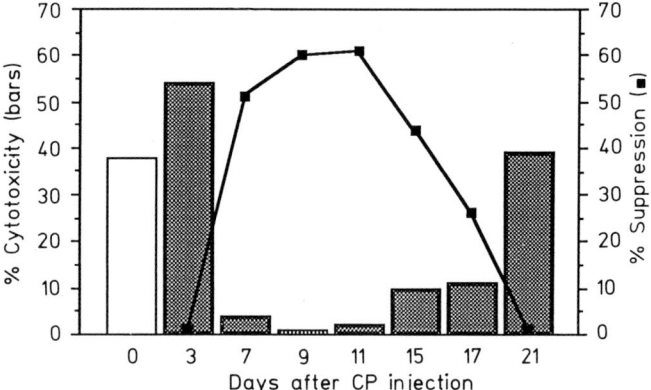

Fig. 3. Suppression of NK cell cytotoxicity by *C. parvum*. Splenic NK cytotoxicity of normal *(open column)* and *C. parvum (CP)*-treated *(screened columns)* B6D2F$_1$ mice was tested in a 16-h ^{51}Cr release assay against YAC-1 at 50:1 E:T ratio. The suppressive effect of CP splenocytes on the cytotoxicity of untreated spleen cells was analyzed in mixing experiments *(superimposed graph)* at 1:1 suppressor: effector ratio

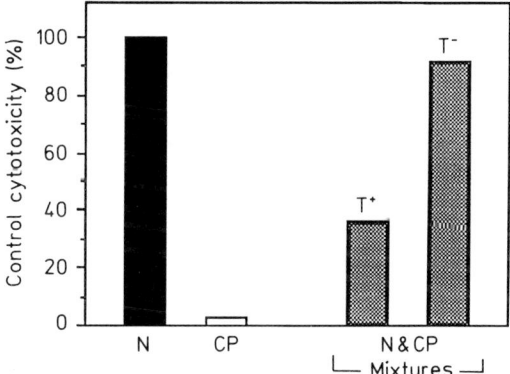

Fig. 4. Suppression of NK cell cytotoxicity by T cells. Splenocytes of normal *(N)* and CP-treated B6D2F$_1$ mice and mixture of both of these populations were tested for cytotoxicity in a 4-h ^{51}Cr release assay against YAC-1 at 50:1, E:T ratio. T^+ and T^- refer to splenocytes from CP-treated mice before and after removal of T cells, respectively

of the "unique" characteristics ascribed to LAK and "apparently" not displayed by NK cells was the ability to kill fresh tumors and cell lines presumably resistant to NK cell lysis (for review see Lotzová and Herberman 1987). This distinction, however, was not scientifically accurate, since the activity of a "putative" population of IL-2-activated lymphocytes was compared to the activity of unstimulated (instead of to IL-2-activated) NK cells. Furthermore, the cell surface characterization of IL-2-activated lymphocytes mediating such activity was incomplete and not reproducible (for review see Lotzová and Herberman 1987; Herberman 1987; Herberman et al. 1987; Lotzová 1987b). Also, the statement that unstimulated NK cells do not display ability to kill fresh tumor cells was quite inaccurate. In fact, it was shown by numerous investigators that highly enriched NK cells exhibit tumoricidal activity in vitro and that malignant cells frequently classified as "NK resistant" are sensitive to NK cell attack in vivo (for review see Lotzová and Herberman 1987; Herberman 1987).

NK Cells Mediate LAK Activity in Leukemia

After noticing this artificial distinction between NK cells and LAK and in view of the therapeutic potential of IL-2-activated lymphocytes in cancer (Rosenberg et al. 1985), we analyzed the LAK phenomenon thoroughly. For these studies we selected patients with leukemia who, as we revealed earlier, displayed an NK cell cytotoxic defect (Fig. 5) (Lotzová et al. 1979, 1985). We postulated that, in addition to clarification of the LAK phenomenon, these studies might contribute to the development of new approaches to the treatment of leukemic patients. Results of these investigations showed that culture of peripheral blood lymphocytes (PBL) or spleen cells of leukemic patients with IL-2 resulted not only in correction of the cytotoxic defect, but also in a significant augmentation of NK cell cytotoxicity (Fig. 6). Of note was the observation that cytotoxic cells were also generated from BM, the compartment vital for the generation and differentiation of NK cells (Lotzová and McCredie 1978) (of both normal donors and leukemic patients), but with low or no cytotoxic function (Lotzová and Savary 1987).

Several observations originating from these studies were of clinical importance. First, the IL-2-generated cytotoxic lymphocytes were effective in destruction of target cells highly resistant to lysis (e.g., Daudi) and, most importantly, acquired the ability to destroy autologous leukemic cells (Fig. 7); secondly, these cytotoxic cells proliferated actively and could be propagated in cultures with IL-2 for at least 2–3 weeks (Fig. 6); thirdly, the lytic activity was also generated from BM and spleen, suggesting that these tissues might represent an alternative source of IL-2-activated killer cells if blood leukopheresis was not possible in some patients. All of these observations show the therapeutic potential of IL-2-activated lymphocytes in the treatment of leukemia and the feasibility of propagating these cells in vitro for therapeutic trials.

Beside these therapeutic considerations, it was of interest to observe that the kinetics of activation of cytotoxic cells from leukemic patients differed from that of normal donors. While 3–7 days of activation with IL-2 were sufficient for induction of cytotoxic cells from PBL of normal donors, 2–3 weeks of culture with IL-2 were required for the generation of an optimal cytotoxic function from PBL of some leukemic patients (Fig. 6). Similarly, the induction of cytotoxic cells from BM (in this instance from both leukemic patients and healthy donors) required a longer period of activation; in contrast, splenic cytotoxicity was induced within the 1st week of culture with IL-2. These data suggest that various degrees of an NK cell defect can be manifested in different tissues of leukemic patients, or that divergent subpopulations of NK cells or NK cells at various stages of activation/differentiation may be present in individual body compartments.

In the light of the importance of IL-2-activated lymphocytes in the destruction of leukemic cells, we considered it essential to identify precisely the population of

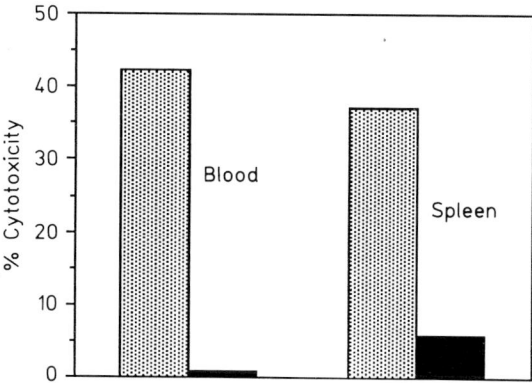

Fig. 5. NK cytotoxicity of normal donors *(screened columns)* and leukemic patients *(solid columns)* against K-562 target. Cytotoxicity was measured at 50:1 E:T ratio in a 3-h ^{51}Cr release assay (Lotzová et al. 1987b) in this and all subsequent experiments

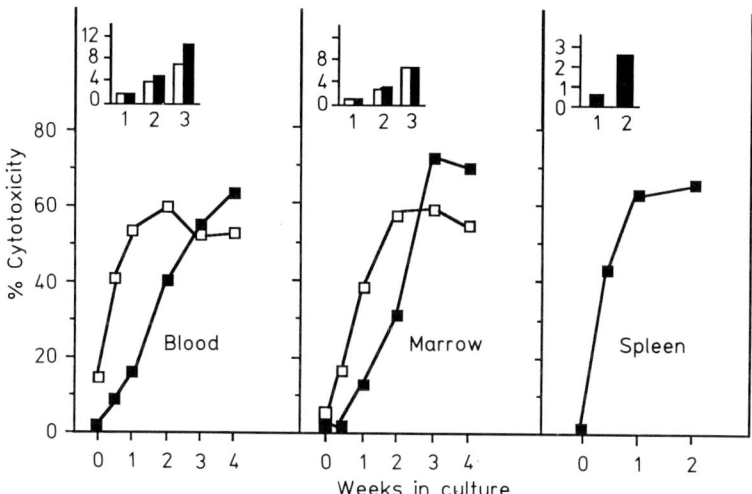

Fig. 6. Lytic activity and growth kinetics of IL-2-activated lymphocytes from normal donors *(open columns)* and leukemic patients *(solid columns)*. Lytic activity was tested against K-562 at E:T of 12:1. IL-2 in this and all subsequent experiments was used in the dose of 10^3 units/ml. *Insets* illustrate cell expansion index *(y axis)* and weeks in culture with IL-2 *(x axis)*

killer cells responsible for this effect. We used the advantage of phenotypic differences between NK cells and T cells and the availability of monoclonal antibodies (MAbs) against these two populations (Leu-1 against CD5 antigen expressed on T cells, and Leu-11 and NKH1/Leu-19 against CD16 and NKH1-Leu-19 antigens expressed primarily on NK cells). After depletion of T cells or NK cells in a complement-dependent cytotoxicity assay, we tested each of these populations for cytotoxic activity against leukemic cells. Results of these investigations, depicted in Fig. 8, demonstrated that the lytic activity against autologous and allogeneic leu-

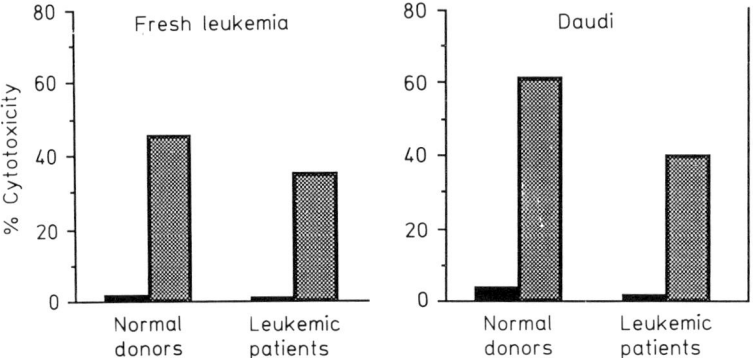

Fig. 7. Generation of NK cell cytotoxicity against fresh leukemia and the Daudi cell line. PBL were tested before *(solid columns)* or after culture with IL-2 *(screened columns, 7-21 days)*. E:T was 12:1 against Daudi and 50:1 against fresh leukemia

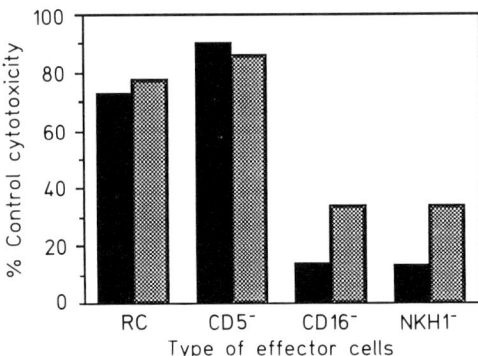

Fig. 8. Characterization of anti-leukemia-directed IL-2-activated lymphocytes. Autologous *(solid columns)* and allogeneic *(screened columns)* PBL were cultured for 7-19 days and then depleted of T or NK cells in a complement *(RC)*-dependent assay. Leu-1 (CD5⁻), Leu-11b (CD16⁻), and NKH1 (NKH1⁻) MAb were used for depletion of T cells and NK cells, respectively (Lotzová et al. 1987b)

kemic cells was abrogated by treatment with MAbs directed against NK cells. In contrast, T cell depletion did not affect the cytotoxic function.

These studies clearly showed that the peripheral blood cytotoxic cells of leukemic patients, generated in culture with IL-2, were NK cells. IL-2-activated cytotoxic cells derived from BM and spleen also expressed NK cell phenotype (Lotzová and Savary 1987, 1989a). Similar characterization studies performed by a number of investigators in a variety of solid cancer models confirmed the role of NK cells in the destruction of cancer cells (for review see Herberman et al. 1987).

Conclusion on LAK

Taken collectively, all the data from our laboratory as well as others show that (a) IL-2-activated NK cells are capable of destroying a variety of tumor cells; (b) most of the cytotoxicity induced by IL-2 from PB, BM, and spleen is mediated by NK cells. Consequently, the tumoricidal function acquired after activation with IL-2 is not a unique property of a new cell population, designated initially as "LAK cells." In fact, LAK should be interpreted as a functional activity and should be redefined as "lymphokine-activated killing." Even though NK cells were shown to be the major effectors of LAK activity, other subsets of lymphocytes may contribute to this phenomenon when LAK is generated from other tissues (for instance thymus) and/or when cytotoxic cells are propagated under atypical conditions (for review see Lotzová and Herberman 1987).

Relationship Between Tumor-Infiltrating Lymphocytes and NK Cells

Tumor-infiltrating lymphocytes (TIL), the population which has been shown to have therapeutic promise in treatment of cancer patients (Skibber et al. 1987; Topalian et al. 1988), are defined as lymphocytes residing within the tumors. These lymphocytes are mostly inactive; however, when activated with IL-2, they are capable of lysing a variety of fresh tumor cells. TIL were originally propagated with the aim of selecting a highly specific population of cytotoxic T lymphocytes for therapeutic application.

We initiated the studies on TIL in order to determine the contribution of NK cells to TIL antitumor effects. Our studies were involved with cytotoxic efficiency and tumor specificity of TIL derived from ascitic and solid human ovarian cancers. We also compared cytotoxic effectiveness of TIL to that of PBL of the same patients. Figure 9 illustrates that high levels of cytotoxicity were manifested by IL-2-activated TIL derived from both ascitic and solid ovarian cancers. These effector cells, however, did not show any pattern of specificity in tumor cell killing. Lytic activity was exhibited against fresh autologous tumors, the ovarian cell line OV-2774, as well as against the erythroleukemia line K-562. Furthermore, when compared to PBL of the same patients, TIL did not show any cytotoxic advantage (Fig. 9). TIL from some patients manifested more rapid growth than PBL; however, this was not a general phenomenon (Lotzová and Savary 1989b).

Characterization studies, illustrated in Fig. 10, showed that TIL derived from solid tumors (similarly to PBL of the same patients) expressed primarily the cell surface phenotype of NK cells, i.e., $CD5^-$, $CD16^+$, $NKH1^+$. Since anti-CD5 MAb might not remove all of the $CD3^+$ cells, minor contribution of MHC-unrestricted T lymphocytes to cytotoxicity cannot be excluded in these studies. Thus, the current methods for TIL production do not result in generation of specific cytotoxic T lymphocytes, as originally intended. The exception in this regard may be represented by a malignant melanoma, where TIL were reported to exhibit more specific, T cell-related antitumor responses (Skibber et al. 1987; Topalian et al. 1988). If further research shows that the specific cytotoxic T lymphocytes are more effective in destruction of certain tumors than are the natural immune effector cells, then more optimal conditions for propagation of these lymphocytes have to

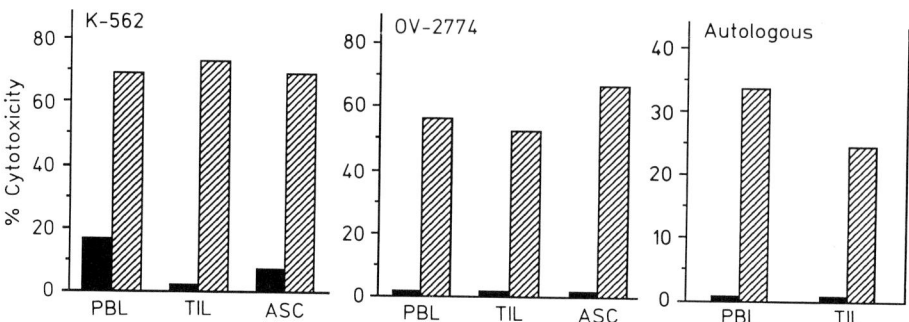

Fig. 9. Augmentation of cytotoxicity of PBL, TIL, and ascitic fluid-associated lymphocytes *(ASC)* of ovarian cancer patients with IL-2. Effector cells were tested before *(solid columns)* and 7 days after *(hatched columns)* culture with IL-2 against various target cells at 25:1 E:T ratio

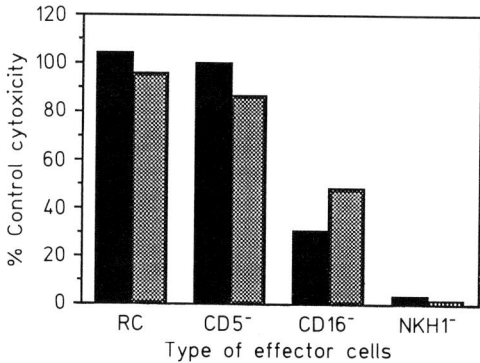

Fig. 10. Characterization of cytotoxic cells in PBL and TIL of ovarian cancer patients. PBL *(solid columns)* and TIL *(screened columns)* were cultured for 14 days with IL-2 and then depleted of T cells or NK cells as indicated in the legend of Fig. 8. Cytotoxicity was tested against the ovarian cell line OV-2774

be developed. In conclusion, our data revealed that NK cells reside within the ovarian tumors and acquire high anticancer cytotoxic potential after activation with IL-2.

Can NK Cells Be Used Clinically?

As shown above, the characterization studies demonstrated that IL-2-activated NK cells are involved in the destruction of leukemia and ovarian cancer. This suggested that adoptive transfer of highly enriched IL-2-activated NK cells may be more effective in treatment of leukemic and ovarian cancer patients than the currently used population of unseparated lymphocytes. Based on this postulation, we investigated whether it was possible to generate and propagate a highly purified, tumoricidal NK cell population in vitro for therapeutic purposes.

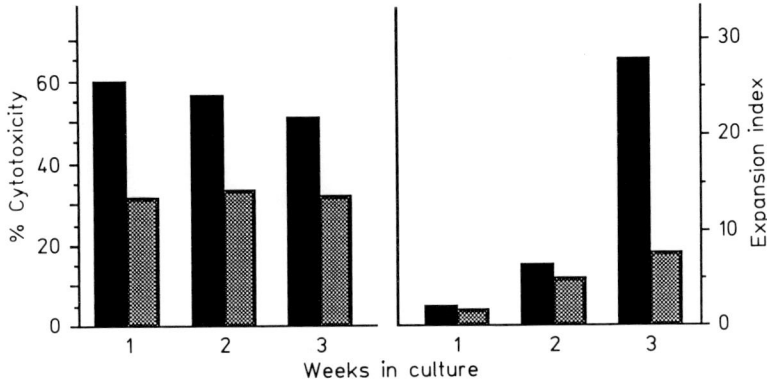

Fig. 11. Cytotoxicity and growth kinetics of NK-enriched and unseparated PBL populations. Percoll density gradient-enriched NK cells *(solid columns)* and nylon wool-filtered PBL *(screened columns)* of normal donors were tested for lysis of K-562 at E:T of 3:1. Proliferation of cultured cells is shown as an expansion index which reflects the growth of cells per culture

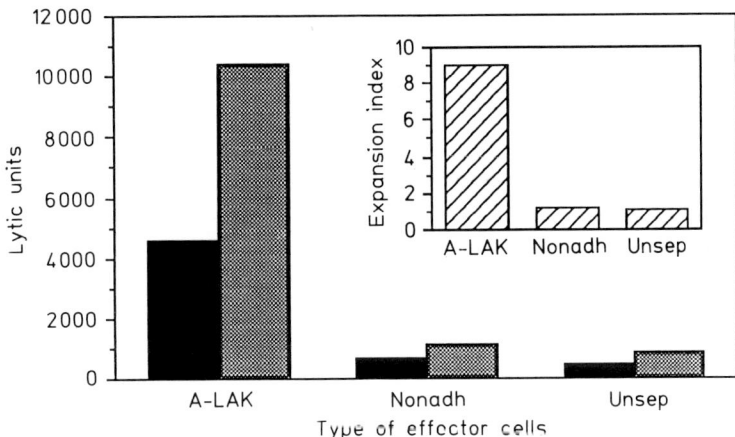

Fig. 12. Lytic activity and growth kinetics of A-LAK. IL-2-activated unseparated, nonadherent, and A-LAK PBL were tested for cytotoxicity against K-562 *(solid columns)* and Daudi *(screened columns)* 7 days after culture with IL-2. Lysis is expressed in lytic units $_{20}/10^7$ cells (Lotzová et al. 1986). *Inset* indicates growth of cells per culture, expressed as an expansion index

In the first study, we enriched NK cells (LGL) by Percoll density gradient (Lotzová et al. 1976) and compared the growth and cytotoxic potency of these cells to unseparated lymphocytes. As Fig. 11 illustrates, the NK cell-enriched population manifested significantly higher levels of cytotoxicity and proliferated more rapidly than unseparated lymphocytes. These data indicated that highly active NK cells do not require the contribution of other lymphocytes (or their products) for acquisition of a cytotoxic function or proliferation. In the second study, we used an alternative approach to NK cell enrichment. Specifically, LGL were separated on the basis of their property to adhere to plastic, shortly (24 h) after activation with IL-2 (Vujanovic et al. 1988). The adherent LGL (designated A-LAK, i.e., adherent

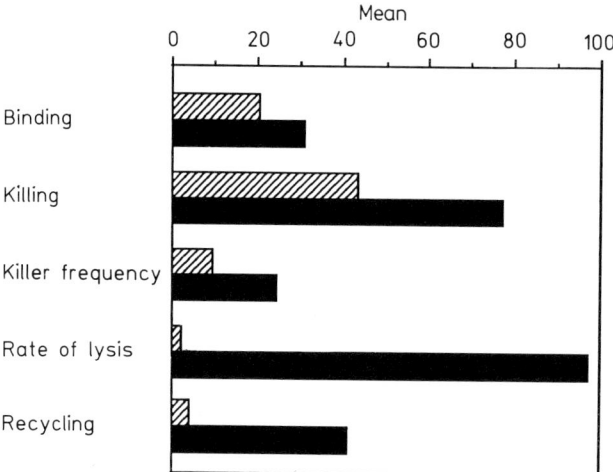

Fig. 13. Comparison of lytic mechanism of NK-enriched and unseparated PBL. Percoll-enriched LGL *(solid columns)* and nylon wool-filtered PBL *(hatched columns)* were tested for various parameters of the lytic mechanism against K-562 target (Lotzová et al. 1987b)

NK cells with LAK activity) were then propagated in vitro, and the growth kinetics and cytotoxic activity of this population was compared to unseparated and plastic-nonadherent lymphocytes (Fig. 12). As shown previously with Percoll-enriched LGL, A-LAK exhibited superior cytotoxicity against K-562 and Daudi in comparison to a nonadherent or unseparated population of lymphocytes. A-LAK also grew more vigorously in culture with IL-2 than the other two populations. Thus, this technique might represent another approach to the propagation of NK cells for clinical trials.

The cytotoxic mechanism of NK cells is not a simple one; it is composed of various steps which, in a simplified way, may be outlined as follows: (a) target cell recognition and binding; (b) effector cell triggering, activation, and granule reorientation; (c) secretion of cytotoxic factor(s); (d) binding of the factor(s) to target cells; (e) target cell death. This cycle is repeated several times by a single NK cell, the phenomenon known as recycling. Since some of these steps of the NK lytic mechanism can be measured experimentally (Lotzová et al. 1987b), we investigated in which step of the cytotoxic mechanisms NK cells surpass unseparated lymphocytes. NK cells showed higher efficiency in all parameters of the lytic mechanism, the most prominent being the rate of lysis and the ability to recycle (Fig. 13). Purified NK cells were capable of destroying ten times more tumor cells (within an 3-h interval) than PBL. These experiments supported our previous postulation that adoptive transfer of highly purified NK cells may result in higher anticancer activity.

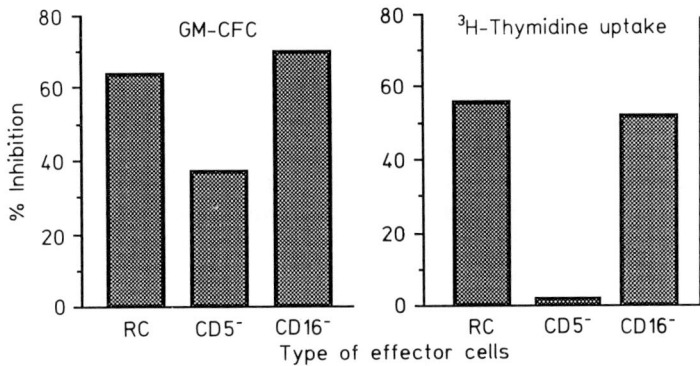

Fig. 14. Inhibition of hematopoietic cells by IL-2-activated T cells. IL-2-activated PBL were depleted of T cells (CD5$^-$) or NK cells (CD16$^-$) by Leu-1 and Leu-11b MAb, respectively, and tested for inhibition of autologous hematopoietic progenitors in GM-CFC assay or for inhibition of BM proliferation in [^{3}H]thymidine incorporation assay (Lotzová et al. 1988). The lymphocytes were mixed with BM cells at 1:1 lymphocyte:BM ratio

Effect of IL-2-Activated Lymphocytes on Hematopoietic Cells

One of the critical questions that has not been investigated thoroughly concerns the effect of IL-2-activated lymphocytes on hematopoietic cells and their progenitors. This information is especially pertinent for patients with leukemia in whom the hematopoietic system is already disturbed. Thus, we investigated whether IL-2-activated NK cells or T cells were involved in the regulation of the clonogenic activity or the growth of hematopoietic cells, using the GM-CFC and [^{3}H]thymidine incorporation assay, respectively (Lotzová et al. 1988). We observed significant inhibition of both GM-CFC and [^{3}H]thymidine incorporation after incubation of BM cells with IL-2-activated lymphocytes. Such inhibitory activity was removed or substantially diminished after depletion of T cells (Fig. 14). On the contrary, removal of NK cells did not affect, in any significant way, the clonogenic potential or proliferation of BM cells. These studies clearly demonstrated that, while the highest antileukemic activity was manifested by IL-2-activated NK cells, the inhibition of normal hematopoietic tissues was displayed primarily by IL-2-activated T lymphocytes. These data also favor the application of a highly enriched NK cell population in an adoptive therapy of leukemia.

Concluding Remarks

As evidenced above, my laboratory has contributed in a meaningful way to the field of natural immunity. It is encouraging to perceive that some of our research data have already been translated to the clinic and resulted in the development of new protocols for treatment of cancer patients.

I have been fortunate to have had the opportunity to conduct research at one of the most dynamic, prestigious, and academically oriented cancer centers in the world. Such a environment, together with my faculty appointment at the Graduate

School of Biomedical Sciences, has also been conducive to my scholarly achievements. I have participated actively in the education of a great number of graduate students, postdoctoral fellows, clinical fellows, residents, and visiting scientists, both nationally and internationally. Recently, I was honored with the Florence Maude Thomas Cancer Research Professorship, awarded to me by the Board of Regents of The University of Texas System for my scientific achievements.

In summary, my professional experience in the United States has been very positive, and I trust that our future research will continue to be fruitful and will allow us to facilitate the understanding of the immunobiology of cancer which would ultimately contribute to a cancer cure.

Acknowledgements. I would like to thank my husband Peter Lotz for his support, inspiration, and continuous encouragement during all these years of our stay abroad. I will always remember and love my parents who so unselfishly supported my independent thinking and decisions. This work was supported by grants CA 39632, CA 21062, and CA 31394 from the National Cancer Institute.

References

Grimm EA, Ramsey KM, Mazumder A et al. (1983) Lymphokine-activated killer cell phenomenon: II. Precursor phenotype is serologically distinct from peripheral T lymphocytes, memory cytotoxic thymus-derived lymphocytes and natural killer cells. J Exp Med 146: 884–897
Herberman RB (1987) Adoptive therapy for cancer with interleukin-2-activated killer cells. Cancer Bull 39: 13–18
Herberman RB, Balch C, Bolhuis R, Golub S, Hiserodt J, Lanier LL, Lotzová E, Phillips JH, Riccardi C, Ritz J, Santoni A, Schmidt RE, Uchida A, Vujanovic N (1987) Lymphokine activated killer cell activity: characteristics of effector cells and their progenitors in blood and spleen. Immunol Today 8: 178–181
Hoffman T, Ferrarini M (1983) A role for natural killer cells in survival: functions of large granular lymphocytes including regulation of cell proliferation. Clin Immunol Immunopathol 29: 323–332
Kasahara T, Djeu JY, Dougherty SF, Oppenheim JJ (1983) Capacity of large granular lymphocytes (LGL) to produce multiple lymphokines: interleukin-2, interferon, and colony-stimulating factor. J Immunol 131: 2379–2385
Kay HD, Sinkovics JG (1974) Cytotoxic lymphocytes from normal donors. Lancet II: 296–297
Kay HD, Bonnard GD, West WH, Herberman RB (1977) A functional comparison of human Fc-receptor-bearing lymphocytes active in natural cytotoxicity and antibody dependent cellular cytotoxicity. J Immunol 118: 2058–2066
Lotze MT, Grimm E, Mazumder A, Strausser JL, Rosenberg SA (1981) Lysis of fresh and cultured autologous tumor by lymphocytes cultured in T-cell growth factor. Cancer Res 41: 4420–4425
Lotzová E (1980) C. parvum-mediated suppression of the phenomenon of natural killing and its analysis. In: Herberman RB (ed) Natural cell-mediated immunity against tumors. Academic, New York, pp 735–752
Lotzová E (1983) Hematopoietic histocompatibility: genetic and immunological aspects. Compendium Immunol 3: 468–493
Lotzová E (1986a) Therapeutic possibilities of virus-modified tumor cell extract and interleukin-2 in human ovarian cancer. Nat Immun Cell Growth Regul 5: 277–282
Lotzová E (1986b) NK cell role in regulation of the growth and functions of hemopoietic and lymphoid cells. In: Lotzová E, Herberman RB (eds) Immunobiology of natural killer cells, vol 2 (6). CRC, Boca Raton, pp 89–105
Lotzová E (1987a) Human natural killer cells. Their role and possible therapeutic application in leukemia. Clin Immunol Newslett 8: 56–60

Lotzová E (1987b) Interleukin-2-generated killer cells, their characterization and role in cancer therapy. Cancer Bull 39: 30-38
Lotzová E, Ades EW (1988) Natural killer cells: definition, heterogeneity, lytic mechanism, functions, and clinical application. Nat Immun Cell Growth Regul 8: 102-110
Lotzová E, Gutterman J (1979) Effect of glucan on natural killer (NK) cells. Further comparison between NK cells and bone marrow effector cells activities. J Immunol 123: 607-611
Lotzová E, Herberman RB (1986a) Immunobiology of natural killer cells, vols I, II. CRC, Boca Raton
Lotzová E, Herberman RB (1986b) Natural immunity, cancer and biological response modification. Karger, Basel
Lotzová E, Herberman RB (1987) Reassessment of LAK phenomonology - a review. Nat Immun Cell Growth Regul 6: 109-115
Lotzová E, McCredie KB (1978) Natural killer cells in mice and man and their possible biological significance. Cancer Immunol Immunother 4: 215-221
Lotzová E, Savary CA (1977) Possible involvement of natural killer cells in bone marrow graft rejection. Biomedicine 27: 341-344
Lotzová E, Savary CA (1984) Stimulation of NK cell cytotoxic potential of normal donors by two species of recombinant alpha interferon. J Interferon Res 4: 201-213
Lotzová E, Savary CA (1986) Regulation of NK cell cytotoxicity by suppressor cells. In: Lotzová E, Herberman RB (eds) Immunobiology of natural killer cells, vol 2 (10). CRC, Boca Raton, pp 163-177
Lotzová E, Savary CA (1987) Generation of NK cell activity from human bone marrow. J Immunol 139: 279-284
Lotzová E, Savary CA (1989a) Function of interleukin-2 activated NK cells in leukemia resistance and treatment. In: Lotzová E (ed) Role interleukin-2 activated killer cells in cancer. CRC, Boca Raton (in press)
Lotzová E, Savary CA (1989b) Growth kinetics, function and characterization of lymphocytes infiltrating ovarian tumors. In: Lotzová E (ed) role interleukin-2 activated killer cells in cancer. CRC, Boca Raton (in press)
Lotzová E, McCredie KB, Muesse L, Dicke KA, Freireich EJ (1979) Natural killer cells in man: their possible involvement in leukemia and bone marrow transplantation. In: Baum SJ, Ledney GD (eds) Experimental hematology today. Springer, Berlin Heidelberg New York, pp 207-213
Lotzová E, Savary CA, Pollack SB (1983) Prevention of rejection of allogeneic bone marrow transplants by NK 1.1 antiserum. Transplantation 35: 490-494
Lotzová E, Savary CA, Keating MJ, Hester JP (1985) Defective NK cell mechanism in patients with leukemia. In: Herberman RB (ed) Mechanism for cytotoxicity by NK cells. Academic, New York, pp 507-519
Lotzová E, Savary CA, Pollack S, Hanna N (1986) Induction of tumor immunity and natural killer cell cytotoxicity by 5-halo-6-phenyl pyrimidinones. Cancer Res 46: 5004-5008
Lotzová E, Savary CA, Freedman RS, Bowen JM (1987a) Natural killer cell antitumor activity in patients with ovarian carcinoma: induction of cytotoxicity by viral oncolysates and interleukin-2. In: Rutledge FM, Freedman RS, Gershenson DM (eds) Diagnosis and treatment strategies for gynecological cancer. University of Texas Press, Austin, pp 123-136
Lotzová E, Savary CA, Herberman RB (1987b) Induction of NK cell activity against fresh human leukemia in culture with interleukin-2. J Immunol 138: 2718-2727
Lotzová E, Savary CA, Dicke KA, Jagannath S (1988) Role of NK cells in tumor cell growth and eradication. In: Baum SJ, Dicke K, Lotzová E, Pluznik DH (eds) Experimental hematology today - 1988). Springer, Berlin Heidelberg New York, pp 15-19
Maximow AA, Bloom W (1947) A textbook of histology, 4th edn. Saunders, Philadelphia, pp 43-45
Pollack SB (1982) Direct evidence for anti-tumor activity by NK cells in vivo: growth of bl6 melanoma in NK 1.1-treated mice. In: Herberman RB (ed) NK cells and other effector cells. Academic, New York, pp 1347-1352
Roder JC, Haliotis T, Klein M, Korec S, Jett JR, Ortaldo J, Herberman RB, Katz P, Fauci AS (1980) A new immunodeficiency disorder in humans involving NK cells. Nature 284: 553-555
Rosenberg EB, McCoy JL, Green SS, Donnelly FC, Siwarski DF, Levine PH, Herberman RB (1974) Destruction of human lymphoid tissue culture cell lines by human peripheral lymphocytes in ^{51}Cr release culture cytotoxicity assays. JNCI 52: 345-353

Rosenberg SA, Lotze MT, Muul LM, Leitman S, Chang AE, Ettinghausen SE, Matory YL, Skibber JM, Shiloni E, Vetto JT, Seipp CA, Simpson C, Reichert M (1985) Special report: observations on the systemic administration of autologous lymphokine-activated killer cells and recombinant interleukin-2 to patients with metastatic cancer. N Engl J Med 23: 1485-1492

Savary CA, Lotzová E (1978) Suppression of natural killer cell cytotoxicity by splenocytes from Corynebacterium parvum-injected, bone marrow-tolerant and infant mice. J Immunol 120: 239-243

Savary CA, Lotzová E (1987) Mechanism of decline of NK cell activity in *Corynebacterium parvum* treated mice: inhibition by erythroblasts and Thyl.2 lymphocytes. JNCI 79: 533-541

Scala G, Djeu JY, Allavena P, Kasahara T, Ortaldo JR, Herberman RB, Oppenheim JJ (1986) Cytokine secretion and noncytotoxic functions of human large granular lymphocytes. In: Lotzová E, Herberman RB (eds) Immunobiology of natural killer cells. CRC, Boca Raton, pp 133-144

Skibber JM, Lotze MT, Muul LM, Uppenkamp K, Ross W, Rosenberg SA (1987) Human lymphokine-activated killer cells: further isolation and characterization of the precursor and effector cell. Nat Immun Cell Growth Regul 6: 291-305

Topalian SL, Solomon D, Avis FP, Chang AE, Freerksen DL, Linehan WM, Lotze MT, Robertson CN, Seipp CA, Simon P, Simpson CG, Rosenberg SA (1988) Immunotherapy of patients with advanced cancer using tumor-infiltrating lymphocytes and recombinant interleukin-2: a pilot study. J Clin Onocol 6: 839-853

Trinchieri G, Matsumoto-Kobayashi M, Clark SC, Seehra J, London L, Perussia B (1984) Response of resting human peripheral blood natural killer cells to interleukin-2. J Exp Med 160: 1147-1169

Vujanovic JD (1988) Lymphokine activated killer cells in rats. III. A simple method for the purification of large granular lymphocytes and their rapid expansion and conversion into lymphokine-activated killer cells. J Exp Med 167: 15-29

Welsh RM (1986) Regulation of virus infections by natural killer cells. A review. Nat Immun Cell Growth Regul 5: 169-199

Allergy to Drugs and Other Chemicals Diagnosed by the Presence of Specific Memory Cells in Human Blood

D. M. V. Stejskal

Introduction

The personality of Professor Milan Hašek greatly contributed to the fact that immunology became a discipline of choice for my university specialization in biology. During 5 years of university studies in biology and chemistry at Charles University in Prague, I worked at Hašek's institute, first as a research assistant, and later on a thesis dealing with antibody production and induction of immunological memory to protein antigens in chickens (Valentova et al. 1966, 1967). This study won the first prize in a competition for the best student scientific work in biology in 1967 and introduced me into a highly qualified immunological society concentrated around Milan at the Institute of Experimental Biology and Genetics (IEBG) at the Czechoslovakian Academy of Sciences in Prague. It is one of the strange coincidences of life that the work summarized in this article deals with the cells carrying immunological memory, this time against drugs and other chemicals in man.

After leaving Czechoslovakia in August 1968, I was given the opportunity to continue my immunological studies at Professor Peter Perlmann's laboratory in Stockholm. During the years 1969–1977 I was drilled in cellular immunology, spending most of my time studying interactions between cytotoxic effector cells and target cells in mouse and man (Stejskal and Perlmann 1976; Stejskal et al. 1973a, b, 1974). In May 1977, I became responsible for building up the immunotoxicology section at Safety Assessment, AB Astra in Södertälje.

During the years 1978–1980 I became aware of occupational hypersensitivity problems in workers handling drugs in pharmaceutical production. As a cellular immunologist, I started to explore the possibility of searching for the presence of drug-specific memory lymphocytes as indicators of drug allergy. The lymphocyte transformation test (LTT) has been used by others for the study of drug allergy in therapeutically treated patients but there were no data available on the use of this test for detection of occupational allergy.

According to general knowledge, all types of immunological reactions start by the induction of sensitized memory T cells with the help of accessory cells such as monocytes and dendritic cells. The role of T lymphocytes in delayed hypersensitivity reactions has been recognized for a long time. Since allergen-specific T lymphocytes also regulate the proliferation of B cells and thus, indirectly, control allergen-specific IgE synthesis, such T cells ought to be present also in patients with immediate hypersensitivity. Hence, LTT could be used to reveal drug allergy in individuals with all types of clinical hypersensitivity.

It is generally recognized that the frequency of antigen-specific lymphocytes is approximately one cell per 100.000 lymphocytes. The successful detection of drug-specific lymphocytes depends on the "cloning" of a few drug-specific lymphocytes with the help of a relevant drug during the 5-day incubation period in vitro.

Under optimal culture conditions, the drug-specific lymphocytes will proliferate, and a significant number of blast cells can be detected in the 5-day cultures. In 1981 we began to establish the conditions necessary to make LTT reproducible and sensitive enough to detect low numbers of drug-specific memory cells. We soon observed that drug-specific lymphoblasts were present in the cultures of subjects with drug-induced hypersensitivity but not in similarly exposed healthy individuals, thus confirming the results of other studies performed on healthy drug-treated patients (Blom et al. 1985; Dewdney 1977; Olive et al. 1980). As reported by Dewdney (1977), a review of the literature suggests that lymphocyte activation correlates, rather better than might have been anticipated, with a state of clinical hypersensitivity. Under these conditions, LTT could be used for the diagnosis of drug allergy.

Table 1. Patients studied by LTT and other established clinical tests during 1981–1988

Patients participating in the study	Clinics responsible for administration/clinical evaluation of patients	Responsible medical personnel
Workers with occupational hypersensitivity to penicillins and other drugs	The Occupational Health Services, AB Astra, Södertälje	H. Freyman, MD R. Olin, MD M. Westberg, nurse
	The Dermatology Clinics, Södersjukhuset, Stockholm	M. Forsbeck, MD
Workers with asthma induced by formaldehyde and chloramine-T	Dept. of Occupational Medicine, Regional Hospital, Linköping	B. Persson, MD
	Dept. of Occupational Medicine, Regional Hospital, Örebro	A. Blomqvist, MD
Nurses with isphagula (psyllium)-induced hypersensitivity	Dept. of Lung Medicine, University Hospital, Uppsala	G. Stålenheim, MD
Patients with dermatitis exhibiting a positive patch test to formaldehyde or isothiazolones	The Dermatology Clinics, Södersjukhuset, Stockholm	M. Forsbeck, MD
Patients with hypersensitivity reactions observed in connection with penicillin therapy	Dept. of allergology, Huddinge Hospital	P. Broman, MD K. Sundell, nurse
	The Institute for Infectious Diseases, Roslagtulls Hospital, Stockholm	L. Lindqvist, MD

Table 2. Allergenic potential of drugs and other chemicals as studied by LTT in vitro

Chemical[a]	Route of exposure	Symptoms	Memory cells in the blood of exposed symptomatic individuals[b]		Other confirmative clinical or in vitro tests (skin test[c], RAST, provocation)
			LTT positive = allergy	LTT negative = pseudoallergy	
Acetylcysteine	Occupational	Conjunctivitis and rhinitis	x		Patch test weakly positive
Azidocillin, bacampicillin, cloxacillin, and flucloxacillin	Occupational	Dermatitis, conjunctivitis, and rhinitis	x	x	Skin test sometimes positive, provocation positive, RAST not available
Alprenolol, clomethiazole, quinidine, terbutaline, and zimelidine	Occupational	Dermatitis	x	x	Skin test mostly positive
Metoprolol	Occupational	Rhinitis		x	Skin test negative
Alprenolol and Metoprolol epoxide	Occupational	Dermatitis	x	x	Skin test positive (test is contraindicated due to strong risk of sensitization)
Isphagula (psyllium)	Occupational	Asthma, conjunctivitis, and rhinitis		x	In LTT positive; skin, RAST, and provocation tests positive. In LTT negative; skin test and provocation negative
Chloramine-T	Occupational	Asthma	x	x	In LTT positive; skin test and provocation positive
Formaldehyde	Occupational	Asthma	x	x	Skin test negative, provocation positive
Formaldehyde	Environmental	Dermatitis	x	x	Skin test positive[d]
Isothiazolones	Environmental	Dermatitis	x	x	Skin test positive[d], provocation seldom positive[e]
Benzylpenicillin and phenoxymethylpenicillin	Therapeutic	Anaphylactic shock, urticaria	x	x	Skin test mostly negative. 2 LTT positive cases were positive by provocation. LTT negative cases were provocation negative. LTT positive cases were often RAST positive
Streptomycin	Therapeutic	Dermatitis, Quincke's oedema	x		Skin test positive
Sulfamethoxypyridazine	Therapeutic	Urticaria	x		Not done

[a] LTT with these chemicals is negative in similarly exposed healthy individuals (they do not have chemical-specific memory lymphocytes). Hence, LTT can be used as a tool for the diagnosis of chemical-induced allergy.
[b] The presence of chemical-specific memory-cells in the blood of hypersensitive individuals is taken as evidence of specific allergy. The absence of such memory cells in clinically ill patients suggests a pseudoallergic nature of hypersensitivity.
[c] Unless otherwise indicated, patch tests were performed on patients with dermatitis and prick test on patients with immediate hypersensitivity symptoms.
[d] In LTT positive patients, positive patch tests confirm allergy. In LTT negative patients positive patch tests indicate to tie effects of chemicals on the skin.
[e] LTT positive patients respond to isothiazolones containing lotion. LTT negative patients are provocation negative

Results and Comments

Blood samples from patients exhibiting various hypersensitive symptoms following drug or clinical exposure were obtained through the cooperation with several highly merited clinics where all clinical tests such as skin tests and provocation tests were performed (Table 1). Since the amount of scientific effort necessary to summarize clinical and laboratory data was considerable, only part of the data have previously been published (Stejskal et al. 1986, 1987). The results are summarized in Table 2.

Penicillins

As previously published (Stejskal et al. 1986, 1987), occupational exposure to penicillins induces hypersensitivity reactions in some of the exposed workers. Bacampicillin was a major offending agent while phenoxymethylpenicillin (PcV) was virtually devoid of allergenic potential. Lymphocyte proliferative responses were side chain specific as shown in Table 3. Thus, a 26-year-old male pharmacist started to

Table 3. LTT with various penicillins in worker suffering from occupational rhinitis due to penicillin dust

Penicillin in culture	Structure	Concentration[a] (µg/ml)	Lymphocyte transformation test[b]		
			Δ cpm	SI	Blasts
Cloxa-cillin		200	5916	14	> 100
Flucloxa-cillin		100	8748	21	> 100
Bacampi-cillin		100	9160	22	> 100
Phenoxy-methyl-penicillin		300	772	1.8	7

[a] A wide range of concentrations has been used (6–300 µg) and the maximal responses at an optimal dose are shown.
[b] Lymphocyte proliferation is expressed by mean Δ cpm and by stimulation index (SI). The number of blast cells per cell smear is also shown. Mean cpm incorporated by control lymphocytes was 416.

Table 4. Lymphocyte proliferation to penicillins and formaldehyde in worker suffering from rhinitis and eczema induced by bacampicillin dust

Drug in culture	Concentration (µg/ml)	Lymphocyte transformation test[a]		
		Δ cpm	SI	Blasts (%)
Bacampicillin	4	7317	1.1	2
	20	20533	3.1	11
	100	17855	3.7	6
Benzylpenicillin	4	−899	0.9	1
	20	1735	1.3	0
	100	6814	2	3
Formaldehyde	0.5	−3739	0.4	0
	1	−3303	0.5	0
	2	−2438	0.6	0
	4	−4040	0.4	0
	40	−6101	0.1	0

[a] Lymphocyte proliferation is expressed as mean Δ cpm or as stimulation index (SI). Increased incorporation by control lymphocytes indicates spontaneous blastogenesis (mean cpm = 6583). Penicillin-specific lymphoblasts in 5-day cultures are also shown. Control cultures contained around 3% of lymphoblasts (subtracted).

work with penicillin powder in a pharmaceutical laboratory and developed rhinitis and conjunctivitis a few months later. His lymphocytes proliferated to flucloxacillin and bacampicillin but not to PcV. Positive LTT was also observed with cloxacillin, a penicillin structurally similar to flucloxacillin. This worker had not been exposed to cloxacillin previously. Therefore, the proliferative response to cloxacillin is an example of immunological cross-reaction at the cellular level.

A 23-year-old operator had noted rhinitis and eczema on the face, neck, and arms following a 4-week period of work in bacampicillin production in March 1985. LTT was performed in late March during the acute illnes period (Table 4). The patient's lymphocytes responded strongly to bacampicillin, but weakly to benzylpenicillin. No proliferation was observed with formaldehyde, another chemical suspected by the patient. Patch and prick tests, performed in May 1988, gave negative results. The patient was relocated to a bacampicillin-free part of the factory and has been symptom free since then.

In another experiment, lymphocytes from this particular patient were separated to T and non-T cell fractions by rosetting with sheep red blood cells (SRBC). Since human T cells have receptors for SRBC, they can be separated from non-rosetting non-T cells on a density gradient (Fig. 1). Bacampicillin-specific proliferation was obtained with T cells containing SRBC-rosetting fraction but not with nonrosetting non-T cells. Thus, bacampicillin-specific lymphocytes belong to the T cell category.

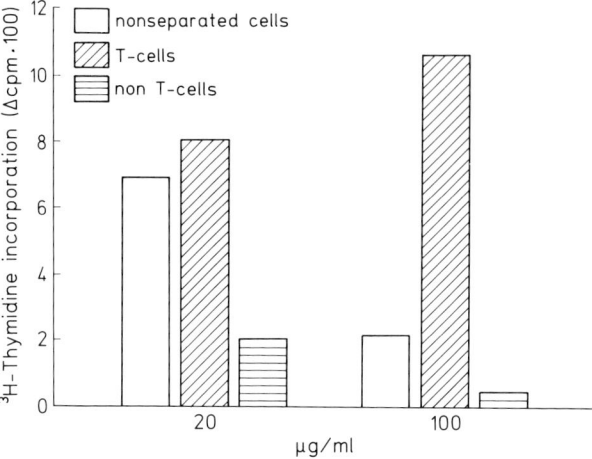

Fig. 1. T cells respond to bacampicillin in vitro. Lymphocytes were separated into T and non-T cell fractions by rosetting with SRBC followed by separation of Ficoll gradient

Nonpenicillin Drugs

Several other drugs induced occupational hypersensitivity in workers exposed to drug dust. A 38-year-old male dragée controller noted the appearance of eczema on his hands in 1975. At that time, he was handling many drugs such as clomethiazole, quinidine, and metoprolol every day. A patch test performed in 1978 was positive to alprenolol and clomethiazole, but negative to quinidine and metoprolol. The patient was then transfered to another job outside drug production, and his eczema cleared. LTT was performed in 1983 and showed the presence of alprenolol-, quinidine- and clomethiazole-specific lymphocytes in the patient's blood (Fig. 2). At this time, a new patch test was made with relevant substances and shown negative. Thus, drug-specific memory lymphocytes circulate in the blood of sensitized subjects long after the sensitization period and may thus be used for allergy diagnosis despite a negative patch test. The greater sensitivity of LTT as compared to the patch test has been described previously (Stejskal et al. 1986).

A 21-year-old process operator developed eczema on the hands after handling terbutaline for several months. The allergic nature of dermatitis was established by terbutaline-positive lymphocyte proliferation (Fig. 3) and by a positive patch test. Since terbutaline is a racemate of two optically active forms (+) and (−), we were curious about the capacity of these isomers to induce terbutaline-specific memory cells (Table 5). The (−)isomer stimulated lymphocytes more vigorously as an original racemate while (+)isomer was not stimulatory. Interestingly, the (−)isomer was found to be about 200 times more potent than the (+)isomer when pharmacological effects of terbutaline were studied in guinea pigs (Wetterlin 1972). Terbutaline-specific lymphocytes were activated with orciprenaline and fenoterol, but no proliferation was observed with salbutamol and isoprenaline. Thus, this experiment indicates the potential of LTT as a tool for the study of allergenic epitopes in

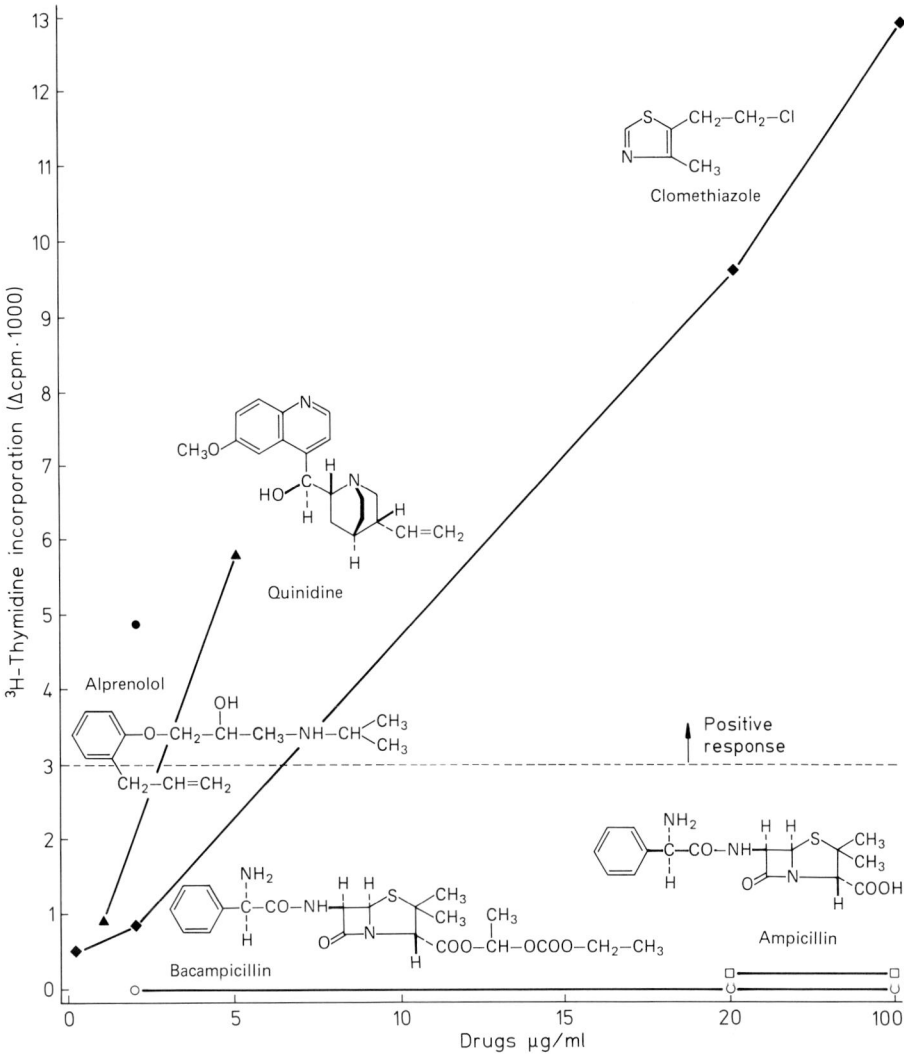

Fig. 2. Lymphocyte proliferation to various drugs in worker with dermatitis induced by drug dust

drug molecules. An increasing knowledge in this field may help to develop safer drugs, devoid of allergic side effects, in the future.

A 38-year-old male process operator, noted the appearance of eczema on the abdomen in connection with the production of zimelidine base in 1982. He then avoided zimelidine and started to work with other drugs such as alprenolol, metoprolol, and clomethiazole. In August 1983, his eczema reappeared, this time on his face, hands, neck, and arms. A patch test for the suspected drugs was performed in October the same year. The patch test was negative with metoprolol, alprenolol, and clomethiazole.

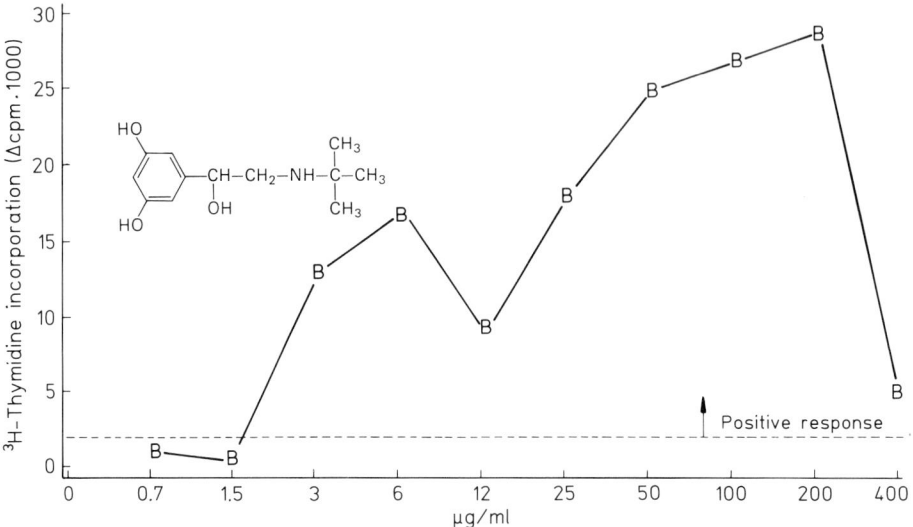

Fig. 3. Lymphocyte proliferation to terbutaline in worker with dermatitis due to terbutaline dust. Patch test weakly positive

Since the patient suspected that his symptoms were connected with his work in metoprolol production, we performed LTT with a pre-stage to metoprolol base, a metoprolol epoxide, and with other drugs (Table 6). Metoprolol epoxide-specific and zimelidine-specific lymphocytes confirmed the occupationally induced dermatitis of the patient. Patch testing with metoprolol epoxide was not performed since there is a definite risk of sensitization by an application of this chemically reactive substance on human skin.

Some of the workers complained about rhinitis and conjunctivitis while working with metoprolol. In recent years the volume of metoprolol production has largely exceeded that of alprenolol. However, until now, we have not been able to detect any metoprolol-specific memory cells in symptomatic workers. Thus, metoprolol-induced symptoms are irritative rather than allergenic in nature, a fact which is confirmed by notoriously negative patch tests.

Formaldehyde

Another example of a chemically reactive substance which often causes hypersensitivity symptoms such as dermatitis or asthma is formaldehyde. Inhalation of formaldehyde by workers using formaldehyde-releasing paints results in occupationally induced asthma. Under other conditions, formaldehyde used ubiquitously as a preservative and disinfectant may cause dermatitis in susceptible individuals. During the years 1983-1988 we tested 15 patients with chronic dermatitis who exhibited positive patch test results to formaline (1% solution of formaldehyde in water). LTT was positive in about half of these patients. A representative experiment is shown in Fig. 4. In November 1986 a female patient noted eczema on the

Table 5. Lymphocyte proliferation to terbutaline and to other structurally related substances in worker with occupational dermatitis due to terbutaline dust

Antigen in culture	Structure	Lymphocyte transformation test[a]		
		µg/ml	Δ cpm	SI
Terbutaline sulfate (racemate)		200	1009	4.4
Terbutaline hydrobromide (+)		200	121	1.4
Terbutaline hydrobromide (−)		200	3835	14
Orciprenaline sulfate		100	1210	5
Fenoterol hydrobromide		6	461	2.5
Salbutamol sulfate		100	−85	0.7
Isoprenaline sulfate		6	57	1.1

[a] The lymphocyte responses were tested over a wide range (1–400 µg/ml) and the maximal responses at an optimal dose are shown. For further explanations see Table 2. Mean cpm incorporated by control of lymphocytes was 299.

back, abdomen, shoulders, arms, and hands after using floorpolish at home in November 1986. The patch test, performed in December 1986, was positive to formaldehyde. LTT, performed in May 1988, demonstrated the presence of formaldehyde-specific memory lymphocytes in her blood. The proliferation was not induced by the toxic effects of the chemical on lymphocyte membranes since acrolein, added to lymphocytes instead of formaldehyde, did not induce lymphocyte proliferation. Formaldehyde-specific proliferation was not observed in a group of 13 painters exposed to formaldehyde-releasing hardeners and suffering from formaldehyde-induced asthma. The painters showed negative results in the formaldehyde prick test. The LTT and skin test results indicate that formaldehyde-induced asthma is caused by irritative (toxic), rather than allergenic, properties of formaldehyde (V. Stejskal, M. Forsbeck, B. Persson, manuscript in preparation).

Table 6. Lymphocyte proliferation to various drugs in worker suffering from occupational dermatitis

Drug in culture	Structure	Concentration[a] (µg/ml)	Lymphocyte transformation test[b]		
			cpm ± SD	SI	Blasts (%)
Alprenolol	(structure)	2, 20, 100	2180 ± 326	1.4	0
Alprenolol epoxide	(structure)	1, 5, *20*, 100, 400	1620 ± 378	1	0
Metoprolol	(structure)	0.04, 0.2, *2*, 5, 20	2245 ± 85	1.4	0
Metoprolol epoxide	(structure)	0.7, *3*, 11, 43	17679 ± 435	11	7
Zimelidine	(structure)	0.1, 1, *10*, 25	6997 ± 284	4.4	3

[a] Concentrations giving maximal proliferative responses are underlined.
[b] Lymphocyte proliferation is expressed as mean cpm ± SD or as stimulation index (SI). Control cpm = 1608 ± 218. Lymphoblasts in 5-day cultures are also shown.

Last but not least, we have elaborated LTT for diagnosis of drug allergy in connection with therapeutic drug treatment. It is common experience that, in some patients with clinical symptoms, drug-specific lymphocytes can be demonstrated, while similarly treated patients without hypersensitive symptoms lack such lymphocytes (Blom et al. 1985; Dewdney 1977; Olive et al. 1980). In apparent paradox to these findings, penicilloyl-specific IgM and IgG antibodies have previously been shown in the majority of penicillin-exposed subjects and even in those who denied ever having penicillin therapy (Weiss and Adkinson 1988). Furthermore,

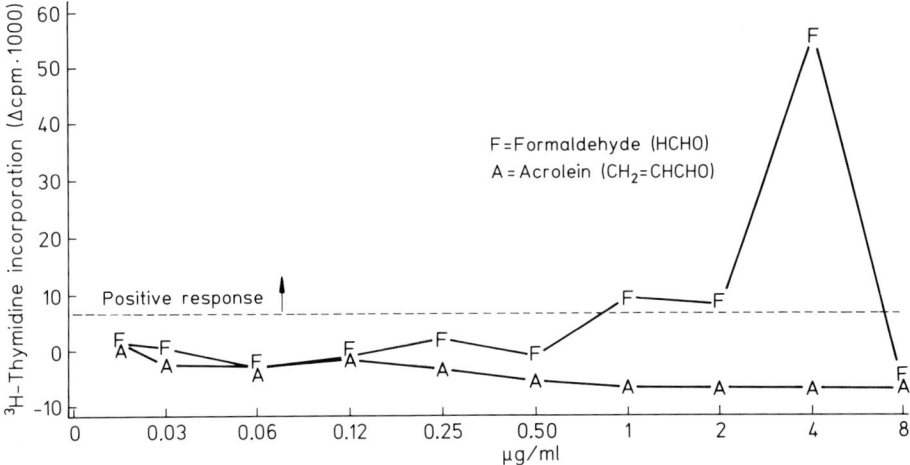

Fig. 4. Lymphocyte proliferation to formaldehyde in patient with eczema induced by floorpolish

the presence of penicilloyl-specific IgM and IgG antibodies did not correlate with the status of clinical hypersensitivity (Dewdney 1977; Lee et al. 1986). The absence of penicillin-specific memory cells in patients with penicilloyl-specific antibodies could be explained if T memory cells responded preferentially to penicillin side chains while antibody-producing B cells recognized mainly penicilloyl determinant. Therefore, we conjugated PcV and benzylpenicillin (PcG) to a nonimmunogenic peptide carrier, poly-L-lysine (PLL), thus artificially creating conjugates with penicilloyl determinant. Both forms of penicillins, conjugated and unconjugated (tentatively called penicillin hapten), were used in LTT.

PcG- and PcV-specific lymphocytes were present in the blood of several patients suffering from anaphylactic shock and/or urticaria after penicillin treatment but not in penicillin-treated symptom-free patients. Positive lymphocyte responses to penicillin haptens agreed remarkably well with the presence of penicillin-specific IgE antibodies as detected in the radio-allergosorbent test (RAST). PcG- and PcV-specific lymphocytes of allergic patients did not cross-react with aminobenzylpenicillins such as bacampicillin or ampicillin. The similar penicillin side chain specificity has been described above (Table 3) and reported previously in workers with occupational hypersensitivity (Stejskal et al. 1986, 1987).

In contrast, lymphocytes from healthy subjects exposed therapeutically or occupationally to penicillins proliferated to penicilloyl-PLL conjugates but not to unconjugated penicillins. Lymphocytes responses to conjugated penicillins lacked side chain specificity and apparently reflected the immunization of subjects with penicillin rather than an allergy.

Taken together, the results in therapeutically treated patients confirmed those obtained in occupationally exposed workers (Stejskal et al. 1986, 1987). Memory cells from allergic subjects respond to penicillin haptens in vitro by side chain-specific proliferative responses. In contrast, covalent binding of penicillin to the protein carrier is necessary for activation of penicilloyl-specific memory cells in healthy immunized subjects. Two patients positive to penicillin haptens in LTT accidentally took the relevant penicillin tablets which resulted in anaphylactic shock. The provocation of six PcV-LTT-negative and PcV-RAST-negative patients with PcV tablets was negative, which indicates the clinical relevance of LTT data. The results of this study will be published in detail in the near future (V.Stejskal, K. Berglund, P. Broman, K. Sundell, L. Lindkuist, manuscript in preparation).

Summary

In summary, after 10 years of experience with LTT, it is my firm belief that it can be used in the diagnosis of allergy in patients with hypersensitivity induced by drugs and other chemicals. Furthermore, it can also be used for the evaluation of allergenic potential of a wide range of chemical substances in humans. The increasing knowledge about the configuration of allergenic epitopes in various chemicals will lead to a better immunotoxic evaluation of new drugs in preclinical and clinical trials and hopefully in avoidance of drug-induced allergic side effects in humans.

Last but not least, the study of cellular mechanisms underlying allergic reactions to low molecular chemicals will result in a better understanding of the allergy phenomenon, which may result in more efficient allergy treatment and finally in the eradication of allergic diseases.

I would like to finish by remembering the last meeting with Milan in spring 1969. He was visiting Peter Perlmann in Stockholm and said to me, "Vera, as long as I am the director of UEBG, the doors of our institute are always open to you." A few weeks later he returned home to find he had lost his position as head of the UEBG. You know, Milan, if I had returned to Prague there would not have been any "rendezvous" with LTT in Södertälje.

Acknowledgements. I thank Prof. Lars Ekman, DVM, head of Safety Assessment, AB Astra, and Jan Larsson, MSc, director of Astra Pharmaceutical Production AB, who have sponsored the LTT project from its very beginning, as well as Civ.ing. Charlotte af Malmborg, director of the Biotechnology Department at The Swedish National Board for Technical Development, who has kindly supported the exploration of LTT for allergy diagnosis in drug-treated patients. We are indebted to the National Chemicals Inspectorate for their support in the project dealing with the use of LTT for the diagnosis of chemical-induced allergy. At the laboratory many people have "tamed" LTT to perform according to our needs. Among others, Karin Berglund, BSc, Nongit Lewin, PhD, and Barbro Emanuelsson have performed LTT with enthusiasm and skill. Last but not least, we are grateful for the assistance of Juhani Weber and Irene Olsén in preparing the manuscript.

References

Blom H, Stolk J, Schreuder HB, von Blomberg-van der Flier M (1985) A case of carbimazole-induced intrahepatic cholestasis: an immune-mediated reaction? Arch Intern Med 145: 1513–1515

Dewdney JM (1977) Immunology of the antibiotics. In: Sela M (ed) The antigens, vol 4. Academic, New York pp 73–245

Lee D, Dewdney JM, Edwards RG, Neftel KA, Wälti M (1986) Measurement of specific IgG antibody levels in serum of patients on regimes comprising high total dose beta-lactam therapy. Int Arch Allergy Appl Immunol 79: 344–348

Olive A, Huguet J, Vich JM, Garcia-Calderon JV, Carcia-Calderon PA (1980) Allergy to penicillin. Comparison of "in vivo" and "in vitro" tests. Allergol Immunopathol 8: 104–111

Stejskal V, Perlmann P (1976) Differential cytotoxicity of activated lymphocytes on allogeneic and xenogeneic target cells. III. Species-specificity of lymphocyte-target cell recognition in vitro. Eur J Immunol 6: 347–352

Stejskal V, Holm G, Perlmann P (1973a) Differential cytotoxicity of activated lymphocytes on allogeneic and xenogeneic target cells. I. Activation by tuberculin and by staphylococcus filtrate. Cellul Immunol 8: 71–81

Stejskal V, Lindberg S, Holm G, Perlmann P (1973b) Differential cytotoxicity of activated lymphocytes on allogeneic and xenogeneic target cells. II. Activation by phytohemagglutinin. Cellul Immunol 8: 82–92

Stejskal V, Härfast B, Holm G, Perlmann P (1974) Cytotoxicity of human lymphocytes induced by pokeweed mitogen or in mixed lymphocyte culture. Specificity and nature of effector cells. Eur J Immunol 4: 126–130

Stejskal V, Olin R, Forsbeck M (1986) The use of lymphocyte transformation test for diagnosis of drug-induced occupational allergy. J Allergy Clin Immunol 77: 411–426

Stejskal V, Forsbeck M, Olin R (1987) Side chain-specific lymphocyte responses in workers with occupational allergy induced by penicillins. Int Arch Allergy Appl Immunol 82: 461–464

Valentova V, Cerny J, Ivanyi J (1966) The characterization of the immunological memory of the IgM type of response in chickens. Folia Biol (Praha) 12: 207–210

Valentova V, Cerny J, Ivanyi J (1967) Immunological memory of IgM and IgG type antibodies. I. Requirements of antigen dose for induction and of time for developement of memory. Folia Biol (Praha) 13: 100–108

Weiss ME, Adkinson NF (1988) Immediate hypersensitivity reactions to penicillin and related antibiotics. Clin Allergy 18: 515–540

Wetterlin K (1972) Resolution of terbutaline, a new sympathomimethic amine. J Med Chem 15: 1182–1183

Contribution of Cytogenetics to Cancer Research: Endometrial Adenocarcinoma

D. Simon

General Introduction

After many decades of speculation that cancer may be initiated by a change in the genetic make up of somatic cells, an idea first introduced by Boveri 1914, we are finally obtaining evidence to support this hypothesis. Cancer cytogenetics has definitely contributed to the discoveries of the past few decades since the original description of the human karyotype (Tjio and Levan 1956). Much progress has been made in the area of hematopoietic tumors. This was originally initiated by Nowell and Hungerford (1960) who carried out cytogenetic studies on chronic myelogenous leukemia (CML) and who first described chromosome abnormality in association with human malignancy. This abnormality, the so-called Ph chromosome, a deletion of a G group chromosome, was later specified as t(9,22). For a long time CML was associated with the Ph chromosome, with no understanding of the biological meaning, but the focus of research on this particular part of the genome has brought better understanding of which particular genes we are dealing with and what is happening at the molecular level. The *abl* proto-oncogene which maps on chromosome 9 is translocated to the site of an unknown gene on chromosome 22; and, by its translocation, a new fusion gene is created which leads to a chimeric protein with high tyrosine kinase activity.

The association of specific chromosome rearrangements with a particular malignancy was a very important step to help focus on certain parts of the genome. This has led to molecular analyses, and the whole picture of the original chromosomal rearrangement begins to be much more meaningful. A classic example is Burkitt's lymphoma, a B cell malignancy, where the original description of the abnormality of chromosome 14 (Manolov and Manolova 1972) initiated a surge in studies of that part of the genome. Today we know that the majority of cases of Burkitt's lymphoma involve the reciprocal translocation of chromosomes 8 and 14, t(8,14), in the region of *myc* proto-oncogene on chromosome 8 and the immunoglobulin heavy chain gene on chromosome 14 (Croce et al. 1987). In the variant translocation chromosome 8,22, t(8,22), and chromosome 8,2, t(8,2), are involved where, instead of the immunoglobulin heavy chain, the light chain is the target site for abnormal joining with *myc*.

CML and Burkitt's lymphoma are the best understood examples of hematopoietic malignancies, first associated with specific chromosome abnormalities. These have led to research focused on particular regions of the genome and finally to a better understanding, at the molecular level, of how rearrangements may alter gene expression. Certain silent genes, after transposition to an actively transcribed site, undergo altered gene expression which results in abnormal proliferation and growth. This alteration of transcription by changes in gene position is not the only known mechanism involved in cellular transformation which leads to malignancies.

In 1971 Knudson introduced a different theory based on the observations in retinoblastoma. This malignancy occurs in two different forms: inherited and sporadic, and it was associated at first with a specific chromosome deletion in 13q14, (Yunis and Ramsay 1978). Knudson proposed the existence of "suppressor genes" involved in cell proliferation and suggested that the loss of both alleles from the same locus leads to uncontrolled proliferation, resulting in retinoblastoma (Knudson 1971, 1986). This theory has been fully confirmed by molecular analysis in the past few years (Cavenee et al. 1985). The loss of heterozygosity in the *rb-1* locus is critical for the development of this tumor. The same mechanism appears to be the case in Wilms' tumor (11p13) and in some adult solid tumors as well, for example, renal carcinoma (3p14) and colon cancer (5q22).

In many solid tumors the situation is far more complex, and much research remains to be done to reach a full understanding. Therefore the focus and interest concerning chromosome abnormalities in solid tumors is more urgent today than ever before. Cytogenetics is a valuable adjunct to other biomedical disciplines in the efforts to solve the puzzle of cancer.

Our Study

In our study we focused on one of the most common gynecological malignancies in the United States, endometrial adenocarcinoma (EC), a malignant proliferation of the glandular epithelial lining of the uterus. Adenocarcinoma of the endometrium predominantly affects postmenopausal women, and the most affected age is 50-60. It is a life-threatening disease, and the only successful surgery is at the early stages of the neoplasm. There are several factors associated with EC, the high risks including obesity and diabetes. Prolonged exogenous estrogen stimulation is believed to be the determining factor which contributes directly to endometrial hyperplasia, finally leading to the development of adenocarcinoma (Gusberg and Frick 1978; Gambrell et al. 1983). The actual causes of cellular transformation from normal secretory epithelial cells to uncontrolled proliferation of invasive adenocarcinoma are not known. So far there are several reports of cytogenetic studies attempting to relate specific chromosome rearrangements in EC to malignancy (Table 1). Unfortunately, there is no clearcut answer. The presence of an abnormality in chromosome 1 has been reported in most of the cases. But this is not recognized as a specific alteration because of its presence in 47.9% of all human malignancies. The molecular data investigating the expression, rearrangement, or amplification of different oncogenes and growth factors have not brought significant new findings.

These earlier reports made us focus on this malignancy with a more complex approach. First, we wanted to determine chromosome abnormalities associated

Table 1. Primary cytogenetic abnormalities in endometrial adenocarcinoma (EA)

Tumor and stage	History of exogenous estrogen treatment	Tissue analyzed	Age (years)	Chromosome range	Modal chromosome number (in 80% of cells)	Chromosomes involved in abberations	Comments	Reference
ND	–	–	–	ND	46XX	1	–	Atkin (1976)
ND	–	–	–	ND	46XX	in D group (13 & 15)	–	Trent and Davis (1979)
EA III	ND	ST	54	ND	46XX	t dic(1,16)	Trisomy 1q	Fujita et al. (1985)
EA IA	ND	ST	57	ND	49XX	i(1q), +2, +10	Trisomy 1q	
EA IB	ND	ST	75	ND	48XX	+1p−, +7	Trisomy 1q	
EA IB	ND	ST	30	ND	47XX	i(1q)	Trisomy 1q	
EA I	ND	ST	60	ND	48XX	+2, +i(1q)	Trisomy 1q	Couturier et al. (1986)
EA I	ND	ST	61	ND	47XX	+10	–	
EA I	ND	ST	62	ND	47XX	+12	–	
EA II	ND	ST	41	ND	46XX	−16, +t(1,16)	Trisomy 1q	
EA II	ND	ST	64	ND	46XX	−21, t(1,21)	Trisomy 1q	
EA II	ND	ST	64	ND	46XX	−21, t(1,21)	Trisomy 1q	
EA IA	ND	ST	60	35–47	ND	t(1,11)	–	Yoshida et al. (1986)
EA IA	ND	Peritoneal fluid	54	44–92	46XX	8p+, q− 12q+, Xp−	Cells with different sizes of minute chromosomes present	Jenkyn and McCartney (1987)
EA IA	⊕	ST	59	ND	48XX	+i(1q), +10	Trisomy 1q	Gibas and Rubin (1987)

ND, not defined; ST, solid tumor.

with this malignancy, looking in direct chromosome preparations for the most representative cytogenetic profile for the tumor. These studies have the potential of establishing an association between the stage and grade of the tumor versus chromosome abnormality. Second, we wanted to perform molecular analyses based on the results of cytogenetic studies, focusing on the region of the genome which was found to be altered. Our long-term goal is to establish cell lines from these original tumors for comparative chromosome studies to confirm the stability or evolution of the given chromosome rearrangements found in direct chromosome preparations. In seven new cases of EC, we report here three cases with an abnormality of chromosome 10. The other four cases show a far more complex rearrangement with very heterogeneous chromosome profiles, probably due to the evolution of a destabilized genome, and these correlate with advanced disease. The simple abnormalities provide direct clues to the primary chromosome changes in a given neoplasia. From this study, we conclude that chromosome 10 is the candidate to become the primary target chromosome for rearrangement in EC, and its role remains to be determined.

Materials and Methods

Tumor specimens were transported on ice within 30 min postoperatively. They were minced mechanically and then digested enzymatically for 1–3 h with a mixture of collagenase and hyaluronidase (Sigma) at 37 °C. Cells were then washed twice with phosphate-buffered saline (PBS) and seeded in culture (a) on an irradiated feeder layer of 3T3 cells; or (b) on a tissue culture dish precoated with 0.5% gelatine. Cultures were grown in RPMI medium (Sigma) with 10% fetal calf serum (FCS) supplemented with 20 g/ml epidermal growth factor (EGF; Sigma).

Chromosome preparations were done within 3, 24, 48, and 72 h postoperatively. From the same specimens some cultures were carried as long-term cultures, pieces of tissue were implanted subcutaneously into nude mice, and the remaining tissue was handled as indicated on the chart showing the experimental strategy (Fig. 1).

Chromosome harvest was performed by standard methods (Simon et al. 1982), using 0.2 g/ml demecolcine for 1–3 h. 0.075 KCl was used as hypotonic solution, and the cells were fixed in methanol:acetic acid (3:1). Conventional slide preparation was followed by a two-step staining process. In the first step, slides were stained in 3% Giemsa. Metaphase spreads were localized and evaluated for morphology and tumor profile in general. In the second step, destained slides underwent banding; G banding with trypsin (GTG) or C banding with Ba(OH) (CBG).

Results

All seven new cases were diagnosed as primary EC, testing positive in vitro for cytokeratins, a typical cytoskeleton marker for epithelial cells (Fig. 2). A survey of the histopathological and cytogenetic findings of all cases is shown in Table 2. Cases 1 and 7 are at the lowest stages of disease by histopathological criteria and

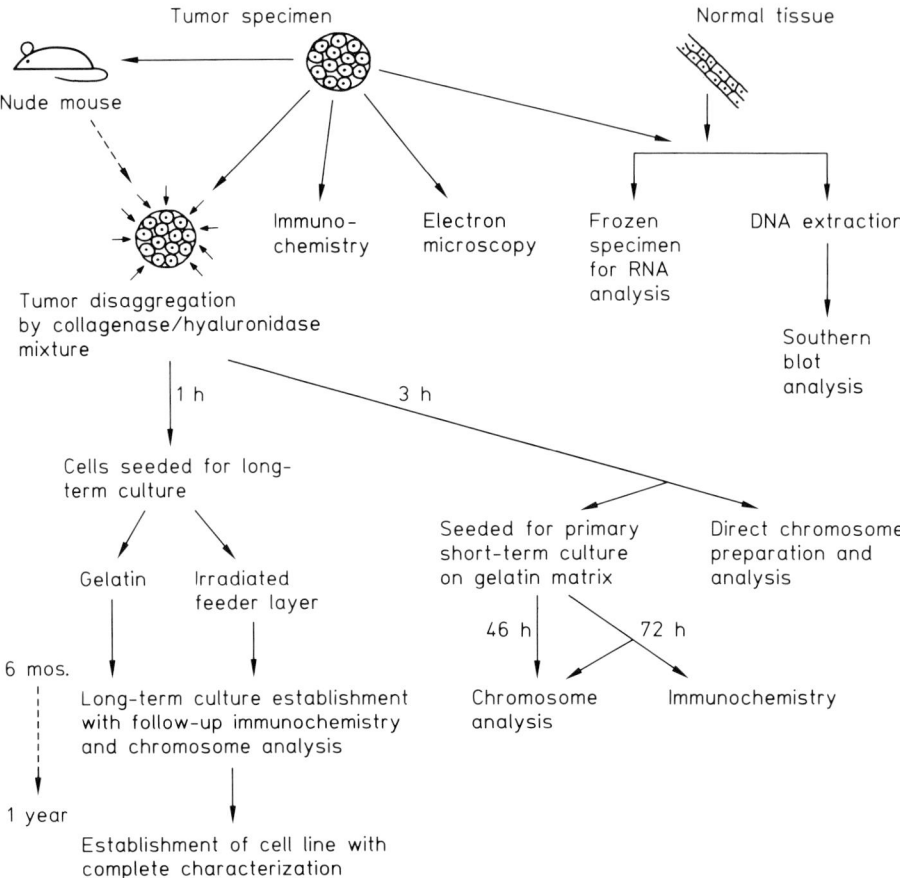

Fig. 1. Experimental strategy for primary tumor handling

they show very minor karyotypical changes. Both tumors fell into the diploid range: case 1, 46 XX, 10p+, with one unbalanced translocation on the short arm of chromosome 10, t(10,?) (p15,?). This was evaluated in different cells as a possibility of t(10,10) (p15,q23), which would make the cell trisomic for 10q23-q25 (Fig. 3). Twenty percent of cells are in the tetraploid configuration due to endoreduplication with the same marker, chromosome 10p+ 2x. Case 7 (Fig. 4) was characteristically very homogeneous in the diploid range, 47 XX, +10, exhibiting only trisomy of chromosome 10 with no other obvious abnormalities. In Case 6, which is a more advanced tumor by clinical and histopathological diagnoses, we found two cytogenetically distinct populations of cells, even in the very limited amount of material available to us. Cells in the diploid range, with a single chromosome rearrangement 46 XX, − 10,16p+, due to t(10,16) (q23,p13), are shown in Fig. 5 which represents the partial karyotype of two representative cells. We also observed spontaneous breakage on different chromosomal sites (Fig. 5). The other subpopulation of cells was very heterogeneous, with minute chromosomes and di-

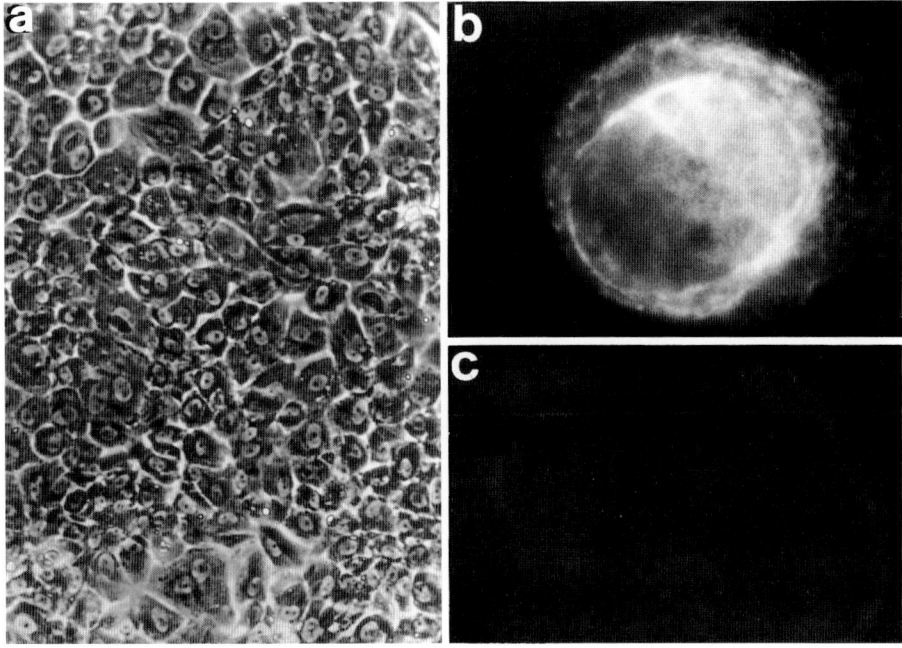

Fig. 2. a Typical epithelial morphology of EC after 3 months in culture. **b** Positive anti-cytokeratine staining. **c** Negative control. **a** ×100; **b, c** ×500

Table 2. Histopathological and cytogenetic findings of EC

Case	Age	Stage/grade	Chromosome analysis						met analyzed	Chromosome range	Karyotype
			Culture								
			3 h	24 h	48 h	72 h	72+ h				
1	59	IA/2				+			30	46/92	46XX, 10 p+
2	72	IB/1	+						30	49–70	Heterogeneous abnormality of chromosomes 1, 3, 4, 6, 7, 10, minutes, HSR, PCC, PCD
3	67	IB/3			+				20	50–70	Heterogeneous, minutes, giant markers, PCD
4	74	IB/1				+			25	50–70	Heterogeneous, minutes, PCD, dicentrics, rings
5	56	II/2		+					15	50–70	Heterogeneous, minutes, rings, dicentrics
6	66	I/2		+					10	46/50–70	46XX, +1 p−, −10, t(10,16)/heterogeneous
7	41	I/1					+		25	47	47XX, +10

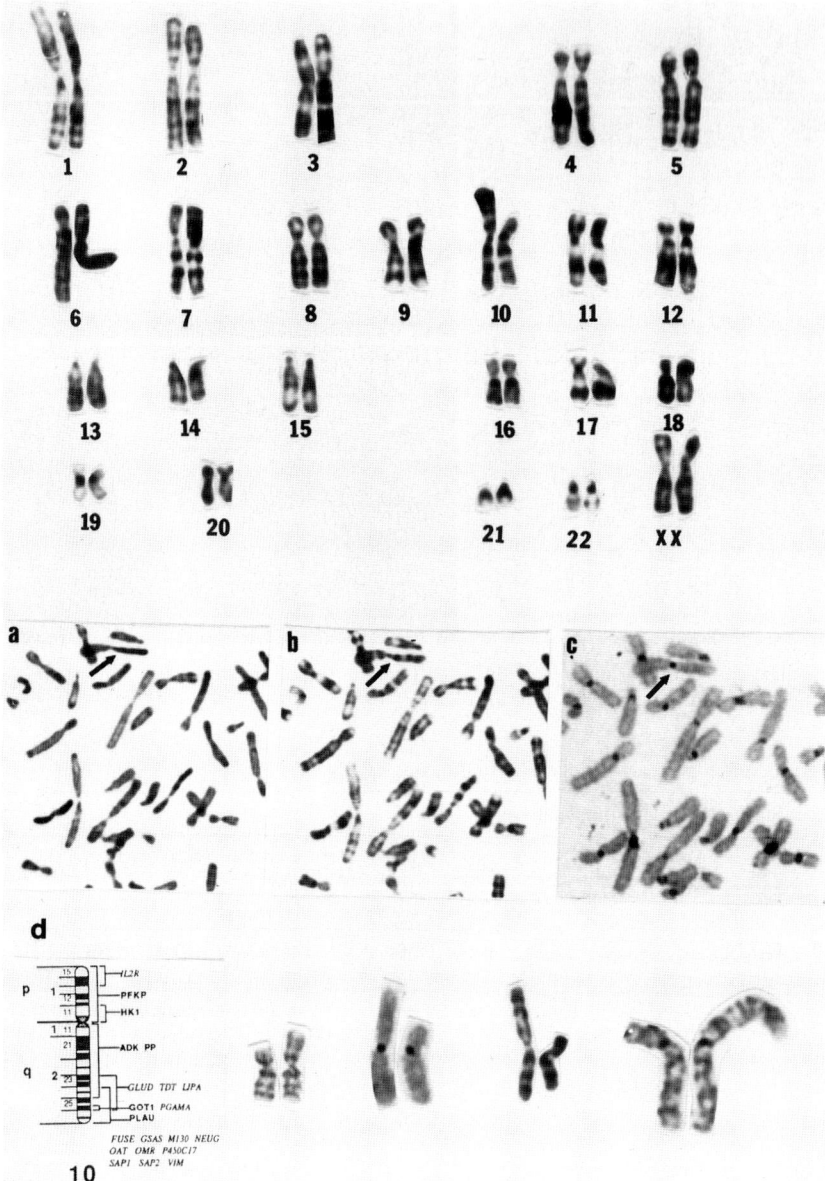

Fig. 3a–d. Representative karyotype of primary EC, case 1: 46XX, 10p+. **a** Giemsa staining; **b** GTG staining; **c** CBG staining of the same metaphase, *arrow* indicates 10p+; **d** chromosome 10 from different cells at different stages of spiralization with strong possibility of t(10,10) (p15,q23)

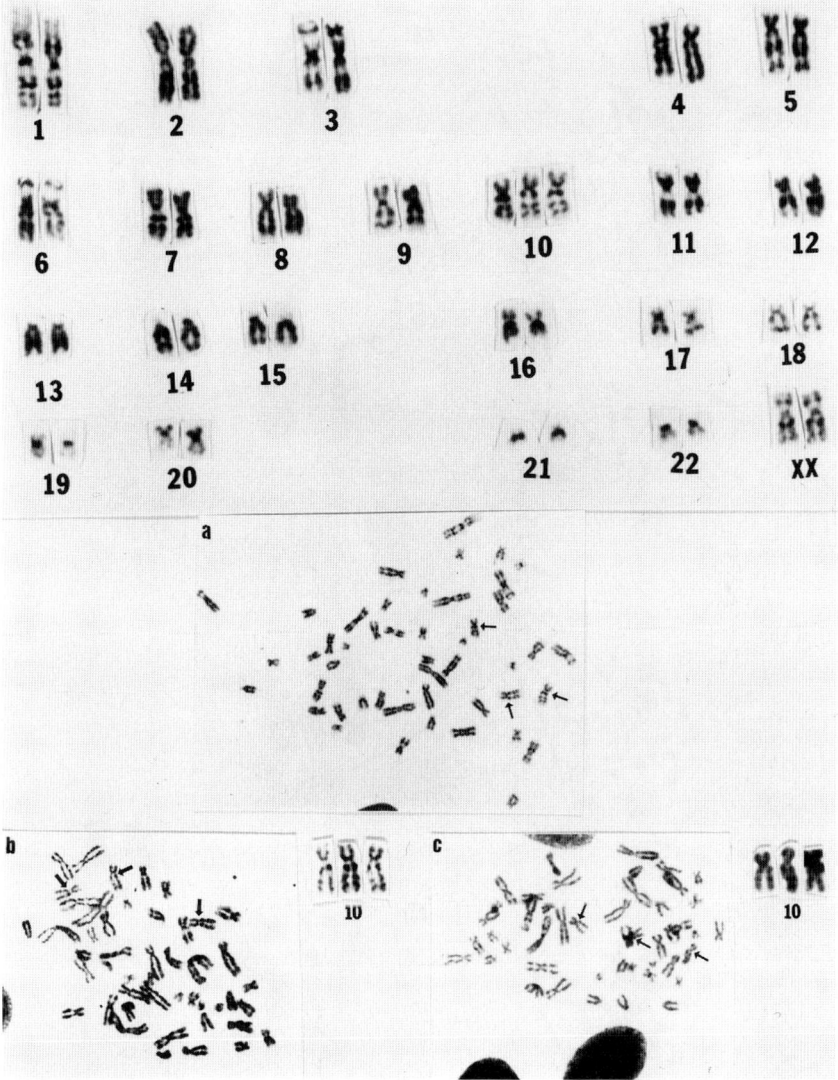

Fig. 4a-c. Representative karyotype of primary EC, case 7: 47XX, +10, GTG banding. **a-c** Three different metaphase spreads; *arrows* indicate chromosome 10

centrics in the chromosome range of 50-70. Cases 2, 3, 4, and 5 were even more advanced neoplasias on the basis of clinical and histopathological criteria. They exhibited very heterogeneous chromosomal profiles, characterized only as pleomorphic, with complex aberrations and abnormalities such as minute chromosomes, rings, homogeneously stained regions (HSR), premature chromosome condensations (PCC), and premature centromere divisions with telomere joinings; examples of these are shown in Fig. 6.

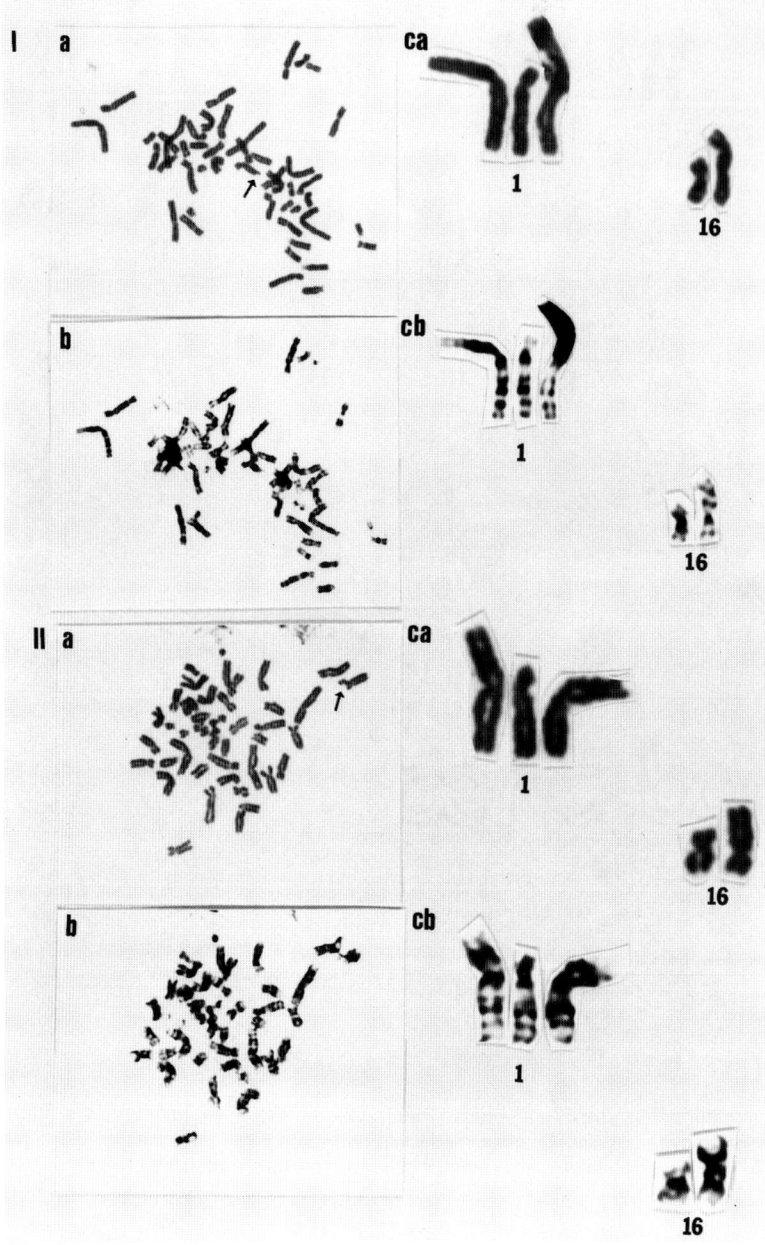

Fig. 5a–c. Two representative cells I and II of primary EC, case 6 with partial karyotype: 46XX, +1p−, −10,16p+. **a** Giemsa stain, *arrow* indicates points of spontaneous breakage; **b** same metaphase after GTG; **c** partial karyotype showing the chromosomes of interest, +1p−, 16p+ which is t(10,16) (q23,p13)

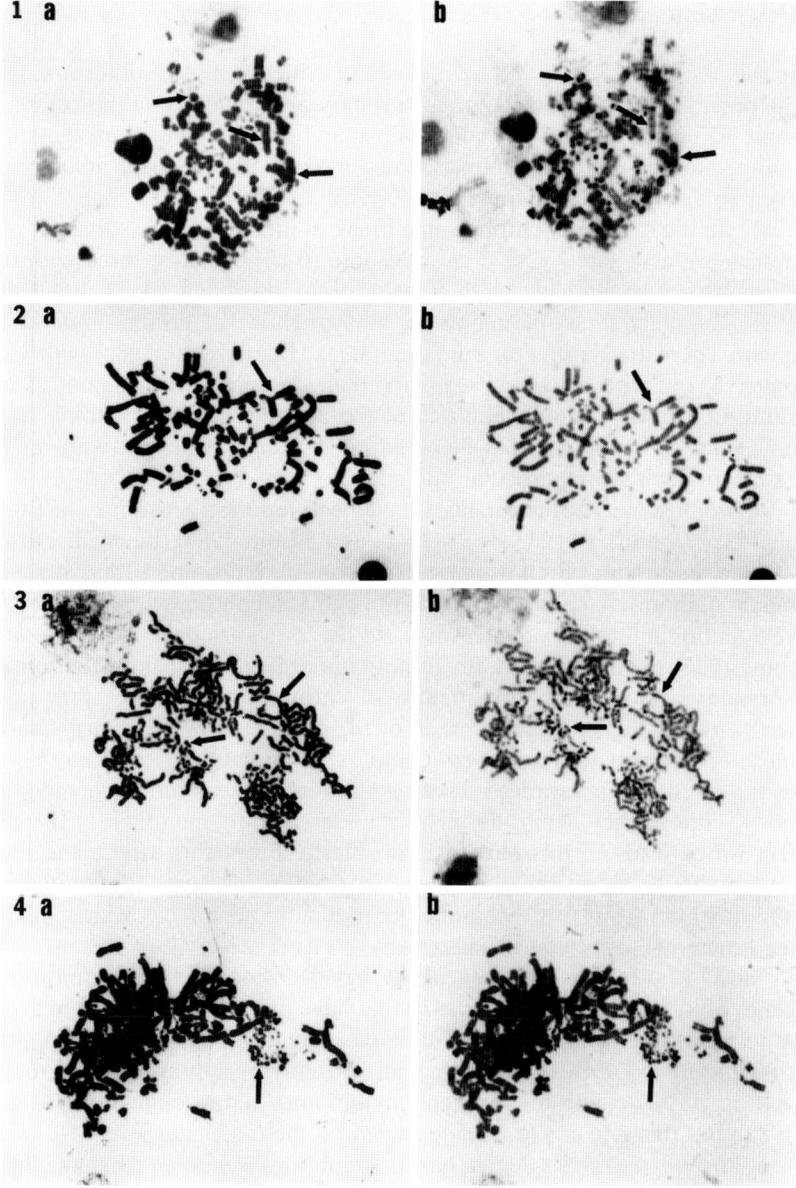

Fig. 6a, b. Four representative metaphase spreads of EC from primary chromosome preparations. *Arrows* indicate some of the phenomena observed in cases 2, 3, 4, and 5: telomere joining, dicentric chromosomes, ring chromosomes, non-sister chromatid joining, minutes, minutes C banding positive, premature centromere division, minute chromosome clustering. **a** Giemsa stain; **b** C banding on the same metaphase spread

Discussion

In the case of EC we have provided some evidence that chromosome 10 might be the possible target chromosome for primary abnormalities in this tumor. Chromosome 10 has not been associated with many malignancies. Linkage studies have mapped multiple familial endocrine neoplasia syndrome to chromosome 10; however, so far there is no functional understanding of the defect (Simpson et al. 1987). In the catalog of chromosome break points in neoplasia five out of 38 melanomas are associated with a chromosome 10 abnormality, three with the loss of chromosome 10, and two with translocations involving 10q24–10q26 (Mitelman 1988). In other types of neoplasia, abnormalities of chromosome 10 are infrequent. There are reports on human gliomas (Bigner et al. 1984) with very similar patterns, but with a higher frequency than described in melanomas. In the few studies on other tumors, neoplasia of the prostate, leiomyosarcoma, and even in leukemia, chromosome 10 is involved in rearrangements, but with no significant association with any particular malignancy.

Chromosome 10 abnormalities have been reported previously in EC (Fujita et al. 1985; Couturier et al. 1986; Gibas and Rubin 1987), but with no higher frequency than other chromosomes. Therefore chromosome 10 has not received as much attention as chromosome 1 within this neoplasia. In this respect it will be very important to reevaluate some of the previous data focusing on chromosome 10. Based on our data, the diploid tumor cell with a simple chromosome abnormality always shows abnormality of chromosome 10. The other cases, which were either a higher stage or grade of the disease show pleomorphism and chromosome heterogeneity with very complex abnormalities, which can be explained as the result of the advanced disease. Although these could be included into diagnostic criteria, they would not help in understanding the origin of the cellular defect which leads to this particular neoplasia. From this aspect, the focus of research should be on the early stages of this malignancy, to obtain the primary abnormalities in EC, to determine the particular gene locus which will lead us to the functional aspects of this neoplasia.

So far, no human proto-oncogene has been mapped to chromosome 10. The genes of interest on chromosome 10 that have been mapped and which could play a potential role in EC are the interleukin 2 receptor on 10 p14–p15, and human cytochrome P-450 PB-1, which has just recently been mapped to chromosome 10 with its physiological role in mephenytoin and steroid oxidations (Meehan et al. 1988). But this remains to be determined on the molecular level.

Cancer cytogenetics, which has its beginnings in human leukemia, has had significant clinical value regarding prognosis; however, its biological value was as the starting point for molecular genetic investigations. Cancer cytogenetics is one of the most rapidly moving fields in cancer research. It holds the promise that what has done for some of the hematopoietic neoplasias is just a beginning for progress in solid tumors. There is the hope of solving the problem of cancer in the near future by understanding some of the changes on chromosomal and genetic levels, and by the close collaboration of cancer cytogenetics, molecular genetics, and other disciplines (Fig. 7).

Contribution of Cytogenetics to Cancer Research

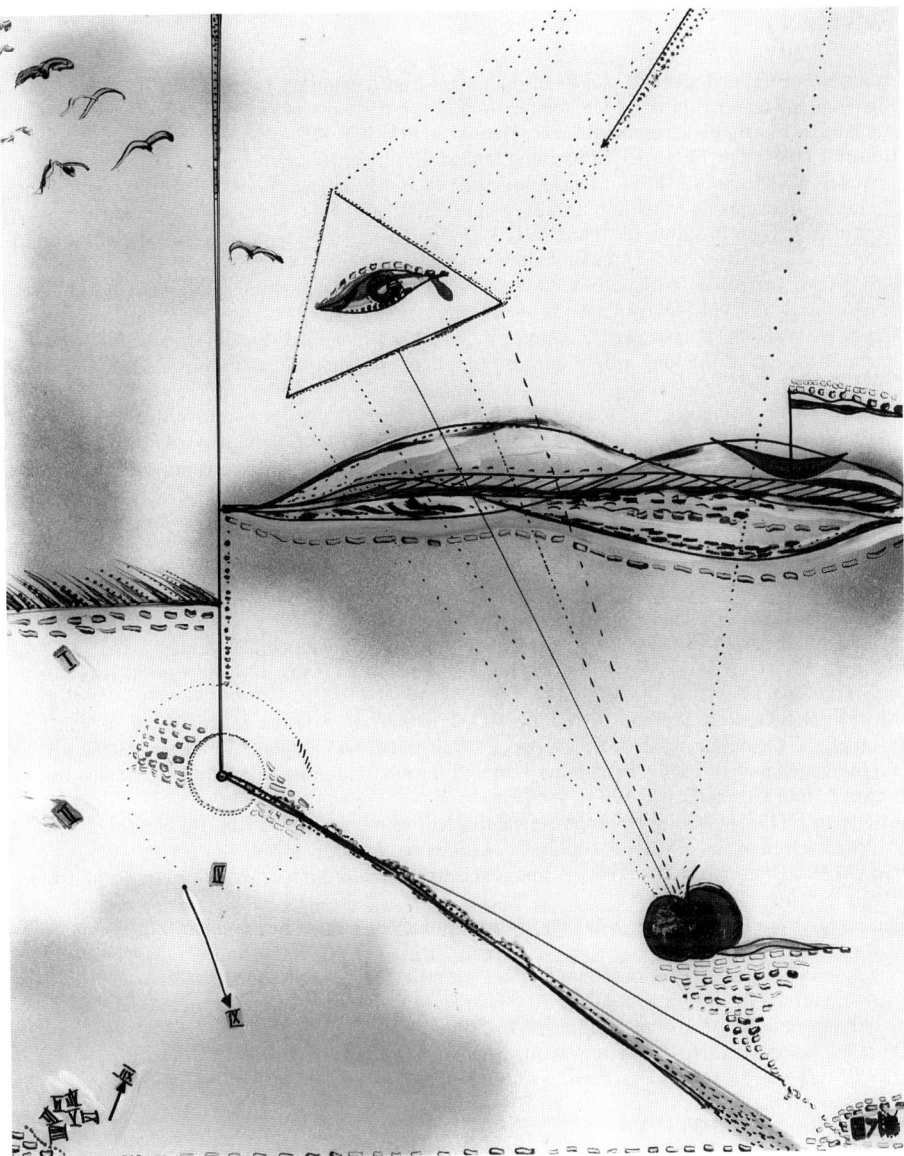

Fig. 7. Daniela Simon. Painting on glass: Me, Him, and DNA in Space and Time, 1987 (dedicated to all participants of the Hašek meeting in Ommen)

References

Atkin NB (1976) Cytogenetic aspects of malignant transformation. Karger, New York
Bigner SH, Mark J, Mahaley MS, Bigner DD (1984) Patterns of the early, gross chromosomal changes in malignant human gliomas. Hereditas 101: 103–113
Boveri T (1914) Zur Frage der Entstehung maligner Tumore. Fischer, Jena
Cavenee WK, Hansen MF, Nordenskjold M, Kock E, Maumenee I (1985) Genetic origin of mutations predisposing to retinoblastoma. Science 228: 501–3
Couturier J, Vielh P, Salmon R, Dutrillaux B (1986) Trisomy and tetrasomy for long arm of chromosome 1 in near-diploid human endometrial adenocarcinomas. Int J Cancer 38: 17–19
Croce CM, Erikson J, Tsujimoto Y, Nowell PC (1987) Molecular basis of human B and T cell neoplasia. Adv Viral Oncol 7: 35–51
Fujita H, Wake N, Kutsuzawa T, Ichione K, Hreshchyshyn MM, Sandberg AA (1985) Marker chromosomes of the long arm of chromosome 1 in endometrial carcinoma. Cancer Genet Cytogenet 18: 283–293
Gambrell RD, Bagnell CA, Greenblatt RB (1983) Role of estrogens and progesterone in the ethiology and prevention of endometrial cancer. Am J Obstet Gynecol 146: 696–707
Gibas Z, Rubin SC (1987) Well differentiated adenocarcinoma of endometrium with simple karyotypic changes: a case report. Cancer Genet Cytogenet 25: 21–26
Gusberg SB, Frick HG II (1978) Gynecologic cancer, 5th edn. Williams & Wilkins, Baltimore
Jenkyn DJ, McCartney AJ (1986) Primary cytogenetic abnormality detected in an endometrial adenocarcinoma. Cancer Genet Cytogenet 20: 149–157
Knudson AG (1971) Mutation and cancer: statistical study of retinoblastoma. Proc Natl Acad Sci USA 68: 820–823
Knudson AG (1986) Genetics of human cancer. Annu Rev Genet 20: 231–251
Manolov G, Manolova Y (1972) Marker band in one chromosome 14 from Burkitt lymphomas. Nature 237: 33–34
Meehan RR, Gosden JR, Rout D, Hastie ND, Friedberg F, Adesnik M, Buckland R, Van Heyningen V, Fletcher J, Spurr NK, Sweeney J, Wolf CR (1988) Human cytochrome P-450 PB-1: a multigene family involved in mephenytoin and steroid oxidations that maps to chromosome 10. Am J Hum Genet 42: 026–037
Mitelman F (1988) Catalog of chromosome aberrations in cancer, 3rd edn. In: Sandberg AA (ed) Progress and topics in cytogenetics, vol 5. Liss, New York, pp 457–467
Nowell PC, Hungerford DA (1960) A minute chromosome in human chronic granulocytic leukemia. Science 132: 1497
Simon D, Aden DP, Knowles BB (1982) Chromosomes of human hepatoma cell lines. Int J Cancer 30: 27
Simpson NE, Kidd KK, Goodfellow PJ, McDermid H, Myers S, Kidd JR, Jackson CE, Duncan AM, Farrer LA, Brasch K et al. (1987) Assignment of multiple endocrine neoplasia type 2A to chromosome 10 by linkage. Nature 328 (6130): 528–530
Tjio JH, Levan A (1956) The chromosome number of man. Hereditas 42: 1–6
Trent JM, Davis JR (1979) D-group chromosome abnormalities in endometrial cancer and hyperplasia. Lancet 2: 361
Yoshida MA, Ohyashiki K, Piver SM, Sandberg AA (1986) Recurrent endometrial adenocarcinoma with rearrangement of chromosomes 1 and 11. Cancer Genet Cytogenet 20: 159–62
Yunis JJ, Ramsay N (1978) Retinoblastoma and subband deletion of chromosome 13. Am J Dis Child 132: 161–163

Bibliography

This bibliography contains the complete list of articles, reviews, and books authored, co-authored, or edited by the participants of the Amsterdam/Ommen meeting, i.e., their work after they left the "Hašek" Institute in Prague. It was not possible to separate papers published in scientific journals from review and proceedings papers. Thus the final list of papers is heterogenous, and there is some overlap between the original contributions and review papers. Abstracts and nonscientific scripts are not included. Incidentally, of the total of almost 1500 articles, 35 were published in *Nature,* 35 in the *Journal of Experimental Medicine,* 45 in the *European Journal of Immunology,* and 110 in the *Journal of Immunology.*

A Book Authors

Festenstein H, Demant P (1978) HLA and H-2: basic immunogenetics, biology and clinical relevance. Arnold, London
Festenstein H, Demant P (1980) HLA e H-2: Principi fondamentali di immunogenetica, aspetti biologici e importanza clinica. Pensiero Scientifico, Rome
Festenstein H, Demant P (1980) Japanese edition of above book. Kindai, Tokyo
Festenstein H, Demant P (1981) Immunogenetica fundamental, biologia y appliccaciones clinicas de HLA y H-2. Manual Moderno, Mexico
Klein J (1975) Biology of the mouse histocompatibility-2 complex. Principles of immunogenetics, applied to a single system. Springer, Berlin Heidelberg New York
Klein J (1982) Immunology. The science of self-nonself discrimination. Wiley, New York
Klein J (1985) Immunogenetics. McGraw-Hill, New York (McGraw-Hill encyclopedia of science and technology)
Klein J (1986) Natural history of the major histocompatibility complex. Wiley, New York
Koldovsky P (1969) Tumor specific transplantation antigen. Springer, Berlin Heidelberg New York
Koldovsky P (1974) Canceroembryonic antigen. Springer, Berlin Heidelberg New York

B Book Editors

Dausset J, Pla M (eds) (1985) HLA, complexe majeur d'histocompatibilité de l'homme. Flammarion, Paris
Dausset J, Pla M (eds) (1989) HLA, complexe majeur d'histocompatibilité de l'homme. Flammarion Paris
Festenstein H, Demant P (eds) (1983) Diversity and polymorphism of the H-2 major histocompatibility complex. Transplant Proc 15 (4)

Ivanyi P (ed) (1988) MHC-X; complex formation and antibody induction. Springer, Berlin Heidelberg New York

Koldovsky P, Koldovsky U, Beck L, Vosteen K-H (eds) (1988) Lymphocytes in cancer therapy. Springer, Berlin Heidelberg New York

Lotzová E, Herberman RB, (eds) (1986) Immunobiology of natural killer cells, vol 1. CRC, Boca Raton

Lotzová E, Herberman RB, (eds) (1986) Immunobiology of natural killer cells, vol 2. CRC, Boca Raton

Lotzová E, Herberman RB (eds) (1986) Natural immunity, cancer and biological response modification. Karger, Basel

Lotzová E (ed) (1988) Role of interleukin-2 activated killer cells in cancer, vol 1. CRC, Boca Raton (in press)

Lotzová E (ed) (1988) Role of interleukin-2 activated killer cells in cancer, vol 2. CRC, Boca Raton (in press)

Baum SJ, Dicke K, Lotzová E, Pluznik DH (eds) (1989) Experimental hematology today 1988. Springer, Berlin Heidelberg New York

Skamene E, Kongshavn P, Landy M (eds) (1980) Genetic control of natural resistance to infection and malignancy. Academic, New York

Skamene E (ed) (1985) Genetic control of host resistance to Infection and malignancy. Liss, New York

C Articles

Adler A, Chervenick PA, Whiteside T, Lotzová E, Herberman RB (1988) Interleukin-2 induced cytotoxicity in peripheral blood and bone marrow of acute leukemia patients. I. Feasibility of large-scale generation of cytotoxic cells in patients with adult leukemia in active stage and in remission. Blood 71: 709–716

Adolph S, Klein J (1981) Robertsonian variation in *Mus musculus* from Central Europe, Spain, and Scotland. J Hered 72: 219–221

Adolph S, Klein J (1983) Genetic variation of wild mouse populations in Southern Germany. I. Cytogenetic study. Genet Res 41: 117–134

Aguayo AJ, Kasarijan J, Skamene E, Kongshavn P, Bray GM (1977) Myelination of mouse nerve fibers by transplanted human Schwann cells. Nature 268: 753

Aihara Y, Bühring H-J, Aihara M, Klein J (1986) An attempt to produce "pre-T" cell hybridomas to identify their antigens. Eur J Immunol 16: 1391–1399

Aihara Y, Klein J (1988) "Autoreactivity" of some hybridomas may be caused by a three-cell interaction. Immunology 63: 389–395

Alexander H, Johnson DA, Rosen J, Jerabek L, Green N, Weissman IL, Lerner RA (1983) Mimicking the alloantigenicity of proteins with chemically synthesized peptides differing in single amino acids. Nature 306: 697

Alter BJ, Schendel DJ, Bach ML, Bach FH, Klein J (1973) Cell mediated lympholysis: Importance of serologically-defined-H-2 regions. J Exp Med 137: 1303–1309

Anderson RJL, Dyer PA, Donnai D, Klouda PT, Jennison R, Braganza JM (1988) Chronic pancreatitis, HLA and auto-immunity. Int J Pancreatol 3: 83–90

Andersson T, Stejskal V, Härfast B (1975) An in vitro method for study of human lymphocyte cytotoxicity against virus-infected target cells. J Immunol 114: 237

Andrews PW, Damjanov I, Simon D, Banting G, Carlin C, Dracopoli NC, Fogh J (1984) Pluripotent embryonal carcinoma clones derived from the human teratocarcinoma cell line Tera-2: Differentiation in vivo and in vitro. Lab Invest 50: 147–162

Andrews PW, Damjanov I, Simon D, Dignazio M (1985) A pluripotent human stem-cell clone isolated from the TERA-2 teratocarcinoma line lacks antigens SSEA-3 and SSEA-4 in vitro, but expresses these antigens when grown as xenograft tumor. Differentiation 29: 127–135

Anthony LSD, Skamene E, Kongshavn PAL (1988) The influence of genetic background on host resistance to experimental murine tularemia. Infect Immun 56: 2089–2093

Anthony LSD, Skamene E, Kongshavn PAL (1985) Genetic regulation of resistance of inbred mouse strains to experimental murine tularemia. Prog Leukocyte Biol 3: 355–360

Anthony LD, Stevenson MM, Skamene E (1984) Enhancement of resistance to *Listeria monocytogenes* infection in mice by pyrimidine analogs. Clin Invest Med 7: 343–348

Aquilera S, Ivanyi J (1978) Acquired heterophile antigens on the surface of human cell lines. Eur J Immunol 8: 446–451

Arden B, Klein J (1982) Biochemical comparison of major histocompatibility complex molecules from different subspecies of *Mus musculus:* Evidence for trans-specific evolution of alleles. Proc Natl Acad Sci USA 79: 2342–2346

Arden B, Wakeland EK, Klein J (1980) Structural comparisons of serologically indistinguishable H-2K-encoded antigens from inbred and wild mice. J Immunol 125: 2424–2428

Arden B, Wakeland EK, Klein J (1982) Minor structural variants of *H-2K*-controlled molecules in wild mice. Immunogenetics 16: 491–493

Armstrong P, Dyer PA, Klouda PT, Harris R (1980) Properdin factor B alleles in pre-eclampsia. Lancet 1: 1145–1146

Asherson GL, Zembala M, Colizzi V, Malkovský M (1983) Lymphokines and antigen-specific T-cell products in contact sensitivity. Lymphokines 8: 143–173

Asherson GL, Colizzi V, Malkovský M, Zembala M (1983) T suppressor cell circuits in contact sensitivity and the role of the acceptor cell which acquires specificity passively (in Russian). Immunologia 1: 27–33

Asherson G, Colizzi V, Malkovský M, Zembala M (1983) Associative recognition in the generation of lymphokines which inhibit the transfer of contact sensitivity and the production of IL-2: requirement for crosslinking of antigen recognition sites and the presence of I-J subregion determinants. In: Oppenheim JJ, Cohen S, Landy M (eds) Interleukins, lymphokines, and cytokines. Academic, New York, pp 359–365

Asherson GL, Colizzi V, Malkovský M, Colonna-Romano G, Zembala M (1985) The role of interleukin-2 as one of the determinants of the balance between immunity and unresponsiveness. Folia Biol (Praha) 31: 387–395

Asjo B, Skoog L, Palminger I, Wiener F, Isaak D, Cerny J, Smith EM (1985) Influence of genotype and the organ of origin on the subtype of T-cell in Moloney lymphomas induces by transfer of preleukemic cells from athymic and thymus-bearing mice. Cancer Res 45: 1040–1045

Aston R, Ivanyi J (1983) Antigenic, receptor-binding and mitogenic activity of proteolytic fragments of human growth hormone. EMBO J 2: 493–497

Aston R, Ivanyi J (1985) Monoclonal antibodies to growth hormone and prolactin. Pharmacol Ther 27: 403–424

Aston R, Young K, van den Berg H, Ivanyi J (1984) Identification of M_r variants of prolactin with monoclonal antibodies. FEBS Lett 171: 192–196

Aston R, Holder AT, Preece MA, Ivanyi J (1986) Potentiation of the somatotropic and lactogenic activity of human growth hormone with monoclonal antibodies. J Endocrinol 110: 381–388

Aston R, Holder AT, Ivanyi J, Bomford R (1987) Enhancement of bovine growth hormone activity in vivo by monoclonal antibodies. Mol Immunol 24: 143–150

Auersperg N, Hudson JB, Goddard EJ, Klement V (1977) Transformation of cultured rat adrenocortical cells by Kirsten Murine sarcoma virus (KiMSV). Int J Cancer 19: 81–89

Ayane M, Klein D, Margetić E, Figueroa F, Klein J (1987) *Neuraminidase-1* variation among mice carrying *t* chromosomes. Immunogenetics 26: 296–298

Bach FH, Widmer MB, Bach ML, Klein J (1972) Serologically defined and lymphocyte defined components of the major histocompatibility complex in the mouse. J Exp Med 136: 1430–1444

Bach FH, Widmer MB, Segal M, Klein J (1972) Genetic and immunological complexity of major histocompatibility regions. Science 176: 1024–1027

Bach ML, Widmer MB, Bach FH, Klein J (1973) Genetic control of the mixed leukocyte cultures, MLC. Transplant Proc 5: 369–375

Balcarová-Staender J, Rother U, Rauterberg E (1981) The attack phase of human complement: differentiation between membrane binding and complex formation by the detectin of neoantigen expression in situ. A morphometric immunoferritin study. J Immunol 127: 1089

Balcarová J, Helenius A, Simons K (1981) Antibody response to spike protein vaccines prepared from Semliki forest virus. J Gen Virol 53: 85

Balcarová-Staender J, Pfeifer S, Fuller SD, Simons K (1984) Development of cell surface polarity in the epithelial Madin-Darby canine kidney (MDCK) cell line. EMBO J 3: 2687

Baranska W, Koldovsky P, Koprowski H (1970) Antigenic study on unfertilized mouse eggs: crossreactivity with SV40 induced antigens Proc Natl Acad Sci USA 67: 73

Barbacid M, Donner L, Ruscetti SK, Sherr CJ (1981) transformation-defective mutants of Snyder-Theilen feline sarcoma virus lack tyrosine-specific protein kinase activity. J Virol 39: 246

Baxevanis CN, Wernet D, Nagy ZA, Maurer PH, Klein J (1980) Genetic control of T-cell proliferative responses to poly(glu^{60}ala^{40}) and poly(glu^{51}lys^{34}tyr^{15}): Subregion-specific inhibition of the responses with monoclonal Ia antibodies. Immunogenetics 11: 617–628

Baxevanis CN, Nagy ZA, Klein J (1981) A novel type of T-T cell interaction removes the requirement for *I-B* region in the H-2 complex. Proc Natl Acad Sci USA 78: 3809–3813

Baxevanis CN, Ishii N, Nagy ZA, Klein J (1982) Role of the E^k molecule in the generation of suppressor T cells in response to LDH$_B$. Scand J Immunol 16: 25–31

Baxevanis CN, Ishii N, Nagy ZA, Klein J (1982) H-2-controlled suppression of T cell response to lactate dehydrogenase B. J Exp Med 156: 822–833

Baxevanis CN, Nagy ZA, Klein J (1983) Mechanism of H-2-controlled interaction between LDH$_B$-specific helper and suppressor T cells. In: Pierce CW, Cullen SE, Kapp JA (eds) Ir genes, past, present, and future. Humana, Clifton, pp 333–337

Baxevanis CN, Nagy ZA, Klein J (1983) The nature of the interaction between suppressor and helper T cells in the response to LDH$_B$. J Immunol 131: 628–632

Baxevanis CN, Ikezawa Z, Klein J, Nagy ZA (1984) Mechanisms involved in the Ir-Gene control of T suppressor cell response to lactate dehydrogenase B. J Mol Cell Immunol 1: 201–210

Befus AD, Skamene E (1986) Host resistance and immunoparasitology. Immunol Today 7: 15–16

Begent RHJ, Birch JA, Clink HM, Hockley A, Jameson B, Kay HEM, Klouda PT, et al. (1974) Bone marrow aplasia after infectious hepatitis treated by bone marrow transplantation. Br Med J 1: 363–364

Behforouz N, Cerny J, Eardley DD (1983) Augmentation of B cell responsiveness by a tumor-activated T cell factor. Cell Immunol 79: 110

Behforouz N, Cerny J, Eardley DD (1983) Activation of T cells in tumor-bearing mice. Cell Immunol 79: 93

Behforouz N, Eardley DD, Cerny J (1983) "Nonspecific" immunoenhancing T cells in tumor-bearing mice include anti-idiotypic subsets. J Immunol 131: 2576

Belosevic M, Faubert G, Skamene E, McLean JD (1984) Susceptibility and resistance of inbred mice to Giardia Muris. Infect Immun 44: 282–286

Ben Porat T, Rakusanova T, Kaplan AS (1971) Early functions of the genome of herpesvirus. II. Inhibition of the formation of cell specific polysomes. Virology 46: 890–899

Ben-Shlomo R, Figueroa F, Klein J (1988) Mhc class II DNA polymorphism within and between chromosomal species of the *Spalax ehrenbergi* superspecies in Israel. Genetics 119: 141–149

Bidwell JL, Champion HM, Champion SN, Klouda PT, Bradley BA (1985) HLA review: Comparative anatomy of HLA class II genes and gene products. Biotest Bull 2: 238–248

Bidwell JL, Jarrold EA, Laundy GJ, Klouda PT, Bradley BA (1986) Molecular genetics of HLA-DR Br: allogenotypes of DR1 and DR Br are indistinguishable. Tissue Antigens 27: 99–101

Bidwell JL, Bidwell EA, Laundy GJ, Klouda PT, Bradley BA (1987) Allogenotypes defined by short DQalfa and DQbeta cDNA probes correlate with and define splits of HLA-DQ serological specificities. Mol Immunol 24: 513–522

Bidwell JL, Bidwell EA, Klouda PT, Goffin RB, Bradley BA, Brenner M (1987) DNA-RFLP typing in the selection of related bone marrow donors. Bone Marrow Transplant 1: 413–414

Bidwell JL, Bidwell EA, Savage DA, Middleton D, Klouda PT, Bradley BA (1988) A DNA-RFLP typing system that positively identifies serologically well-defined and ill-defined HLA-DR and DQ alleles, including DRw10. Transplantation 45: 640–646

Bidwell JL, Sansom DM, Bidwell EA, Klouda PT, Bradley BA (1989) The origin of HLA-DR Br. Exon 2 nucleotide sequence implicates gene conversion of DR1 by DR4-Dw10 or DRw6-Dw18. Hum Immunol (in press)

Bidwell JL, Bidwell EA, Savage DA, Middleton D, Cullen C, Klouda PT, Bradley BA (1989) Identification of Dw2, Dw12 and short DR2 splits with sequential exon-specific Drβ, DQβ and DQα and DNA probes. In: Immunology of HLA, vol 2: Immunogenetics and histocompatibility (in press)

Binet JL, Kinsky RG, Mathe G, Seman G, Amiel JL (1961) Aspects morphologique des cellules immunologiquement compétentes au cours des réactions de greffes allogéniques. Nouv Rev Fr Hematol 1: 887–899

Birnbaum D, Pla M, Colombani M, Colombani J (1982) Serological cross-reactivity between products of separate I regions. Immunogenetics 15: 71–77

Birnbaum D, Pla M, Colombani M, Colombani J (1980) Etude sérologique des antigènes la déterminés aux sous-régions I-A et I-E du complexe H-2 de la souris. C R Acad Sci (Paris) 290: 1313–1316

Bishop D, Demant P, Capel PJA (1980) The blocking effect of antibodies against the products of the H-2 gene complex on lymphocyte complement (C3d) receptors. Complement dependence and specificity. Tissue Antigens 15: 31–39

Blick M, Shin D, Gupta V, Chawla S, Gutterman J, Donner L (1989) Expression of transforming growth factor-alpha, epidermal growth factor receptor and P53 in human sarcomas. Anticancer Res (in press)

Bobé P, Dorić M, Kinsky RG, Voisin GA (1984) Modulation of mouse anti-SRBC antibody response by placental extracts. Cell Immunol 89: 355–364

Bomford R, Aston R, Ivanyi J (1985) Reversal of H-2-restricted hyporesponsiveness to human growth hormone by the use of aluminum hydroxide as adjuvant. Immunogenetics 21: 505–509

Bothamley G, Swanson Beck J, Agusni I, Ilias MI, Kardjito T, Grange JM, Ivanyi J (1987) Antibodies to mycobacterium tuberculosis in leprosy. Lancet 1098

Bothamley GH, Swanson Beck J, Schreuder GMT, d'Amaro J, Ivanyi J (1989) Association of tuberculosis and *M.tuberculosis* specific antibody levels with HLA. J Infect Dis (in press)

Botzenhardt V, Klein J, Ziff M (1978) Primary in vitro cell-mediated lympholysis reaction of NZB mice against unmodified targets syngeneic at the major histocompatibility complex. J Exp Med 147: 1435–1448

Bourassa D, Forget A, Pelletier M, Skamene E, Turcotte R (1985) Cellular immune response to *Mycobacterium bovis* (BCG) in genetically-susceptible and resistant congenic mouse strains. Clin Exp Immunol 62: 31–38

Bourassa D, Forget A, Pelletier M, Skamene E, Turcotte R (1985) Dissociation between different parameters of cell-mediated immunity in genetically susceptible and resistant congenic mouse strains during infection with a low dose of BCG Montreal. Prog Leukocyte Biol 3: 279–284

Boyd RL, Oberhuber G, Hála K, Wick G (1984) Obese strain (OS) chickens with spontaneous autoimmune thyroiditis have a deficiency in thymic nurse cells. J Immunol 132: 718–724

Boyd RL, Hála K, Wick G (1985) Interactions and quantitative analysis of immunoregulatory cells in the chicken thymus. J Immunol 135: 3039–3049

Bowen LD, Isaak DD, Cerny J (1979) Inhibition of in vitro murine leukemia (Friend) infection of activated B cells with concanavalin A. JNCI 62: 1497

Bradley BA, Klouda PT (1983) HLA and immune complexes. In: Dawkins RL, Christiansen FT, Zilko PJ (eds) Immunogenetics in rheumatology. Muskuloskeletal disease and D-penicillamine. Excerpta Medica, Amsterdam, pp 29–33

Bradley BA, Klouda PT, Ray TC, Cope SM (1985) Intelligent mismatching for highly sensitized patients. In: Touraine JL (ed) Transplantation and clinical immunology, vol 17. Elsevier, Amsterdam, pp 139–145

Bradley BA, Klouda PT, Ray TC, Gore SM (1985) Negative crossmatch selection of kidneys for highly sensitized patients. Transplant Proc 17: 2465–2466

Bradley BA, Bidwell JA, Jarrold EA, Goffin RB, Klouda PT (1986) HLA matched unrelated bone marrow transplants: a proposal to speed up donor selection using a DNA bank. Bone Marrow Transplant [Suppl 1] 1: 146–147

Bradley BA, Gilks WR, Gore SM, Klouda PT (1986) A contemporary strategy for matching in kidney transplantation. Transplant Proc 18: 1069–1071

Bradley BA, Gilks W, Gore SM, Klouda PT, Selwood NH (1986) Beneficial HLA matching in centers using cyclosporin A. In: Terasaki P (ed) Clinical transplants 1986. UCLA Tissue Typing Laboratory, Los Angeles, pp 93–98

Bradley BA, Gore SM, Gilks WR, Klouda PT, Selwood NH, Wood RFM, McGeown M (1986) Cyclosporin and graft survival. Lancet 2: 568–569

Bradley BA, Selwood NH, Klouda PT, Gilks WR, Gore SM, Ray TC, Moras D, Riggulsford M (1986) Kidney transplants in the United Kingdom. In: Terasaki P (ed) Clinical transplants 1986. UCLA Tissue Typing Laboratory, Los Angeles, pp 47–51

Bradley BA, Gilks WR, Gore SM, Klouda PT (1987) How many HLA typed volunteer donors for bone marrow transplantation are needed to provide an effective service. Bone Marrow Transplant [Suppl 1] 2: 79

Bradley BA, Bidwell JL, Bidwell EA, Goffin RB, Corbin SA, Klouda PT (1987) DNA probes for acurate HLA-DR and DQ matching in bone marrow transplantation. Bone Marrow Transplant [Suppl 1] 2: 81

Braciale TJ, Mojcik CF, Hauptfeld V (1982) Target cell recognition by cloned lines of influenza virus-specific cytotoxic T lymphocytes. Selective inhibition by a monoclonal H-2 specific antibody. Immunogenetics 15: 41–52

Brandwein SR, Skamene E, Aubut JA, Gervais F, Nesbitt MN (1987) Genetic regulation of lipopolysaccharide-induced interleukin-1 production by murine peritoneal macrophages. J Immunol 138: 4263–4269

Brenner MK, North ME, Chadda HR, Newton CA, Malkovský M, Webster ADB, Farrant J (1984) The role of B cell differentiation factors and specific T cell help in the pathogenesis of primary hypogammaglobulinemia. Eur J Immunol 14: 1021–1027

Breur B, Iványi P (1984) Antigen report: HLA-B27. In: Albert ED, Baur MP, Mayr WR (eds) Histocompatibility testing 1984. Springer, Berlin Heidelberg New York, p 144

Breur-Vriesendorp BS, Huis B, Dekker AJ, Breuning MH, Iványi P (1985) Subtypes of antigen HLA-B27 (B27W and B27K) defined by cytotoxic T lymphocytes: identification of a third subtype (B27C) prevalent in oriental populations. In: Ziff M, Cohen SB (eds) Advances in inflammation research, vol 9. Raven, New York, pp 55–65

Breur-Vriesendorp BS, Ivanyi P (1986) Individual differences in the cytotoxic T-lymphocyte response in man to public HLA determinants. Cell Immunol 103: 252–271

Breur-Vriesendorp BS, Neefjes JC, Huis B, van Seventer G, Ploegh HL, Iványi P (1986) Identification of new B27 subtypes (B27C and B27D) prevalent in Oriental populations. Hum Immunol 16: 163–168

Breur-Vriesendorp BS, Dekker-Saeys AJ, Ivanyi P (1987) Distribution of HLA-B27 subtypes in patients with ankylosing spondylitis: the disease is associated with a common determinant of the various B27 molecules. Ann Rheum Dis 46: 353–356

Breur-Vriesendorp BS, de Waal LP, Ivanyi P (1988) Different linkage disequilibria of HLA-B27 subtypes and HLA-C locus alleles. Tissue Antigens 32: 74–77

Breur-Vriesendorp BS, Post FA, de Waal LP, Blokland E, Pool J, van der Linden S, Dekker-Saeys BJ, Goulmy E, Ivanyi P (1989) Blood lymphocytes from ankylosing spondylitis patients fail to induce disease-specific cytotoxic T lymphocytes. Hum Immunol (in press)

Breuning MH, van Mourik P, Iványi P (1980) Constancy of cross-reactivity patterns in sera of individual mice during the anti-H-2 response. Tissue Antigens 16: 49–55

Breuning M, Iványi P, van Mourik P (1981) Normal mouse sera react specifically with human lymphoblastoid cell lines. Transplant Proc 13: 1962–1965

Breuning MH, Lucas CJ, Breur BS, Engelsma MY, de Lange GG, Dekker AJ, Biddison B, Iványi P (1982) Subtypes of HLA-B27 detected by cytotoxic T lymphocytes and their role in self-recognition. Hum Immunol 5: 259–268

Breuning MH, Breur BS, Engelsma MY, Huis B, Iványi P (1983) Specificity of anti-HLA-B27 cytotoxic T lymphocytes. Tissue Antigens 22: 267–282

Breuning MH, Tekolf WA, Kato S, Breur BS, Engelsma MY, Spits H, Iványi P (1983) High resolution HLA typing by cytotoxic T lymphocytes. Transplant Proc 15: 118–122

Breuning MH, Breur B, Engelsma M, Iványi P (1984) Activation of cytotoxic T lymphocytes in HLA-A-, -B- and -C-identical responder-stimulator pairs. I. Variations in generation of anti-class-II CTL in primary mixed lymphocyte cultures. Tissue Antigens 24: 81–89

Breuning MH, Breur B, Engelsma M, Goulmy E, Iványi P (1984) Activation of cytotoxic T lymphocytes in HLA-A-, -B- and -C-identical responder-stimulator pairs. II. New subtypes of HLA-Bw35. Tissue Antigens 24: 90–97

Breuning MH, Spits H, de Vries JE, Iványi P (1984) A cloned cytotoxic T-lymphocyte (CTL) line recognizing a subtype of HLA-B27. Hum Immunol 9: 231–242

Briles WE, Bumstead N, Ewert DL, Gilmour DG, Hála K, Koch C, Longenecker BM, et al. (1982) Nomenclature for chicken major histocompatibility (B) complex. Immunogenetics 15: 441–447

Britton WJ, Hellqvist L, Ivanyi J, Basten A (1987) Immunopurification of radiolabelled antigens of *Myocbacterium leprae* and *Mycobacterium bovis* (Bacillus Calmette-Guerin) with monoclonal antibodies. Scand J Immunol 26: 149-159

Bruisten SM, Demant P (1989) Regulation of expression of mouse C4 and Slp genes by non-H-2-linked genes. Immunogenetics 29: 6-13

Bruisten SM, Skamene E, Demant P (1989) Haplotype-specific interactions of genetic factors, not linked to H-2, controlling the mouse C4 and Slp protein level. Genetics (in press)

Bryant ML, Klement V (1976) Clonal heterogeneity of wild mouse leukemia viruses. Virology 73: 532-536

Bubenik J, Kieler J, Tromholt V, Indrova M, Lotzová E (1987) Recombinant interleukin-2 inhibits growth of tumor xenografts in congenitally athymic mice. Immunol Lett 14: 325-330

Buchanan TM, Nomaguchi H, Anderson DC, Young RA, Gillis TP, Britton WJ, Ivanyi J, et al. (1987) Characterization of antibody-reactive epitopes on the 65-kilodalton protein of *Mycobacterium leprae*. Infect Immun 55: 1000-1003

Buckspan M, Hojvat S, Skamene E (1977) Immunoprophylaxis toward mammary carcinoma in mice immune to Listeria monocytogenes. Cancer Immunol Immunother 3: 49-56

Bukara M, Vinček V, Figueroa F, Klein J (1985) How polymorphic are class II loci of the mouse *H-2* complex? Immunogenetics 21: 569-579

Buschman E, Skamene E (1988) Genetic background of the host and expression of natural resistance and acquired immunity to M.tuberculosis. In: Friedman H, Bendinelli M (eds) Tuberculosis: Interactions with the immune system, vol 3. Plenum, New York, pp 59-79

Buschman E, Skamene E (1988) Immunological consequences of innate resistance and susceptibility to BCG. Denmark Staten Serum Institut. Immunol Lett 19: 199-210

Buschman E, Apt AS, Nickonenko BV, Moroz AM, Averbakh MH, Skamene E (1988) Genetic aspects of innate resistance and acquired immunity to mycobacteria in inbred mice. Springer Semin Immunopathol 10: 319-336

Bux E, Matsunaga K, Nagatani T, Walden P, Nagy ZA, Klein J (1985) Distribution of alloreactivity among antigenspecific, class II-restricted T-cell clones and hybridomas. Immunogenetics 22: 189-192

Cadman HF, Wallis M, Ivanyi J (1982) The effects of monoclonal antibodies against human growth hormone or hormone-receptor interactions. FEBS Lett 137: 149-152

Calafat J, Demant P, Janssen H (1981) Independence of H-2 and viral antigens on the cell surface and absence of H-2 antigens on murine leukemia virus and mouse mammary tumor virus particles. Immunogenetics 14: 203-220

Calafat J, Janssen H, Demant P, Hilgers J, Zavada J (1983) Specific selection of host cell glycoproteins during assembly of murine leukaemia virus and vesicular stomatitis virus: Presence of Thy-1 glycoprotein and absence of H-2, Pgp-1 and T-200 glycoproteins on the envelopes of these virus particles. J Gen Virol 64: 1241-1253

Calin A, Elswood J, Klouda PT (1989) Destructive arthritis, rheumatoid factor, HLA-DR4. Susceptibility versus severity. Arthritis Rheumatol (in press)

Callahan GN, Ferrone S, Poulik MD, Reisfeld RA, Klein J (1976) Characterization of Ia antigens in mouse serum. J Immunol 117: 1351-1355

Callejas F, Kinsky RG, Voisin GA (1972) Conditions d'action des anticorps cytotoxiques (fixant le complément) dans le rejet des homogreffes tumorales. Ann Inst Pasteur 123: 125-126

Capel PJA, Bishop C, Demant P (1980) Complement dependence of blocking of C3d lymphocyte receptors by anti-H-2 antibodies. Immunobiologe 158: 14-16

Capra JD, Vitetta ES, Klein J (1975) Studies on the murine Ss protein. I. Purification, molecular weight and subunit structure. J Exp Med 142: 664-672

Capra JD, Vitetta ES, Klapper DG, Uhr JW, Klein J (1976) Structural studies on the protein products of the murine chromosome 17. II. The partial amino acid sequence of an $H-2^b$ molecule. Proc Natl Acad Sci USA 73: 3661-3665

Carlin CR, Simon D, Mattison J, Knowles BB (1988) Expression and biosynthetic variation of the EGF receptor in human hepatocellular carcinoma-derived cell lines. Mol Cell Biol 8: 25-34

Caulfield M, Luce KJ, Proffitt MR, Cerny J (1983) Induction of idiotype-specific suppressor T cells with antigen/antibody complexes. J Exp Med 157: 1713

Caulfield M, Cerny J (1988) Specific antigen/antibody complexes induce the in vivo production of a parallel set of nonantigen-binding, idiotype-positive antibodies. Eur J Immunol 18: 439

Caulfield MJ, Cerny J (1980) Cell interactions in leukemia-associated immunosuppression. Suppression of thymus-independent antibody responses by leukemia spleen cells (Moloney) in vitro is mediated by normal T cells. J Immunol 124: 255

Chan C, Kongshavn PAL, Skamene E (1977) Enhanced primary resistance to Listeria monocytogenes in T-cell deprived mice. Immunology 32: 529

Chaouat G, Kinsky RG, Duc HT, Robert P (1979) The possibility of anti-idiotypic activity in multiparous mice. Ann Inst Pasteur Immunol 130: 601–605

Chiang CL, Klein J (1978) Immunogenetic analysis of *H-2* mutations. VII. H-2 associated recognition of minor histocompatibility antigens in $H\text{-}2K^b$ mutants. Immunogenetics 6: 333–342

Chen BP, Malkovský M, Hank JA, Sondel PM (1987) Nonrestricted cytotoxicity mediated by interleukin 2-expanded leukoctes is inhibited by anti-LFA-1 monoclonal antibodies (MoAb), but potentiated by anti-CD3 MoAb. Cell Immunol 110: 282–293

Chandramuki A, Allen PRJ, Keen M, Ivanyi J (1985) Detection of mycobacterial antigen and antibodies in the cerebrospinal fluid of patients with tuberculous meningitis. J Med Microbiol 20: 239–247

Chonmaitree T, Congeni BL, Munoz J, Rakusan TA, Powell KR, Box QT (1984) Twice daily ceftriaxone therapy for serious bacterial infections in children. J Antimicrob Chemother 13: 511–516

Christie JD, Rakusan TA, Martinez MA, Lucia HL, Rajamanan S, Edwards SB, Hayden CK (1986) Hydranencephaly caused by congenital infection with herpes simplex virus. Pediatr Infect Dis 5: 473–478

Chen S-S, Cerny J (1980) Studies on hapten-specific B cell tolerance in vitro. II. Regulation of central tolerance in T-independent B cells by antigen-activated syngeneic T cells. J Immunol 125: 1970

Chen S-S, Cerny J (1980) Studies on hapten-specific B cell tolerance in vitro. I. The inductive phase of central B cell tolerance. J Immunol 125: 1962

Cermakova E, Goerz G, Koldovsky P (1985) Prognostic significance of circulating immuncomplexes in melanoma patients. Tumor Diagn Ther 6: 226

Cerny J (1974) Stimulation of bone marrow hemopoietic stem cells by a factor from activated T cells. Nature 249: 742

Cerny J (1982) The role of anti-idiotypic T cells in cyclical course of antibody response. In: DeLisi C, Hiernaux J (eds) Regulatory implications of oscillatory dynamics in the immune response. CRC, Boca Raton, p 59

Cerny J (1984) Immune regulations by autologous anti-idiotopic T cells. In: Sercarz E, Cantor H, Chess L (eds) Regulation of immune systems. Liss, New York, p 829

Cerny J (1984) Autologous idiotype-specific T cells in regulation of antibody response. In: Greene M, Nisonoff A (eds) The biology of idiotypes. Plenum, New York, p 381

Cerny J (1985) Introduction to immunology. In: Baron S (ed) Medical microbiology, 2nd edn. Addison-Wesley, Menlo Park

Cerny J, Caulfield M (1981) Stimulation of specific antibody-forming cells in antigen-primed nude mice by the adoptive transfer of syngeneic anti-idiotypic T cells. J Immunol 126: 2262

Cerny J, Cronkhite R (1983) An independent regulation of distinct idiotypes of the T15 idiotype by autologous T cells. Ann NY Acad Sci 418: 31

Cerny J, Essex M (1974) Cellular antigen(s) of murine leukemias. Nature 251: 742

Cerny J, Essex M (1979) Immunosuppression by oncogenic RNA viruses. In: Neubauer R (ed) Naturally occurring immunosuppressive factors and their relationship to disease. CRC, Boca Raton, p 233

Cerny J, Halasa J (1973) Antigen binding rosette forming cells in a Friend virus-induced leukemia. Experientia 29: 101

Cerny J, Isaak DD (1979) Interactions of murine leukemia virus (MuLV) with isolated lymphocytes. IV. The role of mitogen-induced cellular DNA synthesis in virus infection and replication. Int J Cancer 23: 260

Cerny J, Kelsoe G (1984) Priority of complementary anti-idiotypic response following antigen stimulation: an artifact or an important network mechanism? Immunol Today 5: 61

Cerny J, Stiller RA (1975) Immunosuppression by spleen cells from Moloney leukemia. Comparison of the suppressive effect on antibody response and on mitogen-induced responses. J Immunol 115: 942

Cerny J, Waner EB (1975) Specific susceptibility of sensitized (memory) B cells to suppression and antigenic alteration by murine leukemia virus. J Immunol 114: 571

Cerny J, McAlack RF, Ceglowski WS, Friedman H (1971) Divergence between immunosuppression and immunocompetence during virus-induced leukemogenesis. Proc Natl Acad Sci USA 68: 1862

Cerny J, McAlack RF, Friedman H (1971) Non-random distribution of vibriolytic foci in the spleen of mice lacking "background" antibody. Proc Soc Exp Biol Med 137: 1021

Cerny J, McAlack RF, Friedman H (1971) Antibody plaque-forming cells: Rapid recruitment and proliferation in the absence of natural antibody background. Experientia 27: 565

Cerny J, McAlack RF, Friedman H (1971) An alternative model of antibody forming cell differentiation. In: Morphological and Functional Aspects of Immunity. Plenum, New York, p 315

Cerny J, McAlack R, Sajid MA, Friedman H (1971) Genetic differences in the immunocyte response fo mice to separate determinants on one bacterial antigen. Nature 230: 247

Cerny J, McAlack RF, Sajid MA, Fronton J, Friedman H (1971) Early accumulation of antibody forming cells in mouse spleen lacking a pre-existing background. J Immunol 106: 1371

Cerny J, McAlack RF, Friedman H (1972) Splenic foci of antibody producing cells to two distinct somatic antigens present on one bacterium. Immunology 22: 573

Cerny J, Essex M, Rich MA, Hardy WD jr (1975) Expression of virus associated antigens and immune cell functions during spontaneous regression of the Friend viral murine leukemia. Int J Cancer 15: 351

Cerny J, Waner EB, Rubin AS (1975) T cell products activating stem cells. Further studies on the origin and action of the factor(s). J Immunol 115: 513

Cerny J, Essex M, Thomas DB (1976) Interactions of murine leukemia virus (MuLV) with isolated lymphocytes. III. Alterations of B and T cells in the spleen of Friend virus-infected mice. Int J Cancer 18: 197-204

Cerny J, Fistel SH, Hensgen PA (1976) Interactions of murine leukemia virus (MuLV) with isolated lymphocytes. I. Virus replication in lymphocytes infected with Friend virus and cultured in diffusion chambers in vivo. Int J Cancer 18: 176-188

Cerny J, Hensgen PA, Fistel SF, Mastalir Demlir L (1976) Interactions of murine leukemia virus (MuLV) with isolated lymphocytes. II. Infection of B and T cells with Friend virus complex in diffusion chambers and in vitro: effect of polyclonal mitogens. Int J Cancer 18: 189-196

Cerny J, Proffitt MR, Essex M (1976) Immunosuppression by Moloney leukemia virus: lack of correlation between virus replication and the immunosuppressive effect. JNCI 56: 819

Cerny J, Grinwich KD, Stiller RA (1977) Immunosuppression by spleen cells from Moloney leukemia. III. Evidence that the suppressor cell is not the leukemic, virus-producing cell. J Immunol 119: 1097

Cerny J, Isaak DD, Hoover EA (1979) Interactions of murine leukemia viruses (Friend and Moloney) with lymphocyte subpopulations. In: Proffitt M (ed) Virus-lymphocyte interactions: implications for disease. Elsevier/North-Holland, New York, p 139

Cerny J, Caulfield MJ, Siat M (1980) Regulation of the T15 idiotypepositive, T-independent immune response to *S.pneumoniae* R36a (Pn). I. Specific suppressor T cells induced by Pn in vitro are antigen-specific and idiotype-positive. Eur J Immunol 10: 661

Cerny J, Heusser C, Wallich R, Hammerling G, Eardley DD (1982) Immunoglobulin idiotopes on T cells. I. Expression of distinct idiotopes detected by monoclonal antibodies on antigen-specific suppressor T cells. J Exp Med 156: 719

Cerny J, Wallich R, Hammerling G (1982) Analysis of T15 idiotypes by monoclonal antibodies. Variability of idiotopic expression on phosphorycholine-specific lymphocytes from individual inbred mice. J Immunol 128: 1885

Cerny J, Cronkhite R, Heusser C (1983) Antibody response of mice following neonatal treatment with anti-receptor antibody. Evidence for B cell tolerance and T suppressor cells specific for different idiotopic determinants. Eur J Immunol 13: 244

Cerny J, Cronkhite R, Stout TS (1986) Rapid changes in the regulatory potential of autologous anti-idiotopic T cells during an antigen-driven primary response. J Immunol 136: 3597

Cerny J, Smith JS, Webb C, Tucker PW (1988) Properties of anti-idiotypic T cell lines propagated with syngeneic B lymphocytes. I. T cells bind intact idiotypes and discriminate between the somatic idiotypic variants in a manner similar to the anti-idiotypic antibodies. J Immunol (in press)

Černý-Provaznik R, Iványi P (1985) Frequency of naturally occurring H-2-specific antibodies in mouse sera monitored by "superreactive" rabbit complement. Tissue Antigens 26: 259-261

Černý-Provaznik R, van Mourik P, Radl J, Leupers T, Limpens JC, Iványi P (1985) Anti-MHC immunity detected prior to intentional alloimmunization. II. Monoclonal H-2-specific antibodies obtained from a normal C57Bl/KaLwRij (H-2b) mouse. Nat Immun Cell Growth Regul 4: 160-168

Černý-Provaznik R, van Mourik P, Limpens J, Leupers T, Iványi P (1985) Anti-MHC immunity detected prior to intentional alloimmunization. III. Natural autoreactive H-2-specific antibodies. Immunogenetics 21: 491-504

Černý-Provaznik R, Radl J, Leupers T, van Mourik P, Brondijk R, de Greeve P, Iványi P (1985) Anti-MHC immunity detected prior to intentional alloimmunization. I. Naturally occurring H-2-specific antibodies in C57Bl/KaLwRij (H-2^b) mice. Nat Immun Cell Growth Regul 4: 138-159

Černý-Provaznik R, Kloosterman T, Verkerk D, Vroom TM, Iványi P (1986) Natural autoreactive H-2-specific serum antibodies in a group of BALB/cBy (H-2^d) mice. Tissue Antigens 27: 106-111

Černý-Provaznik R, Kloosterman T, Verkerk D, van Mourik P, Reboul M, Frangoulis B, Pla M, Ivanyi P (1986) Anti-MHC immunity detected prior to intentional alloimmunization. IV. Natural monoclonal H-2-specific antibodies. J Immunogenet 13: 287-297

Clague RB, Firth S, Holt PJL, Dyer PA, Klouda PT, Harris R (1982) HLA antigens in patients with rheumatoid arthritis and serum antibodies to native type II collagen. Ann Rheum Dis 41: 316

Clarke A, Stewart-Phillips JL, Skamene E (1987) Genetic control of susceptibility to atherosclerosis (with special emphasis on the role of the macrophage). J Clin Invest Med 10: 499-512

Clark JT, Anand R, Akoglut T, McBride JS (1987) Identification and characterisation of proteins associated with the rhoptry organelles of *Plasmodium falciparum* merozoites. Parasitol Res 73: 425-434

Clark JT, Donachie S, Anand R, Wilson CF, Heidrich H-G, McBride JS (1988) 46-53 kDa glycoprotein from the surface of *Plasmodium falciparum* merozoites. Mol Biochem Parasitol (in press)

Coates ARM, Allen BW, Hewitt J, Ivanyi J, Mitchison DA (1981) Antigenic diversity of *Mycobacterium tuberculosis* and *Mycobacterium bovis* detected by means of monoclonal antibodies. Lancet 2: 167-169

Cohen Z, McCulloch P, Leung MK, Mervart H (1981) Histocompatibility antigens in patients with Crohn's disease. In: Pena AS, Weterman IT, Booth CC, Strober W (eds) Recent advances in Crohn's disease. Nijhoff, Hague, pp 186-191 (Developments in gastroenterology, vol 1)

Colizzi V, Malkovský M, Lang G, Asherson GL (1985) In vivo activity of interleukin-2: conversion of a stimulus causing unresponsiveness to a stimulus causing contact hypersensitivity by the injection of interleukin-2. Immunology 56: 653-658

Colizzi V, Asherson GL, James BMB, Malkovský M (1984) T helper factor in contact sensitivity: antigen-specific I-A$^+$ helper factor is made by an Lyt-1$^+$2$^-$, I-A$^+$, I-J$^-$ T cell. Immunology 52: 261-267

Colizzi V, Ferluga J, Garreau F, Malkovský M, Asherson GL (1984) Suppressor cells induced by BCG release non-specific factors in vitro which inhibit DNA synthesis and interleukin-2 production. Immunology 51: 65-71

Colizzi V, Malkovský M (1985) Augmentation of interleukin-2 production and delayed hypersensitivity in mice infected with *Mycobacterium bovis* and fed a diet supplemented with vitamin A acetate. Infect Immun 48: 581-583

Colombani MJ, Pla M, Mouton D, Degos L (1979) H-2 typing of mice genetically selected for high and low antibody production. Immunogenetics 8: 237-243

Colombani J, Pla M (1982) Le modèle murin: H-2. In: Dausset J (ed) HLA 1982, complexe majeur d'histocompatibilité de l'homme. Flammarion, Paris, pp 1-32

Colombatti A, Dux A, Berns A, Demant P, Hilgers J (1979) H-2 dependent regulation of high ecotropic MuLV expression. JNCI 63: 869-873

Congeni BL, Chonmaitree T, Rakusan TA, Box QT (1985) Once daily ceftriaxone therapy of serious bacterial infections in children. Antimicrob Agents Chemother 27: 181–183

Cook RG, Vitetta ES, Uhr JW, Klein J, Wilde CE, Capra JD (1978) Structural studies on protein products of murine chromosome 17. III. Partial amino acid sequence of an H-2K^q molecule. J Immunol 121: 1015–1019

Cook KM, Aston R, Ivanyi J (1985) Topographic and functional assay of antigenic determinants of human prolactin with monoclonal antibodies. Mol Immunol 22: 795–801

Cosimi AB, Skamene E, Bonney W, Russell PS (1970) Experience with large-dose intravenous antithymocyte globulin in primates and man. Surgery 68: 54

Cox JH, Ivanyi J, Young DB, Lamb JR, Syred AD, Francis J (1988) Orientation of epitopes influences the immunogenicity of synthetic peptide dimers. Eur J Immunol (in press)

Cox JH, Ivanyi J (1988) The role of host factors for the chemotherapy of BCG infection in inbred strains of mice. APMIS (in press)

Cronkhite R, Cerny J (1986) A novel idiotopic determinant on phosphorylcholine binding immunoglobulins restricted to isotype and allotype. J Immunol 136: 3729

Cronkhite R, Cerny J, Delisi C (1984) Inhibition of plaque-forming cells with anti-idiotype or hapten: variation due to hapten density on indicator red cells. J Immunol Methods 68: 109

Cronkhite R, Strickland F, Cerny J (1988) Regulation of idiotope expression III. H-2 influences the magnitude and the idiotype of a T-independent antibody response in mice of certain genetic backgrounds. J Immunol 141: 921

Cronkhite R, Schulze D, Cerny J (1989) Regulation of idiotope expression IV. A selective genetic linkage of two D region-dependent T15 idiotopes to the Igh allotype. J Immunol (in press)

Cudkowicz G, Lotzová E (1971) Genetic determinants of hybrid resistance in murine linkage group IX. In: Vojtiskova M, Lengerova A (eds) Immunogenetics of the H-2 system. Karger, Basel, p 76

Cudkowicz G, Lotzová E (1973) Hemopoietic cell-defined components of the major histocompatibility complex of mice. Identification of responsive and unresponsive recipients for bone marrow transplants. Transplant Proc 5: 1399–1405

Cullen SE, Hansen TD, Klein J (1978) Isolation and analysis of H-2 and Ia alloantigens from wild mouse strains. J Immunol 121: 141–148

Czarnomska A, Demant P (1980) H-2 antigenic specificities controlled by the translocation chromosome T190. Transplantation 30: 69–72

Daëron M, Kinsky RG, Voisin GA (1972) Dégranulation anaphylactique de mastocytes in vitro par des anticorps de transplantation chez la souris. CR Acad Sci [D] (Paris) 275: 2571–2573

Daëron M, Duc HT, Kanellopulos J, Le Bouteiller P, Kinsky R, Voisin GA (1975) Allogeneic mast cell degranulation induced by histocompatibility antibodies: an in vitro model of transplantation anaphylaxis. Cell Immunol 20: 133–155

Daëron M, Kanellopoulos J, Duc HT, Kinsky R, Voisin GA (1977) Agents et mécanismes responsables de la dégranulation anaphylactique allogénique directe (DAAD). Ann Inst Pasteur Immunol 128: 61–63

Dalgleish AG, Malkovský M (1987) Group specific component and HIV infection. Lancet 1: 1268

Dalgleish AG, Malkovský M (1988) Advances in human retroviruses. Adv Cancer Res 51: 307–360

Dalgleish AG, Malkovský M (1988) AIDS and the new viruses. In: Webster ADB (ed) Immunodeficiency and disease. Kluwer, London, pp 1–24

Dalgleish AG, Malkovský M, Webster ADB (1986) AIDS, Portugal, and Africa. Lancet 1: 911

Dalgleish AG, Malkovský M (1988) Surgical gloves as a mechanical barrier against human immunodeficiency viruses. Br J Surg 75: 171–172

Dalgleish AG, Malkovský M (1988) Latex gloves off in virus porosity dispute (Letter). Nature 336: 317

Dalgleish AG, Thomson BJ, Chanh LT, Malkovský M, Kennedy RC (1987) Neutralisation of HIV isolates by anti-idiotypic antibodies which mimic the T4 (CD4) epitope: a potential AIDS vaccine. Lancet 2: 1047–1050

Dalgleish AG, Kennedy RC, Sattentau Q, Chanh T, Beverley P, Maddon P, Axel R, Malkovský M (1988) The T4 molecule: its possible use in therapeutic strategies against AIDS. In: Bolognesi D (ed) Human retroviruses, cancer and AIDS: Approaches to prevention and therapy. Liss, New York, pp 283–288 (UCLA symposia on molecular and cellular biology)

David CS, Shreffler DC, Murphy DB, Klein J (1973) Serological cross reaction between H-2D- and H-2K-region antigens. Transplant Proc 5: 287-293

David CS, Klein J, Shreffler DC (1973) Serological homology between H-2 and HL-A systems. Transplant Proc 5: 461-466

Decary F, Ferner P, Giavedoni L, Hartman A, Howie R, Kalovsky E, Laschinger C et al. (1984) An investigation of nonhemolytic transfusion reactions. Vox Sang 46: 277-285

Demant P (1979) H-2K, H-2D, H-2L and H-2G specificities by haplotype of the H-2 gene complex: Mouse. In: Altman P, Katz D (eds) Inbred and genetically defined strains of laboratory animals, part 1: Mouse and rat. Federation of the American Society of Experimental Biology, Bethesda, pp 137-140

Demant P (1980) Histocompatibility genes and their use in genetic control of laboratory mice. In: Proceedings of the 7th ICLAS Symposium, Utrecht, 1979. Fischer, Stuttgart, pp 299-306

Demant P (1985) Corticosteroid-induced cleft palate: Cis interaction of MHC genes and hybrid resistance. Immunogenetics 22: 183-188

Demant P (1986) Histocompatibility and the genetics of tumour resistance (Introductory essay). J Immunogenet 13: 61-67

Demant P, Cleton FJ (1980) Histocompatibility genes and neoplasia. In: Cleton F, Simons J (eds) Genetic origins of tumor cells. Nijhoff, The Hague, pp 109-125

Demant P, Festenstein H (1980) Histocompatibility antigenes, tumors and viruses. J Immunogenet 7: 1-70

Demant P, Hart AAM (1986) Recombinant congenic strains: A new tool for analyzing genetic traits determined by more than one gene. Immunogenetics 24: 416-422

Demant P, Ivanyi D (1981) Further molecular complexities of H-2 K- and D-region antigens. Nature 290: 146-149

Demant P, Neauport-Sautes C (1978) The H-2L locus and the system of H-2 specificities. Immunogenetics 7: 295-311

Demant P, Oudshoorn-Snoek M (1985) H-2 class I antigen expression on mouse teratocarcinoma cell lines. Immunogenetics 22: 543-552

Demant P, Roos MH (1982) Molecular heterogeneity of D-end products detected by anti-H-2.28 sera. I. A molecule similar to Qa-2, detected in the BALB/cBy but not in the BALB/c-H-2dm2 mutant. Immunogenetics 15: 461-466

Demant P, Neauport-Sautes C, Joskowitz M (1977) A three locus model for the 'classical' H-2 antigens. Tissue Antigens 10: 252

Demant P, Ivanyi D, Neauport-Sautes C, Snoek M (1978) H-2.28, an alloantigenic marker allelic to H-2.1, is expressed on all three known types of H-2 molecules. Proc Natl Acad Sci USA 75: 4441-4445

Demant P, Neauport-Sautes C, Ivanyi D, Joskowitz M, Snoek M, Bishop C (1979) System of H-2 specificities: Molecular expression and genetic control. In: Ferrone S, Gorini S, Herberman R, Reisfeld R (eds) Current trends in tumor immunology. Garland, New York, pp 289-298

Demant P, Ivanyi D, Nusse R, Neauport-Sautes C, Snoek M (1979) H-2L locus: Alleles, products, and specificities. Transplant Proc 11: 647-651

Demant P, Ivanyi D, van Nie R (1979) The map position of the rds gene on the 17th chromosome of the mouse. Tissue Antigens 13: 53-55

Demant P, Calafat J, Ivanyi D, Nusse R, Oudshoorn-Snoek M (1981) Antigenic and molecular complexity of K- and D-region products. In: Immunobiology of the major histocompatibility complex. Karger, Basel, pp 11-17

Demant P, Ivanyi D, Oudshoorn-Snoek M (1981) Genetic complexity of H-2 antigens. Transplant Proc 13: 1755-1758

Demant P, Ivanyi D, Oudshoorn-Snoek M, Calafat J, Roos MH (1981) Molecular heterogeneity of H-2 antigens. Immunol Rev 60: 5-22

Demant P, Ivanyi D, Fischer-Lindahl K (1981) Functional heterogeneity of H-2Dk-region products. Immunogenetics 13: 457-461

Demant P, Hart AAM, van Zutphen LFM (1987) Genetic analysis of multigenic traits using recombinant congenic strains. In: Beynen A, Solleveld H (eds) New developments in biosciences – implications for laboratory animals science. Nijhoff, Dordrecht, pp 209-214

Demant P, Oomen LCJM, Oudshoorn-Snoek M (1989) Genetics of tumor susceptibility in the mouse: Major histocompatibility complex and non-MHC genes. Adv Cancer Res (in press)

Degos L, Pla M, Colombani JM (1979) H-2 restriction for lymphocyte homing into lymph nodes. Eur J Immunol 9: 808–814

Degos L, Pla M, Cesar E, Colombani M, Colombani J (1979) Complexe majeur d'histocompatibilité et reconnaissance non immune: passage des lymphocytes du sang dans les ganglions. In: Bernard J (ed) Actualités hématologiques. Masson, Paris, pp 254–259

Deh EM, Klouda PT, Levine M, Harris R, Donnai P (1982) Detection, isolation and characterisation of cell free HLA antigens from human amniotic fluid. Tissue Antigens 20: 260–269

Dembić Z, Singer PA, Klein J (1984) A history of a mutation. EMBO J 3: 1647–1654

Dembić Z, Ayane M, Klein J, Steinmetz M, Benoist CO, Mathis DJ (1985) Inbred and wild mice carry identical deletions in their E_α MHC genes. EMBO J 4: 127–131

Denis M, Forget A, Miailhe A-C, Pelletier M, Skamene E (1985) Evolution of cell types and T-cell subsets in the spleens of *Mycobacterium bovis* BCG-resistant and *M. bovis* BCG-susceptibile strains of mice after infection with *M. bovis* BCG. Infect Immun 49: 253–255

Denis M, Forget A, Pelletier M, Turcotte R, Skamene E (1986) Control of the Bcg gene of early resistance in mice to infections with BCG substrains and atypical mycobacteria. Clin Exp Immunol 63: 517–525

Denis M, Forget A, Pelletier M, Skamene E (1988) Pleiotropic effects of the Bcg gene. I. Antigen presentation in genetically susceptible and resistant congenic mouse strains. J Immunol 140: 2395–2400

Denis M, Forget A, Pelletier M, Skamene E (1988) Pleiotropic effects of the Bcg gene. III. Respiratory burst in Bcg-congenic macrophages. Clin Exp Immunol 73: 370–375

Denis M, Buschman E, Forget A, Pelletier M, Skamene E (1988) Pleiotropic effects of the Bcg gene: Genetic restriction of responses to mitogens and allogeneic targets. J Immunol (in press)

Dev VG, Miller DA, Hasmi S, Warburton D, Miller OJ, Klein J (1972) Cytological identification by quinacrine fluorescence and Giemsa-banding of a biarmed *Mus poschiavinus chromosome*. Genetics 72: 541–543

De Waal LP, Lieder J, DeLange GG, Huis B, Melief CJM, Engelfriet CP, Iványi P (1984) B27 subtypes. In: Albert ED, Baur MP, Mayr WR (eds) Histocompatibility testing 1984. Springer, Berlin Heidelberg New York, pp 418–419

De Waal LP, Krom FEJM, Breur-Vriesendorp BS, Engelfriet CP, Lopez de Castro JA, Ivanyi P (1987) Conventional alloantisera can recognize the same HLA-B27 polymorphism as detected by cytotoxic T lymphocytes. Hum Immunol 20: 265–271

Dicke KA, Lotzová E, Spitzer G, McCredie KB (1978) Immunobiology of bone marrow transplantation. In: Freireich EJ, Hersh EM, Miescher PA, Jaffe ER (eds) Leukemia and lymphoma. Grune and Stratton, New York, pp 227–246

Dicke KA, Lotzová E, Spitzer G, McCredie KB (1978) Immunobiology of bone marrow transplantation. Semin Hematol 15: 263–282

Dicke KA, Spitzer G, Zander AR, Lanzotti VJ, Verma DS, Peters LJ, Valdivieso M, Lotzová E, McCredie KB (1979) Autologous bone marrow transplantation in relapsed adult acute leukemia and solid tumors. Transplant Proc 11: 212–214

Dill O, Kievits F, Koch S, Ivanyi P, Hämmerling GJ (1988) Immunological function of HLA-C antigens in HLA-Cw3 transgenic mice. Proc Natl Acad Sci USA 85: 5664–5668

Dindzans VJ, Skamene E, Levy GA (1986) Susceptibility/resistance to mouse hepatitis virus strain 3 and macrophage procoagulant activity are genetically linked and controlled by two non H-2 linked genes. J Immunol 137: 2355–2360

Dindzans V, Skamene E, Levy GA (1985) Susceptibility/resistance to murine hepatitis virus strain 3 (MHV-3) and monocyte procoagulant activity (PCA) are genetically linked and controlled by 2 non H-2 linked genes. Prog Leukocyte Biol 3: 151–158

Donner LR, Dubbs DR, Kit S (1977) Chromosomal site(s) of integration of herpes simplex virus 2 thymidine kinase gene in biochemically transformed human cell. Int J Cancer 20: 256

Donner L, Turek LP, Ruscetti SK, Fedele LA, Sherr CJ (1980) Transformation-defective mutants of feline sarcoma virus which express a product of the viral *src* gene. J Virol 35: 129

Donner L, Fedele L, Garon CF, Anderson SJ, Sherr CJ (1982) McDonough feline sarcoma virus: Characterization of the cloned provirus and its feline oncogene (v-fms). J Virol 41: 489

Donner L, de Lanerolle P, Costa J (1983) Immunoreactivity of paraffin-embedded normal tissues and mesenchymal tumors for smooth muscle myosin. Am J Clin Pathol 80: 677

Donner L, Triche TJ, Israel MA, Seeger PC, Reynolds CP (1985) A panel of monoclonal antibodies which discriminate neuroblastoma from Ewing's sarcoma, rhabdomyosarcoma, neuroepithelioma, and hematopoietic malignancies. Prog Clin Biol Res 175: 347

Donner LR, Manriquez M, Greene JF Jr (1989) Minimal deviation spindle cell melanoma: unusual histological pattern in an 11-year-old black girl. Pediatr Pathol (in press)

Dorić M, Kinsky RG, Voisin GA (1984) Allogeneic reactivity of maternal lymphoid cells during the course of gestation. Modifications and sex differences in a local GVH assay. J Reprod Immunol 6: 187–195

Dossetor JB, Kovithavongs T, Schlaut J, Pazderka V, Liburd EM, Bettcher KB, Pazderka F (1979) Donor specific immunologic monitoring of transplant patients. Transplant Proc 11: 1235

Dossetor J, Liburd EM, Kovithavongs T, Pazderka F, Bettcher KB (1981) Donor specific suppressor cells in renal allograft recipients: technical aspects and clinical studies. Transplant Proc 12: 1645

Douglass AB, Harris L, Pazderka F (1988) Monozygotic twins concordant for the narcoleptic syndrome. Neurology (in press)

Douvas GS, Kinsky R, Duc HT, Voisin GA (1982) Suppressor cells as an agent of immune facilitation. II. Adoptive transfer of passively induced enhancement of allografted tumors. Cell Immunol 68: 389–401

Douvas G, Kinsky R (1983) The effects of low dose irradiation on the active enhancement of tumor allografts. Transplantation 36: 226–228

Drewinko B, Moskwa P, Lotzová E, Trujillo JM (1986) Successful heterotransplantation of human colon cancer cells to athymic animals is related to tumor cell differentiation and to host natural killer cell activity. Invasion Metastasis 6: 69–82

Duc HT, Kinsky RG, Voisin GA (1973) Efficacité préférentielle des immuns complexes dans la facilitation des allogreffes tumorales. Ann Inst Pasteur Immunol 124: 567–572

Duc HT, Kinsky RG, Kanellopoulos J, Voisin GA (1975) Biological properties of transplantation immune sera. IV. Influence of the course of immunization dilution and complexing to antigen on enhancing activity of Ig classes. J Immunol 115: 1143–1150

Duc HT, Kinsky RG, Voisin GA (1977) Sites antigéniques impliqués dans la facilitation des allogreffes tumorales. Ann Inst Pasteur Immunol 128: 19–20

Duc HT, Kinsky RG, Voisin GA (1978) Ia versus K/D antigens in immunological enhancement of tumor allografts. Transplantation 25: 182–187

Duc HT, Kinsky RG, Voisin GA (1978) Rôle des antigènes codés par les régions H-2 K/D et I (Ia) dans la facilitation immunologique d'allogreffes tumorales. Effets d'anticorps obtenus par absorption-élution ou par immunisation de lignées recombinantes. Ann Inst Pasteur Immunol 129: 747

Duc HT, Kinsky RG, Voisin GA (1979) Ia versus K/D antigens in immunological enhancement of tumor allografts. II. Studies with alloimmune sera prepared in recombinant strains. Ann Inst Pasteur Immunol 130: 461–474

Duc HT, Kinsky RG, Voisin GA (1982) Passive allograft enhancement by subclasses of polyclonal antibodies directed towards restricted regions of the MHC. Transplantation 33: 492–499

Duc HT, Kinsky RG, Monnot P, Voisin GA (1985) Evolution of alloantibodies and suppressor cells in allografted mice treated for passive enhancement. Cell Immunol 95: 180–194

Duc HT, Massé A, Bobé P, Kinsky RG, Voisin GA (1985) Deviation of humoral and cellular alloimmune reactions by placental extracts. J Reprod Immunol 7: 27–39

Dupuy d'Angeac A, Reme T, Pla M, Colombani J (1982) Accessory function of a small radioresistant spleen cell population in the generation of T-cell-mediated cytotoxicity. Cell Immunol 68: 1–15

Dupuy JM, Sparkes BG, Desrosiers M, Skamene E, Micusan VV (1983) Prevention of the enhancing effect of mucin and iron in mouse meningococcal infection. Can J Microbiol 29: 1671–1674

Duncan WR, Wakeland EK, Klein J (1979) Heterozygosity of *H-2* loci in wild mice. Nature 281: 603–605

Duncan WR, Wakeland EK, Klein J (1979) Histocompatibility-2 system in wild mice. VIII. Frequencies of H-2 and Ia antigens in wild mice from Texas. Immunogenetics 9: 261–272

Duncan WR, Klein J (1980) Histocompatibility-2 system in wild mice. IX. Serological analysis of 13 new B10.W congenic lines. Immunogenetics 10: 45–65

Dux A, Demant P (1987) The influence of the MHC on resistance against C3H-MTV induced mammary tumors is predominantly systemic rather than local. Int J Cancer 40: 372–377

Dyer PA, Klouda PT, Harris R, Mallick NP (1980) Properdin factor B alleles in patients with idopathic membranous nephropathy. Tissue Antigens 15: 505–507

Dyer PA, Klouda PT, Harris R (1981) HLA antigens associated with Properdin factor B allotype BfF1. Tissue Antigens 17: 362–367

Dyer PA, Klouda PT, Johnson RWG, Read AP, Mallick NP, Harris R (1981) Matching for Properdin factor B(Bf) in renal transplantation. Transplantation 32: 424–425

Dyer PA, Clague RB, Klouda PT, Firth S, Harris R, Holt PJL (1982) HLA antigens in patients with rheumatoid arthritis and antibodies to native type II collagen. Tissue Antigens 20: 394–396

Dyer PA, Watters EA, Klouda PT, Harris R, Mallick NP (1982) Absence of linkage between adult polycystic kidney disease and the major histocompatibility system. Tissue Antigens 20: 108–111

Ebbers J, Koldovsky P, Vosteen KH (1985) Expression of Ia antigen on NPC xenografted in the nude mice. Arch Otorhinolaryngol 242: 209

Ebbers J, Lindenberger J, Meyer zum Gottesberg A, Koldovsky P, Koldovsky U, Vosteen KH (1986) Xenografting of nasopharyngeal carcinoma into athymic mice. Otolaryngology 48: 1

Evans GH, Ivanyi J (1974) In vitro response of chicken spleen cells to sheep red blood cells Cell Immunol 14: 402–410

Evans G, Ivanyi J (1975) Antibody synthesis by chicken spleen cells in vitro. L. Requirements of B cells at various stages after immunization for T cells, macrophages and antigen. Eur J Immunol 5: 747–752

Ewald SJ, Klein J, Hood LE (1979) Peptide map analysis of mutant transplantation antigens. Immunogenetics 8: 551–559

Ezine S, Jerabek L, Weissman IL (1987) The phenotype of thymocytes derived from a single clonogenic precursor. J Immunol 139: 2195

Faber V, Dalgleish AG, Newell A, Malkovský M (1987) Inhibition of HIV replication in vitro by fusidic acid. Lancet 2: 827–828

Faubert GM, Belosevic M, Skamene E, MacLean JD (1985) Giardiasis: Characteristics of infection in recombinant and male and female mice. Prog Leukocyte Biol 3: 465–470

Faustman D, Hauptfeld V, Davie JM, Lacy PE, Shreffler DC (1980) Murine pancreatic β-cells express H-2K and H-2D but not Ia antigens. J Exp Med 151: 1563–1568

Faustman D, Hauptfeld V, Lacy PE, Davie JM (1981) Prolongation of murine islet allograft survival by pretreatment of islets with antibody directed to Ia determinants. Proc Natl Acad Sci USA 78: 5156–5159

Faustman D, Lacy PE, Davie JM, Hauptfeld V (1982) Prevention of islet allograft rejection in mice by primmunization with donor blood depleted of Ia-bearing cells. Science 217: 157–158

Faustman D, Lacy PE, Davie JM, Hauptfeld V (1982) Demonstration of active tolerance in the maintenance of established islet allografts. Proc Natl Acad Sci USA 79: 4153–4155

Faustman D, Lacy PE, Davie JM, Hauptfeld V (1983) Allograft prolongation by immunization with donor blood depleted of I-A-bearing cells. Transplant Proc 15: 1341–1343

Faustman D, Steinman RM, Gebel H, Hauptfeld V, Davie JM, Lacy PE (1984) Prevention of rejection of murine islet allografts by pretreatment with anti-dendritic cell antibody. Proc Natl Acad Sci USA 81: 3864–3868

Faustman D, Hauptfeld V, Davie J, Lacy P (1985) Prolonged survival of donor skin grafts in mice bearing established islet of Langerhans transplants. Transplantation 40: 216–218

Fedele LA, Even J, Garon CF, Donner L, Sherr CJ (1981) Recombinant bacteriophages containing the integrated transforming provirus of Gardner-Arnstein feline sarcoma virus. Proc Natl Acad Sci USA 78: 4036

Festenstein H, Demant P (1983) New perspectives for the analysis of the major histocompatibility complex (Introduction). Transplant Proc 15: 2007–2008

Figueroa F, Klein J (1986) The evolution of class II Mhc genes. Immunol Today 7: 78–81

Figueroa F, Klein J (1988) Origins of *H-2* polymorphism. In: Davis CS (ed) H-2 antigens, Genes, molecules, function. Plenum, New York, pp 61–76

Figueroa F, Davis WD, Klein J (1981) Ten new monoclonal antibodies detecting antigenic determinants on class I H-2 molecules. Immunogenetics 14: 177–180

Figueroa F, Klein D, Tewarson S, Klein J (1982) Evidence for placing the *Neu-1* locus within the mouse *H-2* complex. J Immunol 129: 2089–2093

Figueroa F, Tewarson S, Neufeld E, Klein J (1982) *H-2* haplotypes of strains DRB7, B10.NZW, NFS, BQ2, STU, TO1, and TO2. Immunogenetics 15: 431–436

Figueroa F, Zaleska-Rutczynska Z, Adolph S, Nadeau JH, Klein J (1982) Genetic variation of wild mouse populations in southern Germany. II. Serological study. Genet Res 41: 135–144

Figueroa F, Zaleska-Rutcznyska Z, Kusnierczyk P, Klein J (1983) Crossreactivity between *Qa-1* region and *H-2K* antigens. Transplantation 35: 391–393

Figueroa F, Tewarson S, Walden P, Nagy ZA, Klein J (1983) *H-2* haplotypes carrying identical *D* but different *L* alleles. Tissue Antigens 21: 24–30

Figueroa F, Golubić M, Nižetić D, Klein J (1985) Evolution of mouse major histocompatibility complex genes borne by *t* chromosomes. Proc Natl Acad Sci USA 82: 2819–2823

Figueroa F, Tichy H, McKenzie I, Hämmerling U, Klein J (1986) Polymorphism of lymphocyte antigens-encoding loci in wild mice. Curr Top Microbiol Immunol 127: 229–235

Figueroa F, Tichy H, Berry RJ, Klein J (1986) The polymorphism in island population of mice. Curr Top Microbiol Immunol 127: 1000–1005

Figueroa F, Kasahara M, Tichy H, Neufeld E, Ritte U, Klein J (1987) Polymorphism of unique noncoding DNA sequences in wild and laboratory mice. Genetics 117: 101–198

Figueroa F, Günther G, Klein J (1988) Mhc polymorphism predating speciation. Nature 335: 265–267

Figueroa F, Neufeld E, Ritte U, Klein J (1988) *t*-Specific DNA polymorphisms among wild mice from Israel and Spain. Genetics 119: 157–160

Figueroa F, Vinček V, Kasahara M, Bell GI, Klein J (1988) Mapping of the Sod-2 locus into the *t* complex on mouse chromosome 17. Immunogenetics 28: 260–264

Fleiszer D, Hilgers J, Skamene E (1988) Multigenic Control of colon carcinogenesis in mice treated with 1,2-Dimethylhydrazine. Curr Tops Microbiol Immunol 137: 243–249

Foppoli JM, Ch'ng LK, Benedict AA, Ivanyi J, Derka J, Wakeland EK (1979) Genetic nomenclature for chicken immunoglobulin allotypes: An extensive survey of inbred lines and antisera. Immunogenetics 8: 385–404

Forger JM III, Cerny J (1976) Thymic hormone modulation of leukemic virus duplication. Cancer Res 36: 2048

Forget A, Skamene E (1985) Genetic regulation of early host defence mechanisms controlling mycobacterial infection. Prog Leukocyte Biol 3: 265–278

Forget A, Skamene E, Gros P, Miailhe AC, Turcotte R (1981) Strain differences in the response to infection with small dispersed doses of mycobacterium bovis BCG among inbred mice. Infect Immun 32: 42

Forget A, Pelletier M, Bourassa D, Gros P, Skamene E (1983) Early resistance and suceptibility of mice to *Mycobacterium bovis* (BCG) infection: immunological and histopathological consequences. In: Keusch G, Wadstrom T (eds) Experimental bacterial and parasitic infections. Elsevier, New York, pp 413–418

Forman J, Klein J (1975) Analysis of *H-2* mutants: Evidence for multiple CML target specificities controlled by the $H-2^b$ gene. Immunogenetics 1: 469–481

Forman J, Klein J (1975) Immunogenetic analysis of *H-2* mutations. II. Cellular immunity to the $H-2^{da}$ mutation. J Immunol 115: 711–715

Forman J, Klein J (1977) Immunogenetic analysis of *H-2* mutations. VI. Crossreactivity in cell-mediated lympholysis between TNP-modified cells from *H-2* mutant strains. Immunogenetics 4: 183–193

Forman J, Klein J, Streilein JW (1977) Spleen cells from animals neonatally tolerant to $H-2^k$ antigens recognize trinitrophenyl modified $H-2^k$ spleen cells. Immunogenetics 5: 561–567

Forman J, Vitetta E, Hart D, Klein J (1977) Relationship between trinitrophenyl and H-2 antigens on trinitrophenyl-modified spleen cells. I. H-2 antigens on cells treated with trinitrobenzene sulfonic acid are derivatized. J Immunol 118: 797–802

Fox N, de Souza L, Simon D, Damjanov I (1983) Male murine embryonal carcinoma cell line selectivity metastatic to the ovaries and adrenals. Virchows Arch 43: 241–251

Frangoulis B, Klein J (1988) High frequency of Mls^a-reactivity among A^b-restricted, H-Y-specific T cell clones. J Immunogenet (in press)

Frangoulis B, Besluau D, Chopin M, Degos L, Pla M (1988) Immune response to H-2 class I antigens on platelets. I. Immunogenicity of platelet class I antigens. Tissue Antigens 32: 46–54

Frangoulis B, Chopin M, Besluau D, Degos L, Pla M (1988) Immune response to H-2 class I on platelets. II. Specific decrease of H-2 class I-specific antibody response induced by treatment with allogeneic platelets. Tissue Antigens 32: 78–86

Fredericksen TL, Longenecker BM, Pazderka F, Gilmour DG, Ruth RF (1977) A T-cell antigen system of chickens: Ly-4 and Marek's disease. Immunogenetics 5: 535

Freedman RS, Bowen JM, Lotzová E, Edwards CL, Lewis E, Katz R (1987) Virus augmentation as a biological modifier approach: Experience with intracavitary virus augmentation therapy. In: Rutledge FM, Freedman RS, Gershenson DM (eds) Diagnosis and treatment strategies for gynecological cancer. UT Press, Austin, pp 137–158

Freedman RS, DelClos L, Atkinson N, Lotzová E, Wharton JT, Edwards CL, Scott W, Patenia R, Bass S (1989) Randomized comparison of viral oncolysates and radiation and radiation alone in uterine cervix carcinoma. Am J Clin Oncology (in press)

Freedman RS, Edwards CL, Bowen JM, Lotzová E, Katz R, Lewis E, Atkinson N, Adams S (1988) Intracavitary viral oncolysates in ovarian cancer. Gynecol Oncol 29: 337–347

Gaddis O Jr, Morrow CP, Klement V, Schlaerth JB, Nalich RH (1983) Treatment of cervical carcinoma employing a template for transperineal interstitial Ir-192 brachytherapy. Int J Radiat Oncol Biol Phys 9: 819–827

Gagnon RF, Gallimore B, Skamene E, Richards GK (1987) Impaired host defense mechanisms in chronic uremia: Conflicting experimental observations? In: Khamna R, Nolph KD, Prowant B, Tmarchorski ZJ, Oreopoulos DG (eds) Advances in continuous ambulatory peritoneal dialysis. University of Toronto Press, Toronto, pp 121–124

Gallagher MT, Lotzová E, Trentin JJ (1976) Genetic resistance to marrow transplantation as a leukemia defense mechanism. In: Battisto JR, Streilein JW (eds) Immuno aspects of the spleen. North-Holand, New York, pp 359–371

Gallagher MT, Lotzová E, Trentin JJ (1976) Genetic resistance to bone marrow transplantation as a leukemia defense mechanism. Biomedicine 25: 1–3

Galton J, Ivanyi J (1977) Immunofluorescent detection of differentiation alloantigens (CA1) in the chicken. Eur J Immunol 7: 241–246

Galton J, Ivanyi J (1977) An immunofluorescent technique for the detection of lymphocyte alloantigens. J Immunol Methods 17: 57–61

Galton J, Ivanyi J (1977) Detection of bursa and thymus-specific alloantigens in the chicken. Eur J Immunol 7: 457–459

Gao L, Malkovský M, Webster ADB, Asherson GL (1985) Impaired lymphokine-activated killer-cell activity in patients with hypogammaglobulinaemia. Lancet 2: 340

Gao L, Asherson GL, Malkovský M (1987) Increased lymphokine activated killer (LAK) activity in the regional lymph nodes of mice following immunization with contact sensitizing agents. Clin Exp Immunol 70: 217–221

Gardell D, Gormley B, Mervart H, Rock G (1987) Is serum the optimal source of HLA antibodies? Vox Sang 52: 89–94

Ghadirian E, Skamene E, Kongshavn PAL (1985) Genetic control of susceptibility to Entamoeba histolytica infection in mice. Prog Leukocyte Biol 3: 559–566

Gardner MB, Klement V, Rongey RR, McConahey P, Estes JD, Huebner RJ (1976) Type-C virus expression in lymphoma-paralysis prone wild mice. JNCI 57: 585–590

Gardner MB, Klement V, Henderson BE, Meier H, Estes JD, Huebner RJ (1976) Genetic control of type-C virus of wild mice. Nature 259: 143–145

Gardner MB, Klement V, Rasheed S, Rongey RW, Brown JC, Pike M, Henderson BE, Huebner RJ (1976) The pathogenesis of lymphoma and paralysis in wild mice. Bibl Haematol 43: 204–208

Gardner MB, Rasheed S, Klement V, Rongey RW, Brown JC, Dworsky R, Henderson BE (1976) Lower motor neuron disease in wild mice caused by indigenous type-C virus and search for a similar etiology in human amyotrophic lateral sclerosis. In: Andrews JM, Johnson RT, Brazier AB (eds) Amyotrophic Lateral sclerosis. Academic, New York, pp 217–234 (Recent research trends, vol 19)

Gardner MB, Klement V, Ester JD, Gilden RV, Toni R, Huebner RJ (1977) Suppression of infectious MuLV in wild mice by passive immunization. JNCI 58: 1855–1857

Gardner MB, Klement V, Henderson BE, Estes JD, Dougherty M, Casagrande J, Huebner RJ

(1977) Efforts to Control Type-C Virus expression in Wild Mice. In: Chirigos MA (ed). Control of neoplasia by modulation of immune system. Raven New York, pp 391–407 (Progress in cancer research and therapy, vol 2)

Gardner MB, McAllister RM, Rasheed S, Klement V, Shimizu S, Rongey RW, Charman HP, et al. (1977) Search for RNA Tumor Virus in Humans. Cold Spring Harbor Conf Cell Proliferation 4: 1235–1251

Gardner MB, Klement V, Henderson BE, Casagrande J, Bryant ML, Dougherty MF, Estes JD (1978) Lymphoma, paralysis and oncorna-viruses in wild mice. In: Severi L (ed) Tumors of early life in man and animals. Perugia University Medical School, Perugia, pp 343–356

Gardner MB, Klement V, Rasheed S, Estes JD, Rongey RW, Dougherty MF, Bryant ML (1978) Persistent MuLV infection in wild mice. ICN UCLA Symp Mol Cell Biol 11: 115–132

Garrido F, Perez M, Iványi P, Schirmacher V (1981) Expression of H-2 antigens in ascitic forms of newly induced BALB/c tumors. Transplant Proc 13: 1824–1827

Garrido F, Perez M, Torres MD, Garcia-Olivares E, Iványi P, Schirmacher V (1979) A syngeneic anti-tumor serum recognizing a complex H-2 alloantigen. Immunobiology 156: 110–120

Geczy AF, van Leeuwen A, van Rood JJ, Ivanyi P, Breur BS, Cats A (1986) Blind confirmation in Leiden of Geczy factor on the cells of Dutch patients with ankylosing spondylitis. Hum Immunol 17: 239–245

Geib R, Poulik MD, Vitetta ES, Kearney JR, Klein J (1976) Relationship between β_2-microglobulin and cellsurface alloantigens of the mouse. J Immunol 117: 1532–1527

Geib R, Goldberg EH, Klein J (1977) Membrane-bound H-2 and H-Y antigens move independently of each other. Nature 27: 352–354

Geib R, Chiang C, Klein J (1978) Evidence for multiple clones of cytotoxic T cells responding to antigenic determinants on the same molecule. J Immunol 120: 340–342

Geib RW, Klein J (1979) MLR blast cells generated in mutant-standard strain combinations bind H-2K and H-2D antigens. Eur J Immunol 9: 135–139

Geiger B, Rosenthal KL, Klein J, Zinkernagel RM, Singer SJ (1979) Selective and unidirectional membrane redistribution of an H-2 antigen with an antibody-clustered viral antigen: Relationship to mechanisms of cytotoxic T-cell interactions. Proc Natl Acad Sci USA 4603–4607

Gelsthorpe K, Smillie D, Klouda PT (1984) HLA-B37 report. In: Albert ED, Baur MP, Mayr WR (eds) Histocompatibility testing 1984. Springer, Berlin Heidelberg New York, pp 145–146

Gervais F, Morris-Hooke A, Tran TA, Skamene E (1986) Analysis of macrophage bactericidal function in genetically resistant and susceptible mice by using the temperature-sensitive mutant of *Listeria monocytogenes*. Infect Immun 54: 315–321

Gervais F, Hébert L, Skamene E (1988) Amyloid-enhancing factor: Production and response in amyloidosis-susceptible and – resistant mouse strains. J Leukocyte Biol 43: 311–316

Gervais F, Stevenson MM, Skamene E (1984) Genetic control of resistance to *Listeria monocytogenes*: Regulation of leukocyte inflammatory responses by the Hc locus. J Immunol 132: 2078–2083

Gervais F, Patel PJ, Skamene E (1988) Increased natural resistance to *Listeria monocytogenes* in senescent mice correlates with enhanced macrophage bactericidal activity. J Gerontol 43: B152–B156

Gervais F, Stevenson MM, Skamene E (1985) Effect of viral infections upon macrophage functions. Prog Leukocyte Biol 1: 241–252

Gervais F, Martel RR, Skamene E (1984) The effect of the non-steroidal anti-inflammatory drug etodolac on macrophage migration in vitro and in vivo. J Immunopharmacol 6: 205–214

Gervais F, Desforges C, Skamene E (1989) The C5-sufficient A/J congenic mouse strain: Inflammatory response and resistance to Listeria monocytogenes. J Immunol (in press)

Gilks WR, Bradley BA, Gore SM, Klouda PT (1985) The relationship between the frequencies of HLA-B locus antigens and their effects on kidney graft survival. Transplant Proc 17: 2242–2244

Gilks WR, Bradley BA, Gore SM, Klouda PT (1987) Substantial benefits of tissue matching in renal transplantation. Transplantation 43: 669–674

Gillet D, Mornet E, Rocca A, Degos L, Cohen D, Pla M (1988) Extensive genomic polymorphism in mouse 21-hydroxylase region. Immunogenetics 27: 133–136

Gill HK, Mustafa AS, Ivanyi J, Harboe M, Godal T (1986) Humoral immune responses to *M. leprae* in human volunteers vaccinated with killed armaadillo-derived *M. leprae*. Lepr Rev [Suppl 2] 57 293–300

Gladman D, Keystone C, Murray B, Lee P, Cand D, Mervart H (1981) Increased frequency of HLA-DR5 in scleroderma. Arthritis Rheum 24: 854–856

Gogusev J, Brun J-L, Hála K, Perramon A, Mongiat F (1980) Distribution des antigènes du complexe majeur d'histocompatibilité (H-B) sur les cellules du sang périphérique et de la moelle osseuse chez des poulets de lignées congéniques. CRAcad Sci [D] (Paris) 291 225–228

Golubić M, Figueroa F, Tosi M, Klein J (1985) Restriction fragment length polymorphism of *C4* genes in mice with *t* chromosomes. Immunogenetics 21: 247–256

Golubić M, Budimir O, Schöpfer R, Kasahara M, Mayer WE, Figueroa F, Klein J (1987) Nucleotide sequence analysis of class II genes borne by mouse *t* chromosomes. Genet Res 50: 137–146

Gorai I, Aihara M, Bixler GS Jr, Atassi Z, Walden P, Klein J (1988) T cell response to myoglobin: a comparison of T cell clones in high-responder and low-responder mice. Eur J Immunol (in press)

Götze D, Reisfeld RA, Klein J (1973) Antibody against Ir-region controlled antigen in mice. Naturwissenschaften 60: 355–356

Götze D, Reisfeld RA, Klein J (1973) Serologic evidence for antigens controlled by the Ir region in mice. J Exp Med 138: 1003–1008

Götze D, Nadeau J, Wakeland EK, Berry RJ, Bonhomme F, Egorov IK, Hjorth JP, et al. (1980) Histocompatibility-2 system in wild mice. X. Frequencies of H-2 and Ia antigens in wild mice from Europe and Africa. J Immunol 124: 2675–2681

Grinwich KD, Alexander TS, Cerny J (1978) Evidence for a role of calcium in immunosuppression in vitro. Cell Immunol 37: 285

Grinwich KD, Alexander TS, Cerny J (1979) Properties of murine leukemia-associated suppressor cells. I. Preferential suppression of thymus-dependent H-2 complex. J Immunol 122: 1108

Gros P, Skamene E, Forget A (1981) Genetic control of natural resistance to mycobacterium bovis (BCG) in mice. J Immunol 127: 2417

Gros P, Skamene E, Forget A, Taylor B (1983) Host response to infection with mycobacterium bovis (BCG) in mice: Genetic study of natural resistance. Adv Exp Med Biol 162: 183–188

Gros P, Skamene E, Forget A (1983) Cellular mechanisms of genetically controlled host resistance to *mycobacterium bovis* (BCG). J Immunol 131: 1966–1972

Gupta GS, Kinsky RG, Duc HT, Voisin GA (1984) Effects of placental extracts on the immune response to histocompatibility antigens: class deviation of alloantibody response and allograft enhancement. Am J Reprod Immunol 6: 117–123

Hajare S, Gibson FB, Rakusan TA, Strunk CL, Kalia A (1989) Laryngeal coccidioidomycosis causing airway obstruction. Pediatr Infect Dis (In press)

Hála K (1987) Inbred lines of avian species. In: Toivanen A, Toivanen P (eds) Avian immunology: Basis and practice, vol 2. CRC Boca Raton, pp 85–99

Hála K (1988) Hypothesis: Immunogenetic analysis of spontaneous autoimmune thyroiditis in Obese strain (OS) chickens: A two-gene family model. Immunobiology 177: 354–373

Hála K, Boyd R, Wick G (1981) Chicken major histocompatibilty complex and disease. Scand J Immunol 14: 607–616

Hála K, Plachy J, Schulmannová J (1981) Role of the B-G-region antigen in the humoral immune response to the B-F-region antigen of chicken MHC. Immunogenetics 14: 393–401

Hála K, Boyd RL, Wolf H, Böck G, Wick G (1984) Functional analysis of B-L(Ia-like) antigen bearing chicken peripheral blood cells. Scand J Immunol 20: 15–19

Hála K, Wick G, Boyd RL, Wolf H, Böck G, Ewert DL (1984) The B-L (Ia-like) antigens of the chicken. Lymphocyte plasma membrane distribution and tissue localization. Dev Comp Immunol 8: 673–682

Hála K, Schauenstein K, Neu N, Krömer G, Wolf H, Böck G, Wick G (1986) A monoclonal antibody reacting with a membrane determinant expressed on activated chicken T lymphocytes. Eur J Immunol 16: 1331–1336

Hála K, Chaussé A-M, Bourlet Y, Lassila O, Hasler V, Auffray C (1988) Attempt to detect recombination between *B-F* and *B-L* genes within the chicken *B* complex by serological typing, in vitro MLR and RFLP analyses. Immunogenetics 28: 433–438

Hall R, McBride JS, Morgan G, Tait A, Zolg JW, Walliker D, Scaife J (1983) Antigens of the erythrocytic stages of the human malaria parasite *Plasmodium falciparum* detected by monoclonal antibodies. Mol Biochem Parasitol 7: 247–265

Hallauer JP, Koldovsky P, Kouros M (1981) Experimentelle Untersuchungen zur Toxicologie eines im Steinkohle verwendeten Netzmittels. Staub Silikosebekämpfung 13: 331

Hammerberg C, Klein J (1975) Evidence for postmeiotic effect of *t* factors causing segregation distortion in the mouse. Nature 253: 137–138

Hammerberg C, Klein J (1975) Linkage disequilibrium between *H-2* and *t* complexes in chromosome 17 of the mouse. Nature 258: 296–299

Hammerberg C, Klein J (1975) Linkage relationships of markers on chromosome 17 of the house mouse. Genet Res 26: 203–211

Hammerberg C, Klein J, Artzt K, Bennet D (1976) Histocompatibility-2 system in wild mice. II. *H-2* haplotypes of *t*-bearing mice. Transplantation 21: 199–212

Hansen TH, Iványi P, Levy RB, Sachs DH (1979) Cross-reactivity among the products of three non-allelic H-2 loci, $H-2L^d$, $H-2D^q$ and $H-2K^k$. Transplantation 28: 339–342

Harboe M, Ivanyi J (1987) Analysis of monoclonal antibodies to *Mycobacterium leprae* by crossed immunoelectrophoresis. Scand J Immunol 25: 133–138

Harder F, Jeannet M, Brunner F, Claudi B, Floersheim GL, Klouda PT, Leski M, et al. (1977) Bluttransfusion und Nierentransplantation. Schweiz Med Wochenschr 107: 694–698

Harder F, Jeannet M, Brunner F, Floersheim GL, Klouda PT, Leski M, Megevand R, et al. (1979) Blood transfusions in cadaver renal transplantations. In: Ferrone S, Curtoni E, Gorini S (eds) HLA antigens in clinical medicine and biology. Garland, pp 167–176

Hardisty RM, Till MM, Lawler SD, Klouda PT, Batchelor JR, Edwards JH, Stuart J, et al. (1971) Data on the linkage relationships of the HL-A and α-haptoglobin loci in man. Ann Hum Genet 35: 161–166

Hardt C, Pfizenmaier J, Röllinghoff M, Klein J, Wagner H (1980) Alloreactive and H-2 restricted Lyt 23 cytotoxic T lymphocytes (CTL) derive from a common pool of antecedent Lyt 123 CTL precursors. J Exp Med 152: 1413–1418

Härfast B, Andersson T, Stejskal V, Perlmann P (1977) Interactions between human lymphocytes and paramyxovirus-infected cells. Adsorption and cytotoxicity. J Immunol 118: 1132

Harmon RC, Clark EA, Klein J, Hildemann WH (1979) H-2D-associated hybrid resistance to EL-4. Transplant Proc 1353–1354

Hartmann W, Hála K, Heil G, Krieg R (1986) Effect of B blood group genotypes on resistance to Mareks disease in Leghorn crosses. In: Larbier M (ed) Proceedings of the 7th European Poultry Conference Paris, vol 1 World's Poultry Science Association pp 216–220

Hauptfeld M, Hauptfeld V, Zeff R, Shreffler DC (1988) Studies on recombination within the mouse H-2 complex: IV. Characterization of new recombinant haplotypes $H-2^{t7}$, $H-2^{t8}$, $H-2^{as2}$ and $H-2^{as3}$. J Mol Cell Immunol 4: 1–8

Hauptfeld V, Klein J (1975) Molecular relationship between private and public H-2 antigens as determined by antigen redistribution method. J Exp Med 142: 288–298

Hauptfeld M, Klein J (1976) The *H-2* complexes of inbred and wild mice are organized in a similar fashion. Immunogenetics 3: 603–607

Hauptfeld V, Klein J (1977) A new histogenetic method for typing of minor histocompatibility antigens. J Immunol 118: 423–426

Hauptfeld V, Klein D, Klein J (1973) Serologic detection of antigens controlled by the Ir region of the H-2 complex in the mouse. Transplant Proc 5: 1811–1813

Hauptfeld V, Klein D, Klein J (1973) Serologic identification of an Ir-region product. Science 181: 167–169

Hauptfeld V, Hauptfeld M, Klein J (1974) Tissue distribution of I region associated antigens in the mouse. J Immunol 113: 181–188

Hauptfeld M, Hauptfeld V, Klein J (1975) A method for detection of Ia antigens in the absence of appropriate *H-2* recombinants. J Immunol 115: 351–355

Hauptfeld M, Hauptfeld V, Klein J (1975) Ia and H-2 antigens on blast cells. Transplantation 19: 528–530

Hauptfeld V, Hauptfeld M, Klein J (1975) Induction of resistance to antibody-mediated cytotoxicity. H-2, Ia, and Ig antigens are independent entities in the membrane of mouse lymphocytes. J Exp Med 141: 1047–1056

Hauptfeld V, Hammerberg C, Klein J (1976) Histocompatibility-2 system in wild mice. III. Mixed lymphocyte reaction and cell mediated lymphocytoxicity with *t*-bearing mice. Immunogenetics 3: 489–497

Hauptfeld V, Braciale TJ, Shreffler DC (1982) Differences in expression of MHC products between several H-2-restricted CTL clones. J Immunol 128: 2026–2031

Hauptfeld V, Hauptfeld M, Nahm M, Trial J, Kapp J, Shreffler DC (1983) Partial characterization of 8 anti-I-J and 3 anti-Ia monoclonal reagents. In: Pierce CW, Cullen SE, Kapp JA, Schwartz BD, Shreffler DC (eds) Ir genes – Past, present and future. (Experimental biology and medicine) Humana, clifton, pp 51–56

Hauptfeld V, Nahm M, Hauptfeld M, Shreffler DC (1984) Monoclonal antibodies to mouse MHC antigens. I. Serological characterization of ten anti-H-2 and and-Ia reagents. Immunogenetics 19: 169–173

Hauptfeld V, Kapp JA, Frederick K, Trial JA, Shreffler DC (1985) Monoclonal antibodies to mouse antigens. II. Characterization of thirtyone anti-I-J reagents. Immunogenetics 21: 193–197

Hauptfeld-Dolejsek V, Shreffler DC (1989) Antigenic properties of thirty six new H-2 congenic strains and four independently derived strains, DDD, BZH, FM, W10LT. Immunogenetics. (in press)

Hauptfeld-Dolejsek V, Shreffler DC (1989) Production of Ia.7 antibody is under Ir gene control. Immunogenetics. (in press)

Hauptfeld-Dolejsek V, Vaidya HC, Shreffler DC (1989) Immune response gene control of the murine antibody response to the human creatine kinase-MM and to the lactate dehydrogenase-1 enzymes. Immunogenetics. (in press)

Henle G, Koldovsky U, Koldovsky P, Henle W (1975) Multiple sclerosis associated agent: neutralisation of the agent by human sera. Infect Immun 12: 1367

Henrotte JG, Santarromana M, Pla M (1987) Genetic factors regulating zinc concentrations in mice spleen and liver: Relationship with the H-2 complex. Immunogenetics 25: 408–410

Herberman RB, Balch C, Bolhuis R, Golub S, Hiserodt J, Lanier LL, Lotzová E, et al. (1987) Most lymphokine activated killer (LAK) activity mediated by blood and splenic lymphocytes is attributable to stimulation of natural killer (NK) cells by interleukin-2. Immunol Today 8: 178–181

Hersh EM, Patt YZ, Gutterman JU, Murphy S, Mavligit G, Richman SP, Maroun J, et al. (1980) Host defense mechanisms in cancer and their modification by immunotherapy. In: Crispen R (ed) Neoplasm immunity: Experimental and clinical. Elsevier/North-Holland, Amsterdam, pp 247–264

Hewitt J, Coates ARM, Mitchison DA, Ivanyi J (1982) The use of murine monoclonal antibodies without purification of antigen in the serodiagnosis of tuberculosis. J Immunol Methods 55: 205–211

Hilgert I, Kinsky RG (1983) Persistence of regulation mechanism responsible for inhibition of allotransplantation reactions in the absence of alloantigen. Folia Biol (Praha) 29: 349–357

Hilgert I, Krištofová H, Angelisová P, Kinsky R, Hořejší V (1983) Adult transplantation tolerance induced by lentil lectin. III. Induction of transplantation tolerance by lentil lectin in mouse strain combinations with different H-2 disparities: tolerogenic effect of H-2D region antigens. J Immunogenet 10: 127–137

Hilkens J, Hilgers J, Demant P, Michalides R, Ruddle F, Nichols E, Holmes R, et al. (1981) Origin and genetic relationships between the mouse inbred strains maintained at The Netherlands Cancer Institute. In: Hilgers J, Sluyser M (eds) Mammary tumors in the mouse. Elsevier, Amsterdam, pp 11–44

Hoeppner VH, Jackett PS, Beck JS, Karjito T, Grange JM, Ivanyi J (1987) Appraisal of the monoclonal antibody based competition test for the serology of tuberculosis in Indonesia. Immunotherapy 1: 69–77

Holder AT, Aston R, Preece MA, Ivanyi J (1985) Monoclonal antibody-mediated enhancement of growth hormone activity in vivo. J Endocrinol 107: R9–R12

Holder AT, Aston R, Rest JR, Hill DJ, Patel N, Ivanyi J (1987) Monoclonal antibodies can enhance the biological activity of thyrotropin. Endocrinology 120: 567–573

Holm G, Stejskal V, Perlmann P (1973) Cytotoxic effects of activated lymphocytes and their supernatants. Clin Exp Immunol 14: 169

Houssaint E, Torano A, Ivanyi J (1983) Ontogenic restriction of colonization of the bursa of Fabricius. Eur J Immunol 13: 590–595

Houssaint E, Torano A, Ivanyi J (1989) "Split tolerance" induced by epithelial thymic rudiments allografted to chicken embryonal recipients. J Immunol (in press)

Houssin D, Pla M (1984) Tolérance des allogreffes hépatiques. Presse Med 13: 1734–1738

Howard RJ, McBride JS, Aley SB, Marsh K (1986) Antigenic diversity of *P. falciparum* antigens in isolates from Gambian patients. II. The schizont surface glycoprotein of molecular weight ~ 200000. Parasite Immunol 8: 57–68

Howard JG, Elson J, Christie GH, Kinsky R (1969) Studies on immunological paralysis. II. The detection and signification of antibody forming cells in the spleen during immunological paralysis with type III pneumococcal polysaccharide. Clin Exp Immunol 4: 41–53

Huang C-M, Klein J (1979) Murine antigen H-2. 7: Its genetics, tissue expression and strain distribution. Immunogenetics 9: 233–243

Huang C-M, Klein J (1979) Murine antigen H-2. 7: In vitro phenotypic conversion of erythrocytes. Immunogenetics 9: 575–581

Huang C-M, Klein J (1980) Murine antigen H-2. 7: Localization of its antigenic determinant to the Ss (C4) molecule. Immunogenetics 11: 605–616

Huang C-M, Geib RW, Klein J (1979) H-2. 7: Phenotypic conversion of erythrocytes in radiation chimeras. Immunogenetics 9: 583–589

Huang C-M, Huang H-JS, Klein J (1979) Serology and polymorphism of H-2L locus encoded antigens. Immunogenetics 9: 173–182

Humphrey D, Tsukamoto-Adey A, Witte ON, Fox R, Jerabek L, Weissman IL (1979) A serological comparison of Moloney lymphoma cell surface and Moloney oncornavirus antigens. J Immunol 123: 412

Ikezawa Z, Baxevanis CN, Nonaka M, Abe R, Tada T, Nagy ZA, Klein J (1983) Monoclonal suppressor factor specific for lactate dehydrogenase B.I. Mechanism of interaction between the factor and its target cells. J Exp Med 157: 1855–1866

Ikezawa Z, Baxevanis CN, Arden B, Tada T, Waltenbaugh CR, Nagy ZA, Klein J (1983) Evidence for two suppressor factors secreted by a single cell suggests a solution to the *J*-locus paradox. Proc Natl Acad Sci USA 80: 6637–6641

Ikezawa Z, Nonaka M, Abe R, Tada T, Nagy ZA, Klein J (1983) Induction of T cell responses in nonresponder mice by abolishing suppression with monoclonal antibodies recognizing a region-controlled, T cell-specific determinants. J Immunol 131: 1646–1649

Ikezawa Z, Arden B, Nagy ZA, Klein J (1984) Feedback regulation of immune suppression by a suppressor factor. Eur J Immunol 14: 681–686

Ikezawa Z, Nagy ZA, Klein J (1984) Manipulation of anti-LDH-B response by T suppressor factors. J Immunol 132: 1605–1607

Ikezawa Z, Walden P, Arden B, Nagy ZA, Klein J (1984) Composition of a suppressor factor that inhibits the immune response to lactate dehydrogenas B Scand J Immunol 20: 113–123

Isaak DD, Price JA, Reinisch CL, Cerny J (1979) Target cell heterogeneity in murine leukemia virus infection. I. Differences in susceptibility to infection with Friend leukemia virus between B lymphocytes from spleen, bone marrow and lymph nodes. J Immunol 123: 1822

Isaak DD, Cerny J (1981) Target cell heterogeneity in murine leukemia virus infection. II. Demonstration of Friend leukemia-virus-permissive and non-permissive subsets of splenic T cells. Int J Cancer 27: 505

Isaak DD, Cerny J (1983) T and B lymphocyte susceptibility to murine leukemia virus Moloney. Infect Immun 40: 977

Isaak DD, Asjo B, Hoover EA, Cerny J (1984) Phenotypic heterogeneity of leukemias associated with Friend MuLV infection: Studies on T-cell lymphomas and null cell leukemias in euthymic and thymus-deficient mice. Leuk Res 8: 617

Isaak DD, Cerny J (1988) T cells inhibit the Fr murine leukemia virus infection of B cells in vitro. Cell Immunol (in press)

Ishii N, Baxevanis CN, Nagy ZA, Klein J (1981) Selection of H-2 molecules for the context of antigen recogniton by T lymphocytes. Immunogenetics 14: 283–292

Ishii N, Baxevanis CN, Nagy ZA, Klein J (1981) Responder T cells depleted of alloreactive cells react to antigen presented on allogeneic macrophages from non-responder strains. J Exp Med 154: 978–982

Ishii N, Nagy ZA, Klein J (1982) Restriction molecules involved in the interaction of T cells with allogeneic antigen-presenting cells. J Exp Med 156: 622–627

Ishii N, Nagy ZA, Klein J (1982) Absence of *Ir* gene control of T cells recognizing foreign antigen in the context of allogeneic MHC molecules. Nature 295: 531–533

Ishii N, Klein J, Nagy ZA (1983) Different repertoires of mouse T cells for bovine insulin presented by syngeneic and allogeneic cells. Eur J Immunol 13: 658–662

Ishii N, Nagy ZA, Klein J (1983) Absence of *Ir* gene control in T-cell responses restricted by allogeneic Mhc molecules. In: Pierce CW, Cullen SE, Kapp JA (eds) *Ir genes-Past, present, and future*. Humana, Clifton, pp 263–267

Ishii N, Nagy ZA, Klein J (1983) In vitro correlate for a clonal deletion mechanism of immune response gene-controlled nonresponsiveness. J Exp Med 157: 998–1005

Ivanyi D, Demant P (1979) Complex genetic effect of B10.D2 (M504) (H-2dm1). Immunogenetics 8: 539–550

Ivanyi D, Demant P (1979) Heterogeneity of H-2D region molecules, recognized by anti H-2.28 seera. Immunogenetics 9: 315

Ivanyi D, Demant P (1981) Serological characterization of previously unknown H-2 molecules identified in the products of the Kd and Dk region. Immunogenetics 12: 397–408

Ivanyi D, Demant P (1982) Private specificity of H-2Ldx molecule detected serologically by a surface antigen redistribution method (capping). Tissue Antigens 20: 274–281

Ivanyi D, Demant P (1982) Molecular heterogeneity of D-end products detected by anti-H-2.28 sera. II. B10.D2(M504) (H-2dm1) mutant fails to express one of the two H-2.4-, 28 + Dd region molecules. Immunogenetics 15: 467–476

Ivanyi D, Demant P (1983) One (H-2D2b) of the three Db region-controlled molecules (H-2D1b, H-2D2b, H-2Lb) is not detected in bm13 mutant. J Immunol 131: 1080–1084

Ivanyi D, Demant P (1983) Capping experiments fail to reveal H-2Rd molecules in Dd region. Transplant Proc 15: 2039–2041

Ivanyi D, Demant P (1984) Five serologically distinguishable Dq region molecules. Immunogenetics 20: 211–216

Ivanyi D, Demant P (1987) New Ly-6 congenic strains. Immunogenetics 25: 271–273

Ivanyi D, Snoek M, Demant P (1979) H-2L: Demonstration of four new allelic products and independence of H-2D and H-2L molecules. Tissue Antigens 14: 233–250

Ivanyi D, Cherry M, Demant P (1982) Molecular heterogeneity of D-end products detected by anti-H-2.28 sera. III. Reactivity of certain anti-H-2.28 alloantisera with Qa-2 antigen. Immunogenetics 15: 477–484

Ivanyi J (1971) The 'informosome'-like particles of lymphoid cells. Biochim Biophys Acta 238: 303–313

Ivanyi J (1972) Recall of antibody synthesis to the primary antigen following successive immunization with heterologous albumins. A two-cell theory of the original antigenic sin. Eur J Immunol 2: 354–359

Ivanyi J (1973) Sequential recruitment of antibody class-committed B lymphocytes during ontogeny. Eur J Immunol 3: 789–793

Ivanyi J (1975) Polymorphism of chicken serum allotypes. J Immunogenetics, 2: 69–78

Ivanyi J (1975) Immunodeficiency in the chicken. I. Disparity in suppression of antibody responses to various antigens following surgical bursectomy. Immunology 28: 1007–1013

Ivanyi J (1975) Immunodeficiency in the chicken. II. Production of monomeric IgM following testosterone treatment or infection with Gumboro disease. Immunology 28: 1015–1021

Ivanyi J (1977) Carbohydrate specificity of T-cell cytophilic chicken anti-SRBC igM antibodies. Cell Immunol 29: 159–164

Ivanyi J (1978) Recombination of C_H genes encoding the M1(IgM) and G1(IgG) chicken allotypes. Nature 276: 166

Ivanyi J (1980) Competition and affinity assay of monoclonal antibodies against human growth hormone. In: Peters H (ed) *Proteins and related subjects*. Pergamon, Oxford, pp 471–474 (Colloquium, vol 28)

Ivanyi J (1980) Prevention of graft versus host reactions and conditioning of recipients for bone marrow transplantation in chickens. In: Thierfelder S, Rodt H, Kolb HJ (eds) *Immunobiology of bone marrow transplantation*. Springer, Berlin Heidelberg New York, pp 219–237

Ivanyi J (1981) Functions of the B-lymphoid system in chickens. In: Rose ME, Payne LN, Freeman BM (eds) *Avian immunology*. British Poultry Science, pp 63–101

Ivanyi J (1982) Study of antigenic structure and inhibition of activity of human growth hormone and chorionic somatomammotropin by monoclonal antibodies. Mol Immunol 19: 1611–1618

Ivanyi J (1982) Analysis of monoclonal antibodies to human growth hormone and related proteins. In: Hurrell JGR (ed) Monoclonal hybridoma antibodies: Techniques and applications. CRC, Baca Raton, pp 59–79
Ivanyi J (1983) Monoclonal antibodies may block sterically or conformationally the antigenic determinants of human growth hormone. In: Celada F, Schumaker VN, Sercarz EE (eds) Protein conformation as an immunological signal. Plenum New york, pp 191–200
Ivanyi J (1984) Application of monoclonal antibodies towards immunological studies in leprosy (Editorial). Leprosy Rev 55: 1–9
Ivanyi J (1986) Pathogenic and protective interactions in mycobacterial infections. Clin Immunol 6: 127–157
Ivanyi J, Cerny J (1969) The significance of antigen dose for immunity and tolerance. Curr Top Microbiol Immunol 49: 114
Ivanyi J, Davies P (1980) Monoclonal antibodies against human growth hormone. Mol Immunol 17: 287–290
Ivanyi J, Davies P (1987) Monoclonal antibodies to human prolactin and chorionic somatomammotropin. In: Peeters H (ed) Proteins and related studies, protides of the biological fluids. Pergamon, Oxford, pp 855–860 (Colloquium, vol 29)
Ivanyi J, Dresser W (1970) Replica analysis of the class of antibodies produced by single cells. Clin Exp Immunol 6: 493–501
Ivanyi J, Dunbar R (1981) Monoclonal antibody based solid phase immunoassay of somatotropic-latogenic hormones. In: Bizollon CA (ed) Physiological peptides and new trends in radioimmunology. Elsevier/North-Holland, Amsterdam, pp 285–292
Ivanyi J, Evans GH (1979) Analysis of the immunoglobulin isotype expression by peripheral blood rosette forming cells in chickens. Immunology 35: 947–952
Ivanyi J, Hudson L (1979) Allelic exclusion of M1 (IgM) allotype on the surface of chicken B cells. Immunology 35: 941–945
Ivanyi J, Lydyard PM (1972) Delineation of chicken lymphocyte populations by specific, anti-thymus and anti-bursa sera. Cell Immunol 5: 180–189
Ivanyi J, Lydyard PM (1975) Segregation of allotypes in a strain of chickens homozygous for the B locus. Immunogenetics 2: 285–289
Ivanyi J, Makings CW (1978) Antagonism between donor and host B cells in allotype congenic chicken chimeras. Transplantation 26: 221–227
Ivanyi J, Makings C (1980) Allotype analysis of B cell chimeric chickens. Transplantation 29: 25–29
Ivanyi J, Moreno C (1977) Isoelectric spectra of antibodies in chickens following recovery from immunological tolerance or bursectomy. In: Solomon JB, Horton JD (eds) Developmental immunobiology. Elsevier/North-Holland, Amsterdam, pp 419–426
Ivanyi J, Morris R (1976) Immunodeficiency in the chicken. IV. An immunological study of infectious bursal disease. Clin Exp Immunol 23: 154–165
Ivanyi J, Moyes L (1980) Acquired α^2 macroglobulin on the surface of human lymphoblastoid cells. Mol Immunol 17: 1545–1551
Ivanyi J, Salerno A (1971) Impairment of humoral antibody response in neonatally thymectomized and irradiated chickens. Eur J Immunol 1: 227–230
Ivanyi J, Salerno A (1972) Cellular mechanisms of escape from immunological tolerance. Immunology 22: 247–257
Ivanyi J, Sharp K (1986) Control by H-2 genes of murine antibody responses to protein antigens of *Mycobacterium tuberculosis*. Immunology 59: 329–332
Ivanyi J, Tempelis CH (1980) Genetic polymorphism of a serum euglobulin of chickens which binds to antigen-antibody complexes. Immunogenetics 10: 83–92
Ivanyi J, Murgatroyd LB, Lydyard PM (1972) Bursal origin of bone marrow cells with competence for antibody formation. Immunology 23: 107–111
Ivanyi J, Fuesalida E, Lydyard PM (1976) Rapid recovery of antigen-binding receptors on chicken B cells following anti-Ig serum treatment. Eur J Immunol 6: 25–30
Ivanyi J, Strudwick L, Makings C (1977) A heterophile carbohydrate moiety common to mammalian IgM and erythrocytes detected by chicken IgM antibody. Eur J Immunol 7: 204–209
Ivanyi J, Krambovitis E, Keen M (1983) Evaluation of a monoclonal antibody (TB72) based serological test for tuberculosis. Clin Exp Immunol 54: 337–345

Ivanyi J, Sinha S, Aston R, Cussell D, Keen M, Sengupta U (1983) Definition of species specific and cross-reactive antigenic determinants of *Mycobacterium leprae* using monoclonal antibodies. Clin Exp Immunol 52: 528–536

Ivanyi J, Morris JA, Keen M (1985) Studies with monoclonal antibodies to mycobacteria. In: Macario ATL, and Macario EC (eds) Monoclonal antibodies against bacteria. Academic, New York, pp 59–90

Ivanyi J, Bothamley GH, Jackett PS (1988) Immunodiagnostic assays for tuberculosis and leprosy. Br Med Bull 44: 635–649

Ivanyi J, Sharp K, Jackett P, Bothamley G (1988) Immunological study of the defined constituents of mycobacteria. Springer Semin Immunopathol (in press)

Iványi P (1978) Some aspects of the H-2 system, the major histocompatibility system in the mouse. Proc R Soc Lond [Biol] 202: 117–158

Iványi P (1981) Interspecies MHS relationship studies by serological and cellular cross-reactions. In: Reisfeld RA, Ferrone S (eds) Current trends in histocompatibility, vol 1. Plenum, New York, pp 133–181

Iványi P (1988) Los subtipos HLA-B27 y la espondilitis anquilosante. Rev Esp Reumatol 15: 1–4

Iványi P, Breur BS (1984) Individual differences in the in-vitro (CTL) immune response to HLA antigens. In: Albert ED, Baur MP, Mayr WR (eds) Histocompatibility testing 1984. Springer, Berlin Heidelberg New York, pp 617–618

Iványi P, Dröes JTPM (1985) HLA: A genetic marker for schizophrenia. Biol Psychol 6: 167–183

Iványi P, de Greeve P (1978) Individual mice of one inbred strain produce anti-H-2 antibodies of different specificities. In: Morse HC (ed) Origins of inbred mice. Academic, New York, pp 633–655

Iványi P, Kievits F (1988) MHC-restricted antibodies: facts and interpretation. In: Iványi P (ed) MHC + X, complex formation and antibody induction. Springer, Berlin Heidelberg New York, pp 119–127

Iványi P, Kloosterman T (1987) Peter Gorer could discover the H-2 complex by naturally occurring human antibodies. In: Chella CS (ed) H-2 antigens: Genes, molecules, function. Plenum, New York, pp 7–10

Iványi P, van Mourik P (1979) Murine anti-H-2I^k sera exhibit a strong cytotoxic effect on human B lymphocytes. Immunogenetics 9: 591–596

Iványi P, van Mourik P, Breuning MH, Melief CJM (1980) Unexpected lympho-cytotoxic reactions of anti-H-2 sera on normal lymph-node cells: are they due to altered H-2 structures on anti-viral antibodies? J Immunogenet 7: 91–97

Iványi P, van Mourik P, Breuning MH, Melief CJM (1980) Anti-H-2 antibodies induced by syngeneic immunization. Immunogenetics 10: 319–332

Iványi P, Melief CJM (1985) Le complexe HLA en immunologie cellulaire. II. La réponse cytotoxique (Detection of HLA antigen polymorphism by cytotoxic T lymphocytes) In: Dausset J, Pla M (eds) HLA complex majeur d'histocompatibilité de l'homme 1984. Flamarion, Paris, pp 209–216

Iványi P, van den Berg-Loonen EM, de Greeve P (1978) Individual mice of one inbred strain produce anti-H-2 and anti-HLA antibodies of different specificities. Tissue Antigens 12: 32–38

Iványi P, van den Berg-Loonen EM, de Greeve P (1978) Anti-H-2D^d antibodies cross-react with HLA-A11 and Aw31. Tissue Antigens 11: 439–442

Iványi P, Melief CJM, de Greeve P, van Mourik P (1979) Individual mice recognize the complex nature of H-2 antigens; an expected reaction (anti-K^k) in anti-BALB/c-H-2^d sera produced in the BALB/c-H-2db mutant. Transplant Proc 9: 642–646

Iványi P, Melief CJM, van Mourik P, Vlug A, de Greeve P (1979) Lymphocytotoxic antibodies produced by H-2 allo-immunisation distinguish between MuLV-positive and -negative substrains of the same H-2 haplotype. Nature 282: 843–845

Iványi P, van Mourik P, de Lange G, Tsuji U, Garrido F (1981) Anti-BROC-A1 (anti-H-2s) antibodies cross-react with HLA-A11. Transplant Proc 13: 1958–1961

Iványi P, van Mourik P, Breuning MH, Kruisbeek AM, Kröse CJM (1982) Natural anti-H-2 antibodies in sera of aged mice. Immunogenetics 15: 95–102

Iványi P, Leupers T, van Mourik P (1983) Naturally occurring cytotoxic human antibodies recognize H-2-controlled murine lymphocyte antigens. Proc Natl Acad Sci USA 80: 4479–4483

Iványi P, Dröes J, Schreuder I, d'Amaro J, van Rood JJ (1983) A search for association of HLA antigens with paranoid schizophrenia: A9 appears as a possible marker. Tissue Antigens 22: 186–193

Iványi P, Černý-Provaznik R, Radl J (1986) Naturally occurring antibodies against antigens of the major histocompatibility complex (H-2) in ageing mice. In: Facchini A, Haaijman JJ, Labo G (eds) Immunoregulation in aging. Eurage, Paris, pp 307–314

Iványi P, Černý-Provaznik R, van Mourik PC (1988) Naturally occurring H-2-specific antibodies. In: Ivanyi P (ed) MHC + X, complex formation and antibody induction. Springer, Berlin Heidelberg New York, pp 7–13

Jakobisiak M, Saidman S, Schlaut J, Pazderka F, Dossetor JB (1986) Elevated natural killer cytotoxicity in HLA-B8 and HLA-DR3 – positive individuals. Immunol Lett 12: 61

James SL, Skamene E, Meltzer MS (1983) Macrophages as effector cells of protective immunity in murine schistosomiasis. J Immunol 131: 948–953

Jardine JH, Jackson HJ, Lotzová E, Savary CA, Small SM (1988) Tumoricidal effect of interleukin-2 activated killer cells in canines. Vet Immunol Immunopathol (in press)

Jeannesson P, Zagury D, Bernard J, Kinsky R, Voisin GA (1975) Caractérisation immuno-cytologique de cellules reconnaissant l'antigène et produisant des anticorps au cours d'immunisation à l'oxalone et au lipopolysaccharide d'E. coli. CR Acad Sci [D] (Paris) 281: 2041–2044

Jeannet M, Klouda PT, Vassalli P, Ramirez E, Legendre C, Speck B (1976) Anomalous MLC and CML tests in human bone marrow transplantation. In: Kissmeyer-Nielsen F (ed) Histocompatibility testing 1975. Munksgaard, Copenhagen, pp 885–892

Jíra M, Malkovský M, Denman AM, Loveland B, Lyons D, Dalgleish AG, Webster ADB (1987) Lymphokine-activated killer cell activity in rheumatoid arthritis. Clin Exp Immunol 68: 535–542

Johny M, Pazderka F, Kovithavongs T, Schlaut J, Dossetor JB (1979) Monocyte specific antigens – detection by antibody dependent cellular cytotoxicity (ADCC) method. Transplant Proc 11: 1970

Juretić A, Nagy ZA, Klein J (1981) Generation of cytotoxic T lymphocytes by the H-2-encoded E molecules. Immunogenetics 14: 73–83

Juretić A, Nagy ZA, Klein J (1981) Detection of CML determinants associated with H-2 controlled E_α and E_β chains. Nature 289: 308–310

Juretić A, Protrka N, Walden P, Nagy ZA, Klein J (1983) Residual minor histocompatibility genes contaminate the B10. AM congenic line: No evidence of C-region-controlled histoincompatibility. Scand J Immunol 18: 515–519

Juretić A, Klein J, Nagy ZA (1983) Correlation between the functional characteristics and expression of molecule E controlled by the major histocompatibility complex in mice. Acta Biol Iugosl 19: 66–69

Juretić A, Nagy ZA, Klein J (1984) Characteristics of E molecules controlled by the *H-2* complex in mice as determined by the CML test. I. A locus in the I-A subregion determinates the private antigenic determinants target cells. Period Biol. 85: 183–185

Juretić A, Vucak I, Malenica B, Nagy ZA, Klein J (1984) H-41, a new minor histocompatibility locus. I. Histogenetic analysis. J Immunol 133: 2950–2954

Juretić A, Juretić E, Nagy ZA, Klein J (1985) Cytotoxic T-cell response to H-Y antigen by B6.C-*H-2*^{bm12} and B10.BR mice. Immunology 55: 671–675

Juretić A, Malenica B, Juretić E, Klein J, Nagy Z (1985) Helper effects required during in vivo priming for a cytolytic response to the H-Y antigen in nonresponder mice. J Immunol 134: 1408–1414

Juretić A, Juretić E, Nagy ZA, Klein J (1985) Analysis of anti-H-Y nonresponsiveness in CAS2 mice after i.p. immunization. Period Biol 87: 9–16

Kanellopoulos J, Kinsky RG, Voisin GA (1975) Isolement et purification d'allo-immunsérums dirigés contre des antigènes de transplantation à l'aide d'immunoadsorbants cellulaires. Ann Inst Pasteur Immunol 126: 90–91

Kaplan JC, Wilbert SM, Collins JJ, Rakusanova T, Zamansky GB, Black PH (1975) Isolation of SV40 transformed inbred hamster cell lines heterogeneous for virus induction by chemicals or radiation. Virology 68: 200–214

Karihaloo AK, Thomsen JJ, Rasmusen BA, Pazderka F, Ruth RF (1972) Normal birth following exteriorization and intravenous injection of the early sheep fetus. Am J Vet Res 33: 1781

Kasahara M, Stojlković I, Mayer WE, Dembić Z, Figueroa F, Klein J (1986) The nucleotide sequence of the mouse $H\text{-}2_aw28$ gene. Immunogenetics 24: 324–327

Kasahara M, Figueroa F, Klein J (1987) Random cloning of genes from mouse chromosome 17. Proc Natl Acad Sci USA 84: 3325–3328

Kasahara M, Figueroa F, Klein J (1987) Molecular cloning of a testis-specific gene from mouse chromosome 17. Transplant Proc 19: 815–816

Kasahara M, Figueroa F, Klein J (1988) Cloning of a testis-specific gene located between *Oa-2* and *Upg-1* on mouse chromosome 17. In: David CS (ed) H-2 antigens. Genes, molecules, function. Plenum, New York, pp 321–325

Kasahara M, Passmore HC, Klein J (1988) A testis-specific gene *Tpx-1* maps between *Pgk-2* and *Mep-1* on mouse chromosome 17. Immunogenetics (in press)

Kato S, Iványi P, Lacko E, Breur B, du Bois R, Eijsvoogel VP (1982) Identification of human CML targets. HLA-B locus (B12) antigen variants defined by CTL's between B-locus-identical (B12) responder-stimulator pairs. J Immunol 128: 949–955

Katz DR, Drzymala M, Turton JA, Hicks RM, Hunt R, Palmer L, Malkovský M (1987) Regulation of accessory cell function by retinoids in murine immune responses. Br J Exp Pathol 68: 343–350

Kau R, Kürten C, Kumazawa H, Koldovsky P (1989) Antibody dependent cell cytotoxicity (ADCC) against tumors of the head and neck region measured by the subrenal capsule assay. Arch Otorhinolaryngol (in press)

Kearney J, Cooper M, Klein J, Abney E, Parkhouse R, Lawton A (1977) Ontogeny of Ia and IgD on IgM-bearing B lymphocytes in mice. J Exp Med 146: 297–301

Kearney JK, Lawton AR, Klein J, Bockman DE, Cooper MD (1977) Mechanism of anti-μ induced suppression of LPS induced immunoglobulin synthesis. In: Regulatory mechanisms in lymphocyte activation. Academic, New York, pp 331–333

Kearny JF, Klein J, Bockman DE, Cooper MD, Lawton AR (1978) B cell differentiation induced by lipopolysaccharide. V. Suppression of plasma cell maturation by anti-μ: Mode of action and characteristics of suppressed cells. J Immunol 120: 158–166

Kelsoe G, Cerny J (1978) Regulation of the immune response. I. Regulatory cell equilibrium in the "virgin" state. Eur J Immunol 8: 176

Kelsoe G, Cerny J (1979) Reciprocal expansions of idiotypic and antiidiotypic clones following antigen stimulation. Nature 279: 333

Kelsoe G, Isaak DD, Cerny J (1980) Thymic requirement for cyclical idiotypic and reciprocal anti-Idiotypic immune response to a T-independent antigen. J Exp Med 151: 289

Kelsoe G, Micelli R, Cerny J, Schulze D (1989) Mapping of antibody specificities to V_H gene families. Eur J Immunol (submitted)

Kettman J, Klein J, Forman J (1977) Immunogenetic analysis of *H-2* mutations. VII. Cells responding to $H\text{-}2^k$ gene products give rise to an allogeneic supernatant. J Immunol 119: 1189–1191

Kievits F, Iványi P (1987) Monomorphic anti-HLA monoclonal antibody (W6/32) recognizes polymorphic H-2 heavy-chain determinants exposed by association with bovine or human but not murine beta-2-microglobuline. Hum Immunol 20: 115–126

Kievits F, Opolski A, Boerenkamp WJ, Pla M, Iványi P (1987) Monoclonal H-2 class-I-specific antibodies isolated after syngeneic immunization with Sendai virus-coated cells. In: Chella CS (ed) H-2 antigens: Genes, molecules, function. Plenum, New York, pp 659–670

Kievits F, Pla M, Opolski A, Limpens J, Leupers T, Rocca A, Leupers T, et al. (1987) Induction of H-2-specific antibodies is triggered by injections with syngeneic Sendai virus-coated cells. Eur J Immunol 17: 27–35

Kievits F, Iványi P, Krimpenfort P, Berns A, Ploegh H (1987) HLA-restricted recognition of viral antigens in HLA-transgenic mice. Nature 329: 447–449

Kievits F, Rocca A, Opolski A, Limpens J, Leupers T, Kloosterman T, Boerenkamp WJ, et al. (1987) Induction of H-2-specific antibodies by injections of syngeneic Sendai virus-coated cells. Eur J Immunol 17: 27–35

Kievits F, Boerenkamp WJ, Iványi P (1988) Exposure of the W6/32-defined determinant on mouse cells is dependent on the interaction of certain H-2 heavy chains with human or bovine β_2-microglobulin. In: Iványi P (ed) MHC+X, complex formation and antibody induction. Springer, Berlin Heidelberg New York, pp 166–170

Kievits F, Boerenkamp WJ, Iványi P (1988) H-2-dependent binding of xenogeneic β_2-microglobulin from culture media. J Immunol 140: 4253–4255

Kievits F, Wijffels J, Lokhorst W, Ivanyi P (1989) Recognition of xeno-(HLA, SLA)-MHC antigens by mouse cytotoxic T cells is not H-2-restricted. A study with transgenic mice. Proc Natl Acad Sci USA 86: 617–620

Kievits F, Boerenkamp WJ, Ivanyi P (1989) Immunization with syngeneic Sendai virus-infected cells induce no MHC-restricted antibodies but antibodies specific for H-2 class-I determinants. Immunogenetics 29: 108–111

Kievits F, Boerenkamp WJ, Ivanyi P (1988) Searching for MHC-restricted antibodies: antibodies induced by injections with syngeneic cells coated with Sendai virus, trinitrophenyl (TNP) and xenogeneic β_2-microglobulin are not restricted by the mouse MHC. In: Ivanyi P (ed) MHC + X, complex formation and antibody induction. Springer, Berlin Heidelberg New York, pp 38–49

Kierszenbaum F, Ivanyi J, Budzko Belia B (1976) Mechanisms of natural resistance to trypanosomal infection. Role of complement in avian resistance to *Trypanosoma crusi* infection. Immunology 30: 1–6

Kingston AE, Ivanyi J (1979) Kinetics of prostaglandin E_2 suppression of mitogeen-stimulated peripheral blood lymphocytes. Biochem Soc Trans 7: 121–122

Kingston AE, Ivanyi J, Kay JE (1984) The effects of indomethacin on T lymphocyte stimulation. Immunol Lett 8: 302–305

Kingston AE, Kay JE, Ivanyi J (1985) The effects of prostaglandin E and I analogues on lymphocyte stimulation. Int J Immunopharmacol 7: 57–64

Kinsky RG, Mitchison NA (1965) Tolerance of skin induced by erythrocytes in poultry. Transplantation 1: 224–231

Kinsky RG (1974) A marked sex difference in the immunization capability of hamsters towards a mouse tumour. Ann Immunol [C] (Paris) 125: 439–443

Kinsky RG (1981) Target-antigen-specific antibodies. In: Mathieu J (ed) Regulation and manipulation of the immune reaction. Roussel Uclaf, Paris, pp 18–20

Kinsky RG, Duc HT (1981) Selective production of rabbit antibodies against mouse suppressor cells. Analogy with mouse anti-IJ sera. Immunol Lett 2: 183–185

Kinsky RG, Chouroulinkov I, Voisin GA (1970) Complete in vivo destruction of allografted sarcoma l cells by circulating antibodies. Transplantation 10: 450–451

Kinsky RG, Voisin GA, Duc HT (1970) Anticorps de transplantation influençant l'évolution d'une homogreffe. Association avec d'autres propriétés biologiques liées à des anticorps de classe Ig connue. Ann Inst Pasteur 119: 136

Kinsky RG, Duc HT, Voisin GA (1971) Présence et rôle d'anticorps facilitants dans le sérum d'animaux hautement tolérants aux cellules vivantes. Ann Inst Pasteur 121: 698–699

Kinsky RG, Voisin GA, Hilgert I, Duc HT (1971) Biological properties of transplantation immune sera. II. PCA in mice with H-2 antigens. Transplantation 12: 171–176

Kinsky RG, Voisin GA, Duc HT (1972) Biological properties of transplantation immune sera. III. Relationship between transplantation (enhancement or inhibition) and serological (anaphylaxis or cytolysis) activities. Transplantation 13: 452–460

Kinsky RG, Voisin GA, Duc HT (1973) La tolérance aux cellules vivantes. Arch Anat Pathol 21: 39–44

Kinsky RG, Voisin GA, Duc HT (1973) Role of IgGl in immunological enhancement facilitation. Adv Exp Med Biol 29: 435–442

Kinsky RG, Hilgert I, Krištofová H (1976) The intersex difference in the production of alloantibodies and growth of tumour allografts in mice. Folia Biol (Praha) 22: 253–263

Kinsky RG, Duc HT, Fuensalida E (1978) Evaluation of in vitro and in vivo activities of isoantibodies directed against idiotypes and recognition structures for transplantation antigens. Folia Biol (Praha) 24: 81–94

Kinsky RG, Duc HT, Chaouat G, Voisin GA (1981) Involvement of suppressor cells in active enhancement of allografted tumors: in vivo (adoptive transfer) and in vitro (MLR) evaluation synergy with enhancing antibodies. Cell Immunol 58: 107–123

Kinsky RG, Witkowski J, Lehmann M, Hilgert I (1986) Modification of suppressor / cytotoxic and helper subsets in lectin pretreated mice. Immunol Lett 13: 51–53

Klein D, Klein J (1972) Polymorphism of the *Apl (Neu-1)* locus in the mouse. Immunogenetics 16: 181–184

Klein J (1970) Histocompatibility-2 (H-2) polymorphism in wild mice. Science 168: 1362–1364

Klein J (1971) Cytological identification of the chromosome carrying the IXth linkage group (including H-2) in the house mouse. Proc Natl Acad Sci USA 68: 1594–1597
Klein J (1971) Private and public antigens of the mouse H-2 system. Nature 229: 635–637
Klein J (1971) Tooth transplantation in the mouse. III. The role of minor (non-H-2) histocompatibility loci in tooth germ transplantation. Transplantation 12: 500–508
Klein J (1972) Histocompatibility-2 system in wild mice. I. Identification of five new H-2 chromosomes. Transplantation 13: 291–299
Klein J (1972) Is the H-2K locus stronger than the H-2D locus? Tissue Antigens 2: 262–266
Klein J (1973) The H-2 system: past and present. Transplant Proc 5: 11–21
Klein J (1973) Polymorphism of the H-2 loci in wild mice. Immunobiol Stand 18: 251–256
Klein J (1974) Genetic polymorphism of the histocompatibility-2 loci of the mouse. Annu Rev Genet 8: 63–77
Klein J (1975) A case of no sex-limitation of Slp in the murine *H-2* complex. Immunogenetics 2: 297–299
Klein J (1975) Many questions (and almost no answers) about the phylogenetic origin of the major histocompatibility complex. Adv Exp Med Biol 64: 467–478
Klein J (1976) An attempt at an interpretation of the mouse *H-2* complex. Contemp Top Immunobiol 5: 297–336
Klein J (1976) The relative importance of *H-2* regions in the development of graft vs. host reactions. Transplant Proc 8: 335–338
Klein J (1977) Allograft reaction against H-2 region antigens. Transplant Proc 9: 847–852
Klein J (1977) A mouse geneticist's impatient waiting for the arival of embryo-freezing techniques. In: Ciba Foundation Symposium on the freezing of mammalian embryos. Elsevier, Amsterdam, pp 305–311
Klein J (1977) Comparison of B-cell activation factors. Cold Spring Harbor Symp Quant Biol 41: 625–626
Klein J (1977) Evolution and function of the major histocompatibility complex: Facts and speculations. In: Götze D (ed) The major histocompatibility system in man and animals. Springer, Berlin Heidelberg New York, pp 339–378
Klein J (1978) Antigens and receptors involved in bone marrow transplantation. Transplant Proc 10: 5–9
Klein J (1978) Contribution of the mouse *H-2* system to the study of the human major histocompatibility complex. Excerpta med Int Congr Ser 411: 316–324
Klein J (1978) Genetics of cell-mediated lymphocytotoxicity in the mouse. Springer Sem. Immunopathol. 1: 31–49
Klein J (1978) *H-2* mutations: Their genetics and effect on immune functions. Adv Immunol 26: 55–146
Klein J (1978) Syrian hamsters: Do they or don't they have an MHC? Fed Proc 37: 2061–2062
Klein J (1978) The unity of genes in the major histocompatibility complex. Arthritis Rheum [Suppl] 21: 590–596
Klein J (1979) Population genetics of the murine chromosome 17. Isr J Med Sci 15: 859–866
Klein J (1979) Allograft reaction: Atavism of immunological tour de force? Cell lineage, stem cells and cell determinants. In: Le Douarin N (ed) Cell lineage, stem cells and cell determination. Elsevier, Amsterdam, pp 241–250
Klein J (1979) Buridan's Ass: One man's view of the immune system. Enzyme defect and immune dysfunction. Ciba Found Ser 68: 19–34
Klein J (1979) Why associative recognition? In: Quastel M (ed) Cell biology and immunology of leukocyte function. Academic, New York, pp 309–413
Klein J (1979) The major histocompatibility complex of the mouse. Science 203: 516–521
Klein J (1980) Generation of diversity at MHC loci: Implications for T-cell receptor repertoires. In: Fougereau M, Dausset J (eds) Immunology 80. Academic, London, pp 239–253
Klein J (1981) The histocompatibility-2 (H-2) complex. In: Foster HL, Small JD, Fox JG (eds) History, genetics, and wild mice. Academic, New York, pp 119–158 (The mouse in biomedical research, vol 1)
Klein J (1982) Evolution and function of the major histocompatibility complex. In: Parham B, Strominger J (eds) Histocompatibility antigens: structure and function. Receptors and Recognition ser B Vol 14. Chapman and Hall, London, pp 221–239

Klein J (1982) Immunogenetics of alloantigens. In: Baron S, Alperin LM (eds) Medical microbiology. Addison-Wesley, Menlo Park, pp 64-69
Klein J (1984) Gene conversion in Mhc genes. Transplantation 38: 327-329
Klein J (1984) What causes immunological nonresponsiveness? Immunol Rev 81: 177-202
Klein J (1985) Is it possible to formulate a unified concept for the biological function of the major histocompatibility complex (MHC)? Vox Sang: 354-367
Klein J (1985) Hegemony of mediocrity in contemporary sciences, particularly in immunology. Lymphology 18: 122-131
Klein J (1985) Big may not be beautiful, but it is necessary. Cell 42: 395-396
Klein J (1986) The major histocompatibility complex. In: Baron S (ed) Medical microbiology, 2nd edn. Addison-Wesley, Menlo Park, pp 16-22
Klein J (1986) Antigen-major histocompatibility complex-T cell receptors: Inquiries into the immunological menage-a-trois. Immunol Res 5: 173-190
Klein J (1986) How many class II immune response genes? A commentary on a reappraisal. Immunogenetics 23: 309-310
Klein J (1986) Gene conversion in Mhc genes: continuation. Transplantation 42: 102-105
Klein J (1986) Seeds of time: Fifty years ago Peter A. Gorer discovered the H-2 complex. Immunogenetics 24: 331-338
Klein J (1987) Genetic control of immune response: New concepts and old misconceptions. J Pediatr 111: 996-999
Klein J (1987) The major histocompatibility complex and protein recognition by T lymphocytes. In: Atassi MZ (ed) T-cell recognition and antigen presentation. Plenum, New York, pp 1-10 (Immunobiology of proteins and peptides, vol 4)
Klein J (1987) Origin of major histocompatibility complex polymorphism: The trans-species hypothesis. Hum Immunol 19: 155-162
Klein J (1987) The major histocompatibility complex and the fugu aspect of immunity. J Dermatol 14: 411-418
Klein J (1988) An essay on the future of H-2 serology. Int Rev Immunol 3: 357-363
Klein J (1988) Unclouded eyes: A short biography of Jack H. Stimpfling. Stimpfling Festschrift. Int Rev Immunol 3: 291-295
Klein J (1988) The evolution, ontogeny, and physiologic function of lymphocytes. In: Bray MA, Morley J (eds) The pharmacology of lymphocytes. Springer, Berlin Heidelberg New York, pp 11-36
Klein J (1988) Brother Juniper's inconclusive experiment: A poetic history of the *H-2* complex. In: David CS (ed) H-2 antigens, genes, molecules function. Plenum, New York, pp 13-28
Klein J (1988) The *Mhc* trans-species hypothesis - in the discussion period. Immunology (in press)
Klein J (1988) Immunologically important loci. In: Lyon MF (ed) Genetic variants and strains of the laboratory mouse, 2nd edn. Oxford University Press, Oxford (in press)
Klein J, Bailey DW (1971) Histocompatibility differences in wild mice. Further evidence for the existence of deme structure in natural populations of the house mouse. Genetics 68: 287-297
Klein J, Chiang C (1976) Ability of *H-2* regions to induce graft-vs-host disease. J Immunol 117: 736-740
Klein J, Chiang CL (1978) A new locus *(H-2T)* at the *D* end of the *H-2* complex. Immunogenetics 6: 235-243
Klein J, Egorov IK (1973) Graft-vs-host reaction with an H-2 mutant. J Immunol 111: 976-979
Klein J, Figueroa F (1981) Polymorphism of the mouse H-2 loci. Immunol Rev 60: 23-57
Klein J, Figueroa F (1986) Evolution of the major histocompatibility complex. CRC Crit Rev Immunol 6: 295-386
Klein J, Figueroa F (1986) The evolution of class I Mhc genes. Immunol Today 7: 41-44
Klein J, Forman J (1976) What can one learn about lymphocytes by studying *H-2* mutations? In: Eijsvoogel, VP Roos D, Zeijlemaker WP (eds) Leukocyte membrane determinants regulating immune reactivity. Academic, New York, pp 443-452
Klein J, Hammerberg C (1977) The control of differentiation by the *T* complex. Immunol Rev 33: 70-104
Klein J, Hauptfeld V (1976) Ia antigens: Their serology, molecular relationships, and their role in allograft reactions. Transplant Rev 30: 83-100

Klein J, Klein D (1972) Position of translocation break T (2;9)138Ca in linkage group IX of the mouse. Genet Res 19: 177-179

Klein J, Klein D (1987) Mouse inbred and congenic strains. Methods Enzymol 150: 163-196

Klein J, Murphy DB (1973) The role of "private" and "public" H-2 antigens in skin graft rejection. Transplant Proc 5: 261-265

Klein J, Nagy ZA (1981) Physiology of alloreactivity: An interpretation. Transplant Proc 13: 918-922

Klein J, Nagy ZA (1982) Trouble in the J-land. Nature 300: 12-13

Klein J, Nagy ZA (1982) Mhc restriction and *Ir* genes. Adv Cancer Res 37: 233-317

Klein J, Nagy ZA (1983) *Ir*-genes: Quo usque tandem? In: Pierce CW, Cullen SE, Kapp JA (eds) Ir genes, past, present, and future. Humana, Clifton, pp 611-617

Klein J, Secosky WR (1971) Tooth transplantation in the mouse. II. The role of the histocompatibility-2 (H-2) system in tooth germ transplantation. Oral Surg Oral Med Oral Pathol 32: 513-521

Klein J, Shreffler DC (1971) The H-2 model for the major histocompatibility systems. Transplant Rev 6: 3-29

Klein J, Shreffler DC (1972) HL-A model of the H-2 system? Tissue Antigens 2: 78-83

Klein J, Shreffler DC (1972) Evidence supporting a two-gene model for the H-2 histocompatibility system of the mouse. J Exp Med 135: 924-937

Klein J, Park MJ (1973) Graft-versus-host reaction across different regions of the *H-2* complex of the mouse. J Exp Med 137: 1213-1225

Klein J, Walden P (1986) Antigen presentation: Paradigm lost? In: Cinader B, Miller RG (eds) Sixth International Congress of Immunology. Academic, Orlando, pp 212-220 (Progress in immunology, vol 4)

Klein J, Zaleska-Rutczynska Z (1977) Histocompatibility-2 system in wild mice. VI. Histogenetic analysis of sixteen B10.W congenic lines. J Immunol 119: 1912-1915

Klein J, Zaleski M (1988) Genetic control of the immune response to the Thy-1 antigens – ten years later (almost). In: Reif AE, Schlesinger M (eds) Thy-1: immunology, neurology, and therapeutic applications. (in press)

Klein J, Klein D, Shreffler DC (1970) H-2 types of translocation stocks T(2;9)138Ca, T(9;13)190Ca, and an H-2 recombinant. Transplantation 10: 309-320

Klein D, Merchant DJ, Klein J, Shreffler DC (1970) Persistence of H-2 and some non-H-2 antigens on long-term-cultured mouse cell lines. JNCI 44: 1149-1160

Klein J, Secosky WR, Klein D (1971) Tooth transplantation in the mouse. I. The use of procion dyes and tritiated proline in a study of syngeneic tooth germ transplantation. Am J Anat 131: 371-385

Klein J, Widmer MB, Segal M, Bach FH (1972) Mixed lymphocyte culture reactivity and H-2 histocompatibility loci differences. Cell Immunol 4: 442-446

Klein J (1973) List of congenic lines in mice. I. Lines with differences at alloantigen loci. Transplantation 15: 137-153

Klein J, Bach FH, Festenstein FJ, McDevitt HO, Shreffler DC, Snell GD, Stimpfling JH (1974) Genetic nomenclature for the *H-2* complex of the mouse. Immunogenetics 1: 184-188

Klein J, Hauptfeld M, Hauptfeld V (1974) Evidence for a third, *Ir*-associated histocompatibility region in the *H-2* complex of the mouse. Immunogenetics 1: 45-56

Klein J, Hauptfeld M, Hauptfeld V (1974) Serological distinction of mutants B6.C(Hzl) and B6.M505 from strain C57BL/6. J Exp Med 140: 1127-1132

Klein J, Hauptfeld V, Hauptfeld M (1974) Involvement of H-2 regions in immune reactions. In: Brent L, Holborow J (eds) Progress in immunology II. North-Holland, Amsterdam, pp 197-206

Klein J, Livnat S, Hauptfeld V, Jerabek L, Weissmann I (1974) Production of anti-H-2 antibodies in thymectomized mice. Eur J Immunol 4: 41-44

Klein J, Hauptfeld M, Hauptfeld V (1975) Splitting of antigen H-2.9 and mapping of its genetic determinants. Tissue Antigens 6: 46-49

Klein J, Hauptfeld V, Hauptfeld M (1975) Evidence for a fifth (G) region in the H-2 complex of the mouse. Immunogenetics 2: 141-150

Klein J, Forman J, Hauptfeld V, Egorov IK (1975) Immunogenetic analysis of H-2 mutations. III. Genetic mapping and involvement in immune reactions of the H-2^{ka} mutation. J Immunol 115: 716-718

Klein J, Chiang C, Lofgreen J, Steinmüller D (1976) Participation of H-2 regions in heart-transplant rejection. Transplantation 22: 384–390

Klein J, Egorov IK, Mantsakanyan YA, Hauptfeld V (1976) Immunogenetic analysis of *H-2* mutations. IV. Mapping of and immune reactions to the H-2^{fa} mutation. Scand J Immunol 5: 521–528

Klein J, Geib R, Chiang C, Hauptfeld V (1976) Histocompatibility antigens controlled by the *I* region of the murine *H-2* complex. I. Mapping of H-2A and H-2C loci. J Exp Med 143: 1439–1552

Klein J, Hauptfeld V, Vitetta ES (1976) Molecular relationships of Ia-antigens controlled by the same and by different subregions of the *I* region. In: Katz DH, Benacerraf B (eds) The role of the products of the histocompatibility gene complex in immune responses. Academic, New York, pp 53–58

Klein J, Hauptfeld M, Geib R, Hammerberg C (1976) Immunogenetic analysis of *H-2* mutations. V. Serological analysis of mutations H-2da, H-2^{fa}, and H-2^{ka}. Transplantation 22: 572–582

Klein J, Chiang CL, Wakeland EK (1977) Histocompatibility antigens controlled by the *I* region of the murine *H-2* complex. III. Blocking with antisera of the in vitro response. Immunogenetics 5: 445–451

Klein J, Chiang CL, Hauptfeld V (1977) Histocompatibility antigens controlled by the *I* region of the murine H-2 complex. II. *K/D* region compatibility is not required for *I*-region cell-mediated lymphocytotoxicity. J Exp Med 145: 450–454

Klein J, Hauptfeld M, Merryman CF, Maurer PH, Gardner MB (1977) Histocompatibility-2 system of wild mice. IV. Ia and Ir typing of two wild mouse populations. Cold Spring Harbor Symp Quant Biol 41: 457–463

Klein J, Duncan WR, Wakeland EK, Zaleska-Rutczynska Z, Huang H-JS, Hsu E (1978) Characterization of *H-2* haplotypes in wild mice. In: Morse HC (ed) Origins of inbred mice. Academic, New York, pp 667–687

Klein J, Flaherty L, VandeBerg JL, Shreffler DC (1978) *H-2* haplotypes, genes regions, and antigens: First listing. Immunogenetics 6: 489–512

Klein J, Götze D, Hämmerling GJ, Lemke H (1979) Nomenclature for H-2 and Ia antigens defined by hybridoma-produced monoclonal antibodies. Immunogenetics 9: 503–507

Klein J, Huang H-JS, Lemke H, Hämmerling GJ, Hämmerling U (1979) Serological analysis of H-2 and Ia molecules with monoclonal antibodies. Immunogenetics 8: 419–432

Klein J, Götze D, Nadeau JH, Wakeland EK (1981) Population immunogenetics of murine *H-2* and *t* systems. In: Berry RJ (ed) Biology of the house mouse. Academic, London, pp 439–453

Klein J, Götze D, Nadeau JH, Arden B, Figueroa F (1981) *H-2* polymorphism. A progress report. In: Zaleski MB, Abeyounis CJ, Kano K (eds) Immunobiology of the major histocompatibility complex. Basel

Klein J, Juretić A, Baxevanis CN, Nagy ZA (1981) The traditional and the new version of the mouse *H-2* complex. Nature 291: 455–460

Klein J, Figueroa F, Klein D (1982) *H-2* haplotypes, genes, and antigens: Second listing. I. Non-*H-2* loci on chromosome 17. Immunogenetics 16: 285–317

Klein J, Marusić M, Nagy ZA (1982) The seven rules of Mhc restriction. Transplant Proc 14: 581–583

Klein D, Tewarson S, Figueroa F, Klein J (1982) The minimal length of the differential segment in *H-2* congenic lines. Immunogenetics 16: 319–328

Klein J, David CS, Démant P, Hämmerling G, McKenzie IFC, Murphy DB, Sachs DH, Tada T (1983) Revised rules for naming class I and class II antigenic determinants controlled by the mouse *H-2* complex. Immunogenetics 17: 597–598

Klein J, Figueroa F, David CS (1983) *H-2* haplotypes, genes, and antigens: Second listing. II. The *H-2* complex. Immunogenetics 17: 533–596

Klein J, Figueroa F, Nagy ZA (1983) Genetics of the major histocompatibility complex: The final act. Annu Rev Immunol 1: 119–142

Klein J, Rammensee H-G, Nagy ZA (1983) Der Haupthistokompatibilitätskomplex und die Unterscheidung zwischen Selbst und Fremd durch das Immunsystem. Naturwissenschaften 70: 265–271

Klein J, Nagy ZA, Baxevanis CN, Ikezawa Z (1984) The histocompatibility complex and the specificity of suppressor T lymphocytes. In: Yamamura Y, Tada T (eds) Progress in Immunology V. Academic, Tokyo, pp 935–947

Klein J, Sipos P, Figueroa F (1984) Polymorphism of *t*-complex genes in European wild mice. Genet Res Camb 44: 39–46

Klein J, Ikezawa Z, Nagy ZA (1985) From LDH-B to J: An involuntary trip. Immunol Rev 83: 61–77

Klein J, Nižetić D, Golubić M, Dembić Z, Figueroa F (1985) Evolution of H-2 genes on t chromosomes. In: Pernis B, Vogel H (eds) Cell biology of the major histocompatibility complex. Academic, New York, pp 97–106

Klein J, Walden P, Nagy JA (1985) Antigen processing: A reevaluation. In: Feldmann M, Mitchison NA (eds) Immune regulation. Humana, Clifton, pp 335–344

Klein J, Golubić M, Schöpfer R, Kasahara M, Figueroa F (1986) On the origin of t chromosomes. Curr Top Microbiol Immunol 127: 239–246

Klein J, Klein D, Figueroa F (1986) Should the *Neuraminidase-1* locus be considered as part of the major histocompatibility complex? Hum Immunol 15: 396–403

Klein D, Zaleska-Rutczynska Z, Davis WC, Figueroa F, Klein J (1987) Monoclonal antibodies specific for mouse class I and class II Mhc determinants. Immunogenetics 25: 351–355

Klein J, Vinček V, Kasahara M, Figueroa F (1988) Is there a *t* complex in man? In: Beard RW, Sharp F (eds) Early pregnancy loss mechanisms and treatment. Royal College of Obstetricians and Gynecologists, London, pp 269–274

Klein J, Vincek V, Kasahara M, Figueroa F (1988) Probing mouse origins with random DNA probes. Curr Top Microbiol Immunol 137: 55–63

Klein J, Tichy H, Figueroa F (1988) On the origin of mice. Chile (in press)

Klement V, McAllister RM (1972) Syncytial cytopathic effect in KB cells of a C-type RNA virus isolated from human rhabdomyosarcoma. Virology 50: 305–308

Klement V, Nicolson MO (1977) Methods for assay of RNA tumor viruses. In: Maramorosch K, Koprowski H (eds) Methods in virology, vol 6. Academic, New York, pp 60–108

Klement V, Hartley JW, Rowe WP, Huebner RJ (1969) Recovery of a hamster-specific focus-forming and sarcomagenic virus from a "non-infectious" hamster tumor induced by the Kirsten mouse sarcoma virus. JNCI 43: 925–934

Klement V, Rowe WP, Hartley JW, Pugh WE (1969) Mixed culture cytopathogenicity: A new test for growth of murine leukemia viruses in tissue culture. Proc Natl Acad Sci USA 63: 753–758

Klement V, Freeman HM, McAllister RM, Nelson-Rees WA, Huebner RJ (1971) Differences in susceptibility of human cells to mouse sarcoma virus. JNCI 47: 65–73

Klement V, Nicolson MO, Huebner RJ (1971) Rescue of the genome of focus forming virus from rat non-productive lines by 5′-bromodeoxyuridine. Nature [New Biol] 234: 12–14

Klement V, Rowe WP, Hartley JW, Pugh WE (1971) Mixed culture cytopathogenicity: A new test for growth of murine leukemia viruses in tissue culture. In: Clark RL, Cumley RW (eds) The year book of cancer. Year Book Medical Publishers, Chicago, pp 422–423

Klement V, Nicolson MO, Gilden RV, Oroszlan S, Sarma P, Rongey R, Gardner MB (1972) Rat C-type virus induced in rat sarcoma cells by 5′-bromodeoxyuridine. Nature [New Biol] 238: 234–237

Klement V, Nicolson MO, Nelson-Rees WA, Gilden RV, Oroszlan S, Rongey RW, Gardner MB (1973) Spontaneous production of C-type RNA virus in rat tissue culture lines. Int J Cancer 12: 654–666

Klement V, Nicolson MO, Gilden RV, Oroszlan S, Sarma P, Rongey R, Gardner MB (1974) Rat C-type virus induced in rat sarcoma cells by 5′-bromodeoxyuridine. In: Tooze J, Sambrook J (eds) Selected papers in tumor virology. Cold Spring Harbor Laboratory Press, Cold Spring Harbor, pp 919–925

Klement V, Gardner MB, Henderson BE, Ihle JN, Estes JD, Stanley AG, Gilden RV (1976) Inefficient humoral immune response of lymphoma-prone wild mice to persistent leukemia virus infection. JNCI 57: 1169–1173

Klement V, Dougherty MF, Roy-Burman P, Pal BK, Shimizu CS, Rongey RW, Nelson-Rees W, Huebner RJ (1978) Endogenous type-C RNA virus of mink (mustela vison). Virology 85: 296–306

Klostergaard J, Lotzová E (1988) Monocyte-mediated cytotoxicity: Role of tumor necrosis factor. Introductory remarks. Nat Immun Cell Growth Regul 7: 249–253

Klouda PT (1980) HLA-B37. Joint Report. In: Terasaki PI (ed) Histocompatibility testing 1980. UCLA Tissue Typing Laboratory, Los Angeles, pp 379–381

Klouda PT, Bidwell JL (1984) Glo typing by isoelectric focusing. In: Albert ED, Baur MP, Mayr WR (eds) Springer, Berlin Heidelberg New York p 603

Klouda PT, Bradley BA (1983) The interface between HLA genes and immunological diseases. In: Thompson R, Rose NR (eds) Recent advances in clinical immunology III. Livingstone, Edinburgh, pp 91–110

Klouda PT, Bradley BA (1985) The role of AB0 blood groups in the sensitization of kidney recipients. In: Touraine JL (ed) Transplantation and clinical immunology XVII. Elsevier, Amsterdam p 241

Klouda PT, Jeannet M (1976) Cold and warm antibodies and graft survival in kidney allograft recipients. Lancet 1: 876–878

Klouda PT, Lawler SD (1972) Another recombination within the HL-A system. Vox Sang 22: 85–88

Klouda PT, Lawler SD (1975) Further analysis of HL-A antigens and antibodies in West Indians. Tissue Antigens 5: 415–419

Klouda PT, Reeves BR (1976) Serial studies of the reactivity of CLL cells with anti-CLL sera. In: Kissmeyer-Nielsen F (ed) Histocompatibility testing 1975. Munksgaard, Copenhagen, pp 697–704

Klouda PT, Lawler SD, Bagshawe KD (1972) HL-A matings in trophoblastic neoplasia. Tissue Antigens 2: 280–284

Klouda PT, Lawler SD, Bagshawe KD (1973) HL-A antibodies in patients with trophoblastic neoplasia I. General survey. Int Symp Ser Immunobiol Stand 18: 268–271

Klouda PT, Lawler SD, Till MM, Hardisty RM (1974) Acute lymphoblastic leukaemia and HL-A: A prospective study. Tissue Antigens 4: 262–265

Klouda PT, Lawler SD, Oliver RTD, Powles RL, Grant CK (1975) HL-A antibody response in patients with AML treated by immunotherapy. Transplantation 19: 245–249

Klouda PT, Werner O, Vassalli P, Legendre C, Ramirez E, Jeannet M (1977) Antibody responses in kidney transplant recipients and graft survival. Transplant Proc 9: 747–750

Klouda PT, Johnson RWG, Harris R, Mallick NP, Orr WMcN (1979) HLA matching in kidney transplantation: Experience of a single centre. Transplant Proc 11: 1293–1294

Klouda PT, Harris R, Price DA (1978) HLA and congenital adrenal hyperplasia. Lancet 2: 1046

Klouda PT, Manos J, Acherson EJ, Dyer PA, Goldby FS, Harris R, Lawler W, et al. (1979) Strong association between idiopathic membranous nephropathy and HLA-DRw3. Lancet 2: 770–771

Klouda PT, Harris R, Price DA (1980) Linkage and association between HLA and 21-hydroxylase deficiency. J Med Genet 17: 337–341

Klouda PT, Donnai D, Harris R (1981) HLA study in a live born infant with triploidy of paternal origin. Tissue Antigens 17: 240–242

Klouda PT, Williams E, Okoye RC, Ollier WER, Festeinstein H, Bradley BA (1983) Properdin factor B (Bf) polymorphism in three nigerian tribes. Dis Markers 1: 19–23

Klouda PT, Corbin S, Bradley BA, Ahern MJ, Maddison PJ (1983) HLA antigens in Felty's syndrome. Ann Rheum Dis 43: 120

Klouda PT, Syrbopoulos EK, Entwhistle CC, Goffin RB, Easty DL, Bradley BA (1983) HLA and keratoconus. Tissue Antigens 21: 397–399

Klouda PT, Ollier WER, Al Hilali A, Bacchus RS (1984) Properdin factor B (Bf) polymorphism in Saudi Arabs. A high frequency of a rare allele BfSo. 7. Hum Hered 34: 269–272

Klouda PT, Ray TC, Bowerman P, Bradley BA (1985) The prediction of a negative crossmatch in highly sensitized patients. Transplant Proc 17: 2467–2468

Klouda PT, Corbin SA, Bidwell JL, Bradley BA, Ahern MJ, Maddison PJ (1986) Felty's syndrome and HLA-DR antigens. Tissue Antigens 27: 122–113

Klouda PT, Harrison R, Corbin SA, Bradley BA, Easty DL (1986) HLA-A,B and DR antigens in patients with keratoconus. Tissue Antigens 27: 114–115

Klouda PT, Bidwell JL, Bodmer JG, Wasik A, Maddison PJ (1986) A possible haplotype association in Felty's syndrome. Dis. Markers 4: 27–28

Klouda PT Corbin SA, Bradley BA, Cohen BJ, Woolf AD (1986) HLA and acute arthritis following human parvarious infection. Tissue Antigens 28: 318–319

Klouda PT, Porter SR, Scully C, Corbin SA, Bradley BA, Smith R, Davies RM (1986) Association between HLA-A9 and rapidly progressive perioclonitis. Tissue Antigens 28: 146–149

Klouda PT, Ray YC, Gore GM, Bradley BA (1987) Organ sharing for highly sensitized patients. Transplant Proc 19: 731–733

Klouda PT, Ray TC, Kirkpatrick J, Bradley BA (1987) Graft survival in highly sensitized patients. Transplant Proc 19: 3744-3745

Knight SC, Krejčí J, Malkovský M, Colizzi V, Gautam A, Asherson GL (1985) The role of dendritic cells in the initiation of immune responses to contact sensitizers. I. In vivo exposure to antigen. Cell Immunol 94: 427-434

Knowles G, Davidson WL, McBride JS, Jolley D (1984) Antigenic diversity found in isolates of *Plasmodium falciparum* from Papua New Guinea by using monoclonal antibodies. Am J Trop Med Hyg 33: 204-211

Kohn HI, Klein J, Melvold RM, Nathenson SG, Pious D, Shreffler DC (1978) First *H-2* mutant workshop. Immunogenetics 7: 279-294

Koldovsky P (1970) The significance of immunology in oncology. In: Textbook of general pathology, vol 8. Springer, Berlin Heidelberg New York

Koldovsky P, Axler D (1970) Production of heterologous cytotoxic antibodies in vitro. Nature 228: 1323

Koldovsky P, Weinstein J (1973) Presence of organ and embryo specific antigens in human tumors. NCI Monogr 37: 33

Koldovsky P, Turano A, Fadda G (1969) Attempts to produce in vitro reaction of immunologically competent cells of C57BL/6 origin to Balb/c embryo fibroblasts. J Cell Physiol 74: 31

Koldovsky P, Turano A, Fadda G (1969) Specific transplantation resistence against mouse tumors induced by mouse sarcoma virus (Harvey). Folia Biol (Praha) 15: 224

Koldovsky P, Sawicki W, Koprowski H (1972) Crossreactivity between mouse eggs and SV40 transformed cells. In: Nowotny A (ed) Cell surface antigens. Springer, Berlin Heidelberg New York

Koldovsky P, Koldovsky U, Hummeler K (1974) Immunological studies on Wilms' tumor. Miami Symp Cancer 10: 254

Koldovsky P, Stark M, Idel H, Schlipköter HW (1978) Vergleich der immunobiologischen Eigenschaften von menschlichen Tumoren, gezüchtet in vitro und in nu/nu Mäusen. Z Immunitätsforsch Immunobiol 155: 26

Koldovsky U, Koldovsky P, Henle G, Henle W (1975) Multiple sclerosis associated agent: transmission to animals and some properties of this agent. Infect Immun 12: 1355

Koldovsky P, Koldovsky U, Ebbers J, Vosteen KH (1986) Stimulation of peripheral blood lymphocytes from laryngeal carcinoma patients with autologous tumor and serum derioved fractions. Arch Otorhinolaryngol 243: 309

Koltay M, Kinsky RG, Arnason BG, Schaffner JB (1965) Immunoglobulins and antibody formation in mice during the graft versus host reaction. Immunology 581-590

Koltay M, Kinsky R, Arnason B, Schaffner J (1965) Immunoglobulin levels in mice undergoing the GVH reaction. Nature 205: 509-510

Kongshavn PAL, Sadarangani C, Skamene E (1980) Cellular mechanisms of genetically determined resistance to listeria monocytogenes. In: Skamene E, Kongshavn PAL, Landy M (eds) Genetic control of natural resistance to infection and malignancy. Academic, New York, pp 149-163

Kongshavn PAL, Sadarangani C, Skamene E (1980) Genetically-determined differences in antibacterial activity of macrophages are expressed in the environment in which the macrophage precursors mature. Cell Immunol 53: 341-349

Kongshavn PAL, Skamene E (1984) The role of natural resistance in protection of the murine host from listeriosis. Clin Invest Med 7: 253-257

Kongshavn PAL, Vargas F, Skamene E, Ghadirian E (1985) Genetic control of resistance to infection with trypanosoma musculi. Prog Leukocyte Biol 3: 517-522

Koprowski H, Sawicki W, Koldovsky P (1971) Immunological crossreactivity between antigen of unfertilized mouse eggs and mouse cells transformed by simian virus 40. JNCI 46: 1317

Kovithavongs T, Schlaut J, Pazderka V, Lao V, Pazderka F, Bettcher KB, Dossetor JB (1978) Posttransplant immunologic monitoring with special consideration of technique and interpretation of LMC. Transplant Proc 10: 547

Kovithavongs T, Ferrone S, Thorsby E, Schlaut J, Pazderka F, Dossetor JB (1978) ADCC detects a public B-cell specificity broader than DRw3 and DRw6. Transplant Proc 10: 829

Kovithavongs T, Marchuk L, Schlaut J, Pazderka F, Dossetor JB (1983) Perturbation of immune function by lithium: a possible explanation for an irreversible renal transplant rejection. Transplant Proc 15: 1832

Kovithavongs T, Schlaut J, Marchuk L, Bettcher KB, Pazderka F, Dossetor JB (1982) Beneficial effect of blood transfusion in HLA, identical and haploidentical renal allografts. Transplant Proc 14: 690

Krömer G, Sundick RS, Schauenstein K, Hála K, Wick G (1985) Analysis of lymphocyte infiltrating the thyroid gland of obese strain chickens. J Immunol 135: 2452-2457

Krömer G, Faessler R, Hála K, Boeck G, Schauenstein K, Brezinschek H-P, Neu N, et al. (1988) Genetic analysis of extrathyroidal features of obese strain (OS) chickens with spontaneous autoimmune thyroiditis. Eur J Immunol 18: 1499-1505

Kürten C, Kau R, Kumazawa H, Koldovsky P (1989) Antitumoral effect of in vitro with tumor stimulated autologous peripheral blood lymphocytes measured by subrenal capsule assay. Arch Otorhinolaryngol (in press)

Kvist S, Klein J, Peterson PA (1980) Genetic control of the serum concentration of an H-2 antigen-like polypeptide chain. Immunogenetics 10: 499-507

Lai C-H, Babu UM, Matsunaga K, Nagy ZA, Klein J, Turchini HA, Maurer PH (1986) Complementation of class II A alleles in the immune response to (Glu Lys Tyr) polymers. Exp Clin Immunogenet 3: 38-48

Lamb JR, Iványi J, Rees A, Young RA, Young DB (1986) The identification of T cell epitopes in *Mycobacterium tuberculosis* using human T lymphocyte clones. Lepr Rev [Suppl 2] 57: 131-137

Lamb JR, Iványi J, Rees ADM, Rothbard JB, Howland K, Young RA, Young DB (1987) Mapping of T cell epitopes using recombinant antigens and synthetic peptides. EMBO J 6: 1245-1249

Landais D, Beck BN, Buerstedde J-M, Degraw S, Klein D, Koch N, Murphy D, et al. (1986) The assignment of chain specificities for anti-Ia monoclonal antibodies using L cell transfectants. J Immunol 137: 3002-3005

Lannigan R, Skamene E, Kongshavn PAL, Duguid WP (1979) Morphology of liver lesions in experimental listeriosis in splenectomized mice. J Reticuloendothel Soc 25: 457

Laundy GJ, Raffoux CM, Schreuder I, Klouda PT (1984) Bu and SV (HLA-Bw70, w71, w72) report. In: Histocompatibility testing 1984. Albert ED, Baur MP, Mayr WR (eds) Springer Verlag, pp 173-175

Laundy GJ, Middleton D, Klouda PT (1985) A new DQw1 associated antigen: HLA-DR Br. Tissue Antigens 26: 210-211

Lawler SD, Klouda PT (1973) West Indian negroes immigrant in the United Kingdom. In: Dausset J, Colombani J (eds) Histocompatibility testing 1972. Munksgaard, Copenhagen, pp 415-419

Lawler SD, Klouda PT (1973) Hodgkin's disease in a Caucasian population. In: Dausset J, Colombani J (eds) Histocompatibility testing 1972. Munksgaard, Copenhagen, pp 555-557

Lawler SD, Klouda PT, Bagshawe KD (1971) The HL-A system in trophoblastic neoplasia. Lancet 2: 834-837

Lawler SD, Klouda PT, Hardisty RM, Till MM (1971) Histocompatibility and acute lymphoblastic leukaemia. Lancet 1: 699

Lawler SD, Klouda PT, Hardisty RM, Till MM (1971) The HL-A system in lymphoblastic leukaemia: A study of patients and their families. Br J Haematol 21: 595-605

Lawler SD, Klouda PT, Bagshawe KD (1973) HL-A antibodies in patients with trophoblastic neoplasia II, after molar pregnancies. Symp Ser Immunobiol Stand 18: 272-275

Lawler SD, Klouda PT, Bagshawe KD (1974) Immunogenicity of molar pregnancies in the HL-A system. Am J Obstet Gynecol 120: 875-861

Lawler SD, Klouda PT, Smith PG, Till MM, Hardisty RM (1974) Survival and the HL-A system in acute lymphoblastic leukaemia. Br Med J 1: 547-548

Le Bouteiller P, Vujanović N, Duc HT, Kinsky RG, Voisin GA (1974) Ultrastructure des lymphocytes d'aspect thymique et d'aspect médullaire de la souris: identification par marquage immuno-enzymatique. Ann Inst Pasteur Immunol 125: 445-450

Le Bouteiller P, Kinsky R, Vujanović N, Duc HT, Voisin GA (1976) Morphological differences between thymus and bone-marrow derived lymphocytes. II. An electron microscopic and experimental study in unstimulated mice. Differentiation 6: 125-141

Le Bouteiller P, Kinsky R, Righenzi S, Voisin GA (1978) Electron microscopic study of thymus and bone marrow derived mouse lymphocytes. III. Morphological differences and evolution of surface markers before and after in vitro mitogenic stimulation. Ann Inst Pasteur Immunol 129: 635-651

Lemieux S, Lusignan Y, Skamene E (1985) NK cell activity in recombinant inbred mice: Selection of a model useful for in vivo studies. Prog Leukocyte Biol 3: 763–768

Lemieux S, Stevenson MM, Skamene E (1989) Genetic factors in natural immunity. In: Nelson DS (ed) Natural immunity. Academic, New York (in press)

Leski M, Favre H, Volanthen M, Chatelanat F, Milli JC, Garcia T, Klouda PT, et al. (1977) Rejet hyperaigu d'un rein transplanté de cause non-immunologique. J Urol Nephrol (Paris) 83 (9): 728–730

Levi-Strauss M, Tosi M, Steinmetz M, Klein J, Meo T (1985) Multiple duplications of complement $C4$ gene correlate with H-2-controlled testosterone-independent expression of its sexlimited isoform, C4-Slp. Proc Natl Acad Sci USA 82: 1746–1750

Lilly F, Klein J (1973) An H-2^g-like recombinant in the mouse. Transplantation 16: 530–532

Liu R, Pazderka F, Singh B, Dossetor JB (1984) Detection of IgG in supernatants of pokeweed mitogen-stimulated human lymphocyte cultures by one step solid-phase radioimmunoassay (SPIRA). Immunol Commun 13: 105

Livnat S, Klein J, Bach FH (1973) Graft-versus-host reaction in H-2 identical mice. Nature [New Biol] 243: 43–44

Longenecker BM, Pazderka F, Law GRJ, Ruth RF (1972) Genetic control of graft-versus-host competence. Transplantation 14: 424

Longenecker BM, Pazderka F, Law FRJ, Ruth RF (1973) The graft-versus-host reaction to minor alloantigens. Cell Immunol 8: 1

Longenecker BM, Pazderka F, Stone AH, Gavora JS, Ruth RF (1975) In ovo assay for Marek's disease virus and turkey herpes virus. Infect Immun 11: 922

Longenecker BM, Pazderka F, Ruth RF (1975) Modification by herpes virus of hereditary GVHR competency. J Immunol 2: 59

Longenecker BM, Pazderka F, Gavora JS, Ruth RF (1976) Lymphoma induced by herpes virus: resistance associated with a major histocompatibility gene. Immunogenetics 3: 401

Longenecker BM, Menezes J, Sanders EJ, Pazderka F, Ruth RF (1977) A new class of infectious agents detectable by the production of choriollantoic membrane lesions by human lymphoblastoid cell lines and their culture supernatants. JNCI 58: 853

Lotzová E (1977) Induction of unresponsiveness to bone marrow grafts. J Immunol 119: 543–547

Lotzová E (1977) Resistance to parental, allogeneic and xenogeneic hemopoietic grafts in irradiated mice. Exp Hematol 5: 215–235

Lotzová E (1977) Involvement of MHC-linked hemopoietic-histocompatibility genes in allogeneic transplantation in mice. Tissue Antigens 8: 148–152

Lotzová E (1980) Several aspects of natural killer cell-mediated cytotoxicity in normal individuals and cancer patients. Cell Mol Biol 26: 423–431

Lotzová E (1980) Centrifugal elutriation allows enrichment of natural killing and separates xenogeneic and allogeneic reactivity. In: Herberman RB (ed) Natural cell-mediated immunity against tumors. Academic, New York, pp 131–137

Lotzová E (1980) C. parvum-mediated suppression of the phenomenon of natural killing and its analysis. In: Herberman RB (ed) Natural cell-mediated immunity against tumors. Academic, New York, pp 735–752

Lotzová E (1980) Analogy between rejection of hemopoietic transplants and natural killing. In: Herberman RB (ed) Natural cell-mediated immunity against tumors. Academic, New York, pp 1117–1120

Lotzová E (1981) Experimental radiation and immune defense interactions. In: Prasad N (ed) Radiotherapy and cancer immunology. CRC, Boca Raton, pp 1–15

Lotzová E (1981) Leukemia: Whole body irradiation and reconstitution. In: Prasad N (ed) Radiotherapy and cancer immunology. CRC, Boca Raton, pp 93–107

Lotzová E (1982) Bone marrow transplantation. Surv Immunol Res 1: 37–39

Lotzová E (1982) Natural bone marrow graft rejection phenomenon in mice. Surv Immunol Res 1: 155–161

Lotzová E (1983) Hematopoietic histocompatibility: Genetic and immunological aspects. Compend Immunol 3: 468–493

Lotzová E (1983) Function of natural killer cells in various biological phenomena. Surv Synth Pathol Res 2: 41–46

Lotzová E (1984) Natural immunity. History, present and future. Nat Immun Cell Growth Regul 3: 1-6
Lotzová E (1984) The role of natural killer cells in immune surveillance against malignancies. Cancer Bull 36: 215-226
Lotzová E (1984) Relevance of natural killer cells in autologous bone marrow transplantation. In: Dicke KA, Spitzer G, Zander AR (eds) Proceedings of the first international symposium on bone marrow transplantation. MD Anderson Hospital, Houston, pp 301-303
Lotzová E (1985) Effector immune mechanisms in cancer. Nat Immun Cell Growth Regul 4: 293-304
Lotzová E (1986) Role of NK cells in defense against cancer, microbial infection and regulation of hemopoiesis. In: Lotzová E, Herberman RB (eds) Natural immunity, cancer and biological response modification. Karger, Basel, pp 309-312
Lotzová E (1988) Cytotoxicity and clinical application of activated NK cells. Med Oncol Tumor Pharmacother (in press)
Lotzová E (1986) NK cell role in regulation of the growth and functions of hemopoietic and lymphoid cells. In: Lotzová E, Herberman RB (eds) Immunobiology of natural killer cells, vol 2. CRC, Boca Raton, pp 89-105
Lotzová E (1987) Human natural killer cells. Their role and possible therapeutic application in leukemia. Clin Immunol Newslett 8: 56-60
Lotzová E (1987) Possible application of natural killer cells and interleukin-2 therapy of human leukemia. In: Truitt RL, Gale RP, Bortin MM (eds) Cellular immunotherapy of cancer. Liss, New York, pp 259-266
Lotzová E (1988) Natural immunity mechanisms stimulated by immunomodulators. Adv Biosci 68: 193-201
Lotzová E (1985) Natural immunity and biological response: Introduction. Nat Immun Cell Growth Regul 4: 233-234
Lotzová E (1986) Effector immune mechanisms in cancer. Curr Cancer Contents 9: 17
Lotzová E (1986) Therapeutic possibilities of virus-modified tumor cell extract and interleukin-2 in human ovarian cancer. Nat Immun Cell Growth Regul 5: 277-282
Lotzová E (1987) Interleukin-2 generated killer cells, their characterization and role in cancer therapy. Cancer Bull 39: 30-38
Lotzová E (1987) Role of interleukin-2 and interleukin-2-activated killer cells in cancer therapy. Cancer Bull 39: 5
Lotzová E (1988) Ovarian tumor-infiltrating lymphocytes: Phenotype and antitumor activity. Nat Immun Cell Growth Regul 7: 226-229
Lotzová E (1988) Immune surveillance and natural immunity. In: Cooper EL (ed) Developmental immunology. Oxford University Press, Oxford (in press)
Lotzová E (1988) Role of natural killer cells in defense against leukemia: Therapeutic considerations. Nat Immun Cell Growth Regul 7: 170-179
Lotzová E, Ades EW (1988) Natural killer cells: Definition, heterogeneity, lytic mechanism, functions, and clinical application. Nat Immun Cell Growth Regul (in press)
Lotzová E, Cudkowicz G (1971) Hybrid resistance to parental NZW bone marrow grafts: Association with the D end of H-2. Transplantation 12: 130-138
Lotzová E, Cudkowicz G (1972) Hybrid resistance to parental WB/Re bone marrow grafts. Association with genetic markers of linkage group IX. Transplantation 13: 256-264
Lotzová E, Cudkowicz G (1973) Resistance of irradiated F_1 hybrid and allogeneic mice to bone marrow grafts of NZB donors. J Immunol 110: 791-800
Lotzová E, Cudkowicz G (1974) Abrogation of resistance to bone marrow grafts by silica particles. Prevention of the silica effect by the macrophage stabilizer poly 2-vinylpyridine N-oxide. J Immunol 113: 798-803
Lotzová E, Dicke KA (1987) Possible therapeutic value of NK cells in suppression of residual leukemia after autologous marrow transplantation. Proceedings, 3rd International Symposium on Autologous Bone Marrow Transplantation. Dicke KA, Spitzer G, Jagannath S, Favrot M, Peters W (eds), The Univ. of Texas, MD Anderson Tumor and Cancer Institute, Houston: 669-673
Lotzová E, Gutterman J (1979) Effect of glucan on natural killer (NK) cells. Further comparison between NK cells and bone marrow effector cells activities. J Immunol 123: 607-611

Lotzová E, Herberman RB (1987) Reassessment of LAK phenomonology – a review. Nat Immun Cell Growth Regul 6: 109–115

Lotzová E, Herberman RB (1987) Natural resistance to tumors and mechanism of killing. Cancer Bull 39: 260–261

Lotzová E, McCredie KB (1978) Natural killer cells in mice and man and their possible biological significance. Cancer Immunol Immunother 4: 215–221

Lotzová E, Richie E (1977) Promotion of incidence of adenovirus 12 transplantable tumors by carrageenan, a specific anti-macrophage agent. JNCI 58: 1171–1172

Lotzová E, Savary CA (1977) Possible involvement of natural killer cells in bone marrow graft rejection. Biomedicine 27: 341–344

Lotzová E, Savary CA (1981) Parallelism between the effect of cortisone acetate on hybrid resistance and natural killing. Hematol 9: 766–774

Lotzová E, Savary CA (1983) Natural resistance to foreign hemopoietic transplants: A possible model of leukemia surveillance. Proc. Thirteenth International Cancer Congress, Part C. Mirand EA, Hutchinson WB, Mihich E (eds). Liss, New York, 3: 125–135

Lotzová E, Savary CA (1984) Stimulation of NK cell cytotoxic potential of normal donors by two species of recombinant alpha interferon. J Interferon Res 4: 201–213

Lotzová E, Savary CA (1986) Interleukin-2 corrects defective NK activity of patients with leukemia. Comp Immunol Microbiol Infect Dis 9: 169–175

Lotzová E, Savary CA (1986) Pyrimidinones: Inducers of NK cell activity and antitumor immunity. Comp Immunol Microbiol Infect Dis 9: 185–191

Lotzová E, Savary CA (1986) Augmentation of natural immunity against neoplasia by pyrimidinones. In: Lotzová E, Herberman RB (eds) Natural immunity, cancer and biological response modification. Karger, Basel, pp 160–172

Lotzová E, Savary CA (1986) Regulation of NK cell cytotoxicity by suppressor cells. In: Lotzová E, Herberman RB (eds) Immunobiology of natural killer cells, vol 2. CRC, Boca Raton, pp 163–177

Lotzová E, Savary CA (1987) Generation of NK cell activity from human bone marrow. J Immunol 139: 279–284

Lotzová E, Savary CA (1988) Function of interleukin-2 activated NK cells in leukemia resistance and treatment. In: Lotzová E (ed) Role interleukin-2 activated killer cells in cancer, vols 1, 2. CRC, Boca Raton (in press)

Lotzová E, Savary CA (1988) Growth kinetics, function and characterization of lymphocytes infiltrating ovarian tumors. In: Lotzová E (ed) Role interleukin-2 activated killer cells in cancer, vols 1, 2. CRC, Boca Raton (in press)

Lotzová E, Savary CA, Herberman RB, McCredie KB, Barlogie B (1987) The role of natural killer cells in resistance to leukemia: Generation of antileukemia activity in NK-deficient leukemic patients. Novel Approaches in Cancer Therapy, 14th International Cancer Congress. Lapis K, Eckhardt S (eds), S. Karger AG, Basel, Switzerland 5: 305–312

Lotzová E, Tsubura E (1988) Effector functions of cytokines in cancer. 4th International Congress on Immunopharmacology. Pergamon, Oxford (in press)

Lotzová E, Gallagher MT, Trentin JJ (1975) Involvement of macrophages in genetic resistance to bone marrow grafts. Studies with two specific antimacrophage agents, carrageenan and silica. Biomedicine 22: 387–392

Lotzová E, Gallagher MT, Trentin JJ (1975) Genetic control of resistance to rat bone marrow grafts in mice. Biomedicine 23: 335–336

Lotzová E, Gallagher MT, Trentin JJ (1976) Macrophage involvement in genetic resistance to bone marrow transplantation. In: Dupont B, Good RA (eds) Immunobiology of bone marrow transplantation. Grune and Stratton, New York, pp 151–156

Lotzová E, Dicke KA, Trentin JJ, Gallagher MT (1977) Genetic control of bone marrow transplantation in irradiated mice. Classification of mouse strains according to their responsiveness to bone marrow allografts and xenografts. Transplant Proc 9: 289–292

Lotzová E, McCredie KB, Maroun JA, Dicke KA, Friereich EJ (1979) Some studies on natural killer cells in man. Transplant Proc 11: 1390–1392

Lotzová E, Maroun JA, McCredie KB, Drewinko B, Dicke KA (1979) Studies on natural killer cell-mediated cytotoxicity in normal individuals and cancer patients. Adv Med Oncol Res Educ 6: 149–154

Lotzová E, McCredie KB, Muesse L, Dicke KA, Friereich EJ (1979) Natural killer cells in man: Their possible involvement in leukemia and bone marrow transplantation. In: Baum SJ, Ledney GD (eds) Experimental hematology today. Springer, Berlin Heidelberg New York, pp 207–213

Lotzová E, Pollack SB, Savary CA (1982) Direct evidence for the involvement of natural killer cells in bone marrow transplantation. In: Herberman RB (ed) NK cells and other natural effector cells. Academic, New York, pp 1535–1540

Lotzová E, Savary CA, Gutterman JU, Hersh EM (1982) Natural killer cell-mediated cytotoxicity: Modulation by partially purified and cloned interferon-α. Cancer Res 42: 2480–2488

Lotzová E, Savary CA, Gutterman JU, Quesada JR, Hersh EM (1983) Regulation of human natural killer cell cytotoxicity by recombinant leucocyte inferferon clone A. J Biol Response Mod 2: 482–496

Lotzová E, Savary CA, Gutterman JU, Quesada JR, Hersh EM (1983) Analysis of natural killer cell cytotoxicity in recombinant interferon-treated cancer patients. JNCI 71: 903–910

Lotzová E, Savary CA, Keating MJ (1983) Leukemia diseased patients exhibit multiple defects in natural killer cell lytic machinery. Exp Hematol 10: 83–95

Lotzová E, Savary CA, Stringfellow DA, Drewinko B, Gray KN, Raulston GL, Jardine JH (1983) Analysis of natural killer cell activity in random-bred Rowett athymic rats. Proceedings of the fourth international workshop on immune deficient animals, Chexbres. Karger, Basel, pp 53–59

Lotzová E, Savary CA, Stringfellow DA (1983) Modulation of murine NK cell cytotoxicity in vitro and antitumor immunity in vivo by low molecular weight interferon inducers. In: Crispen RG (ed) Cancer: Etiology and prevention. Elsevier, New York, pp 199–211

Lotzová E, Savary CA, Stringfellow DA (1983) 5-halo-6-phenyl pyrimidinones: New molecules with cancer therapeutic potential and interferon-inducing capacity are strong inducers of murine natural killer cells. J Immunol 130: 965–969

Lotzová E, Savary CA, Pollack SB (1983) Prevention of rejection of allogeneic bone marrow transplants by NK 1.1 antiserum. Transplantation 35: 490–494

Lotzová E, Savary CA, Khan A, Stringfellow DA (1984) Stimulation of natural killer cells in two random-bred strains of athymic rats by interferon-inducing pyrimidinone. J Immunol 132: 2566–2570

Lotzová E, Savary CA, Freedman RS, Bowen JM (1984) Natural killer cell cytotoxic potential of patients with ovarian carcinoma and its modulation with virus-modified tumor cell extract. Cancer Immunol Immunother 17: 124–129

Lotzová E, Savary CA, Stringfellow DA, Drewinko B, Gray KN, Raulston GL, Jardine JH (1984) Analysis of natural killer cell activity in random-bred Rowett athymic rats. Exp Cell Biol 52: 53–59

Lotzová E, Savary CA, Hersh EM, Khan AA, Rosenblum M (1984) Depression of murine natural killer cell cytotoxicity by isobutyl nitrite. Cancer Immunol Immunother 17: 130–134

Lotzová E, Savary CA, Gray KN, Raulston GL, Jardine JH (1984) Natural killer cell profile of two randombred strains of athymic rats. Exp Hematol 12: 633–640

Lotzová E, Savary CA, Keating MJ, Hester JP (1985) Defective NK cell mechanism in patients with leukemia. In: Heberman RB (ed) Mechanism for cytotoxicity by NK cells. Academic, New York, pp 507–519

Lotzová E, Savary CA, Freedman R, Bowen JM (1986) Natural immunity against ovarian tumors. Comp Immunol Microbiol Infect Dis 9: 269–275

Lotzová E, Savary CA, Lowlachi M, Murasko DM (1986) Cytotoxic and morphological profile of endogenous and pyrimidinone-activated murine NK cells. J Immunol 136: 732–740

Lotzová E, Savary CA, Pollack, S, Hanna N (1986) Induction of tumor immunity and natural killer cell cytotoxicity in mice by 5-halo-6-phenyl pyrimidinones. Cancer Res 46: 5004–5008

Lotzová E, Savary CA, Herberman RB, Dicke KA (1986) Can NK cells play a role in therapy of leukemia? Nat Immun Cell Growth Regul 5: 61–64

Lotzová E, Savary CA, Pollack S, Hanna N (1986) Induction of tumor immunity and natural killer cell cytotoxicity by 5-halo-6-phenyl pyrimidinones. Cancer Res 46: 5004–5008

Lotzová E, Savary CA, Herberman RB (1986) Impaired NK cell profile in leukemia-diseased patients. In: Lotzová E, Herberman RB (eds) Immunobiology of natural killer cells, vol 2. CRC, Boca Raton, pp 29–53

Lotzová E, Savary CA, Herberman RB (1986) Antileukemia reactivity of endogenous and IL-2 activated NK cells. In: Lotzová E, Herberman RB (eds) Natural immunity, cancer and biological response modification. Karger, Basel, pp 177-195

Lotzová E, Savary CA, Herberman RB (1987) Induction of NK cell activity against fresh human leukemia in culture with interleukin-2. J Immunol 138: 2718-2727

Lotzová E, Savary CA, Herberman RB (1987) Inhibition of clonogenic growth of fresh leukemia cells by unstimulated and IL-2 stimulated NK cells of normal donors. Leuk Res 11: 1059-1066

Lotzová E, Savary CA, Herberman RB (1987) Augmentation of antileukemia lytic activity by OKT3 monoclonal antibody: Synergism OKT3 and interleukin-2. Nat Immun Cell Growth Regul 6: 218-223

Lotzová E, Savary CA, Freedman RS, Bowen JM (1987) NK cell antitumor activity of patients with ovarina carcinoma. Induction of cytotoxicity by viral oncolysates and interleukin-2. In: Rutledge FM, Freedman RS, Gershenson DM (eds) Diagnosis and treatment strategy for gynecological cancer. UT, Austin, pp 123-126

Lotzová E, Savary CA, Pollack S, Hanna N (1987) Induction of tumor immunity and natural killer cell cytotoxicity in mice by 5-halo-6-phenyl pyrimidinone. In: Hickey R, et al. (eds) 1987 yearbook of cancer. Saunders, Philadelphia, pp 438-439

Lotzová E, Savary CA, Freedman RS, Edwards CL, Wharton JT (1988) Recombinant IL-2 activated NK cells mediate LAK activity against ovarian cancer. Int J Cancer 42: 225-231

Lotzová E, Savary CA, Dicke KA, Jagannath S (1988) Role of NK cells in tumor cell growth and eradication. In: Baum SJ, Dicke KA, Lotzová E, Pluznik DH (eds) Experimental hematology today. Springer, Berlin Heidelberg New York (in press)

Loveland B, Hunt R, Malkovský M (1986) Autologous lymphoid cells exposed to recombinant interleukin 2 in vitro in the absence of antigen can induce the rejection of long-term tolerated skin allografts. Immunology 59: 159-161

Lubenko A, Iványi J (1986) Epitope specificity of blood group A reactive murine monoclonal antibodies. Vox Sang 51: 136-142

Lydyard P, Iványi J (1971) Suppression of graft-versus-host-reactive lymphocytes by heterologous antithymus serum in vitro. Transplantation 12: 493-499

Lydyard PM, Iványi J (1974) The role of opsonization in antithymocyte globulin-induced suppression of graft-versus-host reaction in chick embryos. Transplantation 17: 400-404

Lydyard PM, Iványi J (1975) Immunodeficiency in the chicken. III. Hypoplasia of bursal follicles following intravenous injection of embryos with lipopolysaccharide or allogenic lymphocytes. Immunology 28: 1023-1031

Lydyard PM, Iványi J (1975) Chimaerism of immunocompetent cells in allogeneic bone marrow-reconstituted lethally irradiated chickens. Transplantation 20: 155-162

Maisel J, Klemen V, Lai M, Duesberg P (1973) Ribonucleic acid components of murine sarcoma and leukemia viruses. Proc Natl Acad Sci USA 70: 3536-3540

Malkinson AM, Nesbitt MN, Skamene E (1985) Analysis of lung tumor susceptibility differences using the AXB and BXA recombinant inbred strains of mice. Prog Leukocyte Biol 3: 805-810

Malkinson AM, Nesbitt MN, Skamene E (1985) Susceptibility to urethan-induced pulmonary adenomas between A/J and C57BL/6J mice: Use of AXB and BXA recombinant inbred lines indicating a three-locus genetic model. JNCI 75: 971-974

Malkovský M (1985) Stimulation of interleukin 2 production by purified protein derivative (PPD) in spleen cells from control or retinyl acetate-fed mice infected with Bacille Calmette-Guérin (BCG). Ciba Found Symp Ser 113: 126-131

Malkovský M (1987) Is T cell help involved in establishment of tolerance? Theory and experiment. In: Matzinger P, Flajnik M, Nemazee D, Rammensee H-G, Rolink T, Stockinger G, Nicklin L (eds) Tolerance workshop 1986, vol 2. Roche, Basel, pp 73-79

Malkovský M (1988) Immunological tolerance. Applications. In: Matzinger P, Flajnik M, Nemazee D, Rammensee H-G, Rolink T, Stockinger G, Nicklin L (eds) Tolerance workshop 1986, vol 3. Roche, Basel, pp 216-217

Malkovský M (1988) The relativity of immunological information. Proceedings of the 9th European Congress on Immunology, Rome. Pensiero, pp 14-17

Malkovský M, Dalgleish AG (1988) Immunopathology of HIV infection. In: Salerno A (ed) Cellular proliferation and differentiation. Proceedings of 19th Congress of the Italian Society for Pathology, Oct. 19-22, Palermo, pp 467-470

Malkovský M, Medawar PB (1984) Is immunological tolerance (non-responsiveness) a consequence of interleukin 2 deficit during the recognition of antigen? Immunol Today 5: 340–343

Malkovský M, Medawar PB (1984) Retinoids and in vivo immunity to transplantable tumours: a terra relatively incognita. Immunol Today 5: 178–180

Malkovský M, Sondel PM (1987) Interleukin-2 and its receptor: structure, function and therapeutic potential. Blood Rev 1: 254–266

Malkovský M, Asherson GL, Stockinger B, Watkins MC (1982) Nonspecific inhibitor released by T acceptor cells reduces the production of interleukin-2. Nature 300: 652–655

Malkovský M, Doré C, Hunt R, Palmer L, Chandler P, Medawar PB (1983) Enhancement of specific antitumor immunity in mice fed a diet enriched in vitamin A acetate. Proc Natl Acad Sci USA 80: 6322–6326

Malkovský M, Edwards AJ, Hunt R, Palmer L, Medawar PB (1983) T-cell-mediated enhancement of host-versus-graft reactivity in mice fed a diet enriched in vitamin A acetate. Nature 302: 338–340

Malkovský M, Asherson GL, Chandler P, Colizzi V, Watkins MC, Zembala M (1983) Nonspecific inhibitor of DNA synthesis elaborated by T acceptor cells. I. Specific hapten- and I-J-driven liberation of an inhibitor of cell proliferation by Lyt-1^-2^+ cyclophosphamide-sensitive T acceptor cells armed with a product of Lyt-1^+2^+ specific suppressor cells. J Immunol 130: 785–790

Malkovský M, Hunt R, Palmer L, Doré C, Medawar PB (1984) Retinyl acetate-mediated augmentation of resistance to a transplantable 3-methylcholanthrene-induced fibrosarcoma: the dose response and time course. Transplantation 38: 158–161

Malkovský M, Medawar P, Hunt R, Palmer L, Doré C (1984) A diet enriched in vitamin A acetate or in vivo administration of interleukin-2 can counteract a tolerogenic stimulus. Proc R Soc Lond [Biol] 220: 439–445

Malkovský M, Medawar PB, Thatcher DR, Toy J, Hunt R, Rayfield LS, Doré C (1985) Acquired immunological tolerance of foreign cells is impaired by recombinant interleukin-2 or vitamin A acetate. Proc Natl Acad Sci USA 82: 536–538

Malkovský M, Jira M, Gao L, Loveland B, Malkovska V, Dalgleish AG, Webster ADB (1986) Reduced expression of interleukin-2 receptors in hypogammaglobulinaemia: a possible cause of higher cancer incidence. Lancet 1: 1442–1443

Malkovský M, Brenner MK, Hunt R, Rastan S, Doré C, North ME, Asherson GL (1986) T-cell depletion of allogeneic bone marrow prevents acceleration of graft-versus-host disease induced by exogenous interleukin-2. Cell Immunol 103: 476–480

Malkovský M, Colizzi V, Asherson GL, Krejčí J, Bacon T, Watkins MC, Zembala M (1986) Nonspecific inhibitor of DNA synthesis elaborated by T acceptor cells. II. Requirements for its production and action. Cell Immunol 98: 114–124

Malkovský M, Jira M, Madar J, Malkovska V, Asherson GL (1987) Generation of lymphokine-activated killer cells does not require DNA synthesis. Immunology 60: 471–473

Malkovský M, Loveland B, North M, Asherson GL, Gao L, Ward P, Fiers W (1987) Recombinant interleukin-2 directly augments the cytotoxicity of human monocytes. Nature 325: 262–265

Malkovský M, Sondel PM, Strober W, Dalgleish AG (1988) The interleukins in acquired disease. Clin Exp Immunol 74: 151–161

Malkovský M, Newell A, Dalgleish AG (1988) Inactivation of HIV by nonoxynol-9. Lancet 1: 645

Malkovský M, Philpott K, Dalgleish AG, Mellor AL, Patterson S, Webster ADB, Edwards AJ, Maddon PJ (1988) Infection of B lymphocytes by the human immunodeficiency virus and their susceptibility to cytotoxic cells. Eur J Immunol 18: 1315–1321

Malkovský M, Sondel PM, Strober W, Dalgleish AG (1988) The interleukins. In: Cohen RD, Alberti KGMM, Lewis B, Denman AM (eds) The metabolic and molecular basis of acquired disease. Bailliere Tindall, London (in press)

Mark C, Figueroa F, Nagy ZA, Klein J (1982) Cytotoxic monoclonal antibody specific for the Lyt-1.2 antigen. Immunogenetics 16: 95–97

Maron R, Klein J, Cohen IR (1982) Mutations of *H-2K* or *H-2D* alter immune response phenotype of autoimmune thyroiditis. Immunogenetics 15: 625–627

Marshall WM, Barnard JM, Churchill D, Farid NR, Grandy R, Larsen B, Payne RH, et al. (1984) Study of alleles of the second complement component (C2) on Canadian HLA haplotypes. Tissue Antigens 23: 229–239

Marusić M, Nagy ZA, Koszinowski U, Klein J (1982) Involvement of Mhc loci in immune responses that are not *Ir*-gene controlled. Immunogenetics 16: 471–483

Masihi KN, Lange W, Lotzová E (1987) Immunomodulators and nonspecific defense against microbial infections. Nat Immun Cell Growth Regul 6: 213–218

Mauff G, Alper CA, Awdeh Z, Batchelor JR, Bertrams J, Bruun-Petersen G, Dawkins RL, et al. (1983) Statement on the nomenclature of human C4 complement. Immunobiology 164: 184–191

Mayer WE, Jonker M, Klein D, Iványi P, van Seventer GA, Klein J (1988) Nucleotide sequences of chimpanzee MHC class-I alleles: evidence for trans-species mode of evolution. EMBO J 7: 2765–2774

McAlack RF, Cerny J, Allen JL, Friedman H (1970) Vibriolytic antibody forming cells: A new application of the Pfeiffer phenomenon. Science 168: 141

McAlack RF, Cerny J, Sajid MA, Friedman H (1971) Cellular formation of vibrolytic antibody by mouse immunocytes: cytokinetics and specificity. J Immunol 107: 1751

McAllister RM, Peer M, Gilden RV, Klement V, Landing B (1974) Tumors formed by human rhabdomyosarcoma cells in chorioallantoic membrane of embryonated hens' eggs. Int J Cancer 13: 886–890

McAllister RM, Isaacs H, Gardner MB, Klement V (1975) Transplantation of human rhabdomyosarcoma cells in heterologous hosts: tumors formed and viruses recovered. In: Ito Y, Dutcher RM (eds) Comparative leukemia research, 1973. Leukemogenesis. University of Tokyo Press, Tokyo; Karger, Basel, pp 659–662

McBride JS (1983) Monoclonal antibodies and applications to parasitisms. In: Guardiola J, Luzzatto L, Trager W (eds) Molecular biology of parasites. Raven, New York, pp 173–184

McBride JS, Heidrich H-G (1987) Fragments of the polymorphic M_r 185 000 glycoprotein from the surface of isolated *Plasmodium falciparum* merozoites from an antigenic complex. Mol Biochem Parasitol 23: 71–84

McBride JS, Micklem HS (1977) Immunosuppression in murine malaria. II. The primary response to ovine serum albumin. Immunology 33: 253–259

McBride JS, Micklem HS (1981) Immunodepression of thymus-independent response to dextran in mouse malaria. Clin Exp Immunol 44: 74–81

McBride JS, Micklem HS, Ure JM (1977) Immunosuppression in murine malaria. I. Response to type III pneumococcal polysaccharide. Immunology 32: 635–644

McBride JS, Walliker D, Morgan G (1982) Antigenic diversity in the human malaria parasite *Plasmodium falciparum*. Science 217: 254–257

McBride JS, Welsby PD, Walliker D (1984) Serotyping *Plasmodium falciparum* from acute human infections using monoclonal antibodies. Trans R Soc Trop Med Hyg 78: 32–34

McBride JS, Newbold CI, Anand R (1985) Polymorphism of a high molecular weight schizont antigen of the human malaria parasite *Plasmodium falciparum*. J Exp Med 161: 160–180

McDevitt HO, Deak BD, Shreffler DC, Klein J, Stimpfling JH, Snell GD (1972) Genetic control of the immune response. Mapping of the *Ir-1* locus. J Exp Med 135: 1259–1278

McGrath MS, Pillemer E, Kooistra DA, Jacobs S, Jerabék L, Weissman IL (1980) T-lymphoma retroviral receptors and control of T-lymphoma cell proliferation. Cold Spring Harbor Symp Quant Biol 44: 1297

McGrath MS, Jerabék L, Pillemer E, Steinberg RA, Weissman IL (1981) Receptor mediated murine leukemogenesis: monoclonal antibody induced lymphoma cell growth arrest. Haematol Blood Transfus 26:

McGrath MS, Jerabék L, Weissman IL (1982) Receptor mediated leukemogenesis: retrovirus receptors on B and T lymphomas share idiotypic determinants. In: Baum S, Ledney GD, Thierfelder S (eds) Experimental hematology today. Karger, Basel, pp 93–100

Melief CJM, de Waal LP, van der Meulen MY, de Greeve P, Iványi P (1979) Target specificity of cytotoxic T cells directed against H-2L. Immunogenetics 9: 324–325

Melief CJM, de Waal LP, van der Meulen MY, Iványi P, Melvold RW (1981) Fine specificity of cytotoxic T lymphocytes directed against H-2L^d. Immunogenetics 12: 74–88

Meltzer MS, Nacy CA, Stevenson MM, Skamene E (1982) Macrophages in resistance to Rickettsial infections: genetic analysis of susceptibility to lethal effects of Rickettsia Akari infection and development of activated, cytotoxic macrophages in A and B10. A mice. J Immunol 129: 1719–1723

Mekori T, Kinsky RG (1983) The ability of placental extracts to modulate a direct PFC response to SRBCs in mice. Immunol Lett 6: 21–24

Merchant JA, Klouda PT, Soutar CA, Parkes WR, Lawler SD, Turner-Warwick M (1975) The HL-A system in asbestos workers. Br Med J 1: 189–191

Mervart H, Moore BPL (1983) HLA typing in Canada: production and free distribution of tissue-typing trays. Can Med Assoc J 129: 689–690

Mervart H, Tibensky D (1980) Possible new C locus antigen T11. In: Terasaki PI (ed) Histocompatibility testing 1980. UCLA Tissue Typing Laboratory, Los Angeles, p 791

Mervart H, Mosely P, Tibensky D (1980) HLA-A29. In: Terasaki PI (ed) Histocompatibility testing 1980. UCLA Tissue Typing Laboratory, Los Angeles, pp 320–322

Mervart H, Kalovsky E, Moore BPL (1983) Splits of the HLA DR2 antigen. Tissue Antigens 22: 29–31

Mervart H, Taylor C, Ting A (1984) HLA-Bw41. In: Albert ED, Baur MP, Mayr WR (eds) Histocompatibility testing 1984. Springer, Berlin Heidelberg New York, p 149

Miettinen-Baumann A, Strych W, McBride J, Heidrich H-G (1988) A 46 000 dalton *Plasmodium falciparum* merozoite surface glycoprotein not related to the 185–195 000 dalton schizont precursor molecule: isolation and characterization. Parasitol Res 74: 317–323

Milas L, Hunter N, Ito H, Lotzová E, Stringfellow DA (1983) Studies on the antitumor activities of pyrimidinone-interferon inducers. II. Potentiation of antitumor resistance mechanism. Clin Exp Metastas 1: 213–222

Miller K, Maisey J, Malkovský M (1984) Enhancement of contact sensitization in mice fed a diet enriched in vitamin A acetate. Int Arch Allergy Appl Immunol 75: 120–125

Mobraaten LE, Forman J, Klein J, Cherry M, Bailey DW (1978) Genetic mapping and immunogenetic characterization of the H-2^{fb} mutation in the mouse. Immunogenetics 7: 41–50

Modabber F, Bear SE, Cerny J (1976) The effect of cyclophosphamide on the recovery from a local chlamydial infection: guinea pig inclusion conjunctivitis. Immunology 30: 929

Mölders HH, Breuning MH, Iványi P, Ploegh HL (1983) Biochemical analysis of variant HLA-B27 antigens. Hum Immunol 6: 111–117

Moll R, Achstatter T, Becht E, Balcarova-Stander J, Ittensohn M, Franke W (1988) Cytokeratins in normal and malignant transitionel epithelium. Am J Pathol 132: 123

Montaraz JA, Novotny P, Iványi J (1985) Identification of a 68-kilodalton protective protein antigen from *Bordetella bronchiseptica*. Infect Immun 47: 744–751

Moore MJ, Iványi J (1988) Idiotype vaccines. In: Liew E (ed) Vaccines in tropical diseases. (In press)

Morello D, Neauport-Sautes C, Demant P (1977) Topographical relationships among H-2 specificities controlled by the D region. Immunogenetics 4: 349–364

Morgan K, Holmes TM, Schlaut J, Marchuk L, Kovithavongs T, Pazderka F, Dossetor JB (1980) Genetic variability of HLA in the Dariusleut Hutterites. A comparative genetic analysis of the Hutterites, the Amish and other selected caucasian populations. Am J Hum Genet 32: 246

Morgan K, Holmes TM, Pazderka F, Dossetor JB (1986) Segregation of HLA A, B haplotypes and the distribution of antigen mismatches between mother and offspring in Hutterite families. Am J Hum Genet 38: 971

Morris JA, Iványi J (1985) Immunoassays of field isolates of *Mycobacterium Bovis* and other mycobacteria by use of monoclonal antibodies. J Med Microbiol 19: 367–373

Mortensen RF, Gervais F, Skamene E, Rae D, Stevenson M (1985) Acute phase reactants and host resistance: Role of mouse serum amyloid P-component. Prog Leukocyte Biol 3: 585–594

Munk Z, Skamene E (1979) Goodpasture's syndrome – Effects of plasmapheresis. Clin Exp Immunol 36: 244

Mwatha J, Moreno C, Sengupta U, Sinha S, Iványi J (1988) A comparative evaluation of serological assays for lepromatous leprosy. Lepr Rev 59: 195–199

Myerson D, Scheinberg D, Klement V, Strand M, August JT (1979) Characterization of a defective pseudotype particle of Kirsten sparcoma virus. Virology 95: 536–549

Nacy CA, Meltzer MS, Leonard EJ, Stevenson MM, Skamene E (1983) Activation of macrophages for killing of Rickettsiae: Analysis of macrophage effector function after Rickettsial inoculation of inbred mouse strains. Adv Exp Med Biol 162: 335–353

Nadeau JH, Klein J (1981) Wild-derived alleles of five allozyme-encoding loci in B10.W mice. Immunogenetics 13: 173–176

Nadeau JH, Wakeland, EK, Götze D, Klein J (1981) The population genetics of the *H-2* polymorphism in European and North African populations of the house mouse *Mus musculus* L.). Genet Res 37: 17–31

Nadeau JH, Collins A, Klein J (1982) Organization and evolution of the mammalian genome. I. Polymorphism of *H-2* linked loci. Genetics 102: 583–598

Nagy ZA, Kusnierczyk P, Klein J (1981) Terminal differentiation of T cells specific for mutant H-2K antigens. Conversion of Lyt-1, 2 cells into Lyt-2 but not Lyt-1 cells, in vitro. Eur J Immunol 11: 167–172

Nagy ZA, Baxevanis CN, Ishii N, Klein J (1981) Ia antigens as restriction molecules in Ir-gene controlled T-cell proliferation. Immunol Rev 60: 59–83

Nagy ZA, Baxevanis CN, Klein J (1982) Haplotypespecific suppression of T cell response to lactate dehydrogenase B in (responder × nonresponder) F_1 mice. J Immunol 129: 2608–2611

Nagy ZA, Baxevanis CN, Klein J (1983) Cross-reactivity of suppressor T cells specific for lactate dehydrogenase B and IgG2a myeloma protein. J Immunol 130: 1498–1499

Nagy ZA, Ikezawa Z, Marusić M, Baxevanis CN, Ishii N, Klein J (1983) Ia antigens as restriction molecules in *Ir*-gene controlled T-cell proliferation. In: Pierce CW, Cullen SE, Kapp JA (eds) *Ir* genes, past, present, and future. Humana, Clifton, pp 425–431

Nagy ZA, Servis C, Walden P, Klein J, Goldberg E (1985) Fine specificity analysis of lactate dehydrogenase B-specific proliferating T cell clones: Implications for the mechanisms of alloreactivity. Eur J Immunol 15: 814–821

Nagy ZA, Servis C, Klein J (1987) Immunogenicity of lactate dehydrogenase B for helper and suppressor cells. In: Sercarz EE, Berzofsky JA (eds) Immunogenicity of protein antigens: repertoire and regulation, vol 2. CRC, Boca Raton, pp 91–96

Nauciel C, Ronco E, Guenet L-L, Pla M (1988) Role of H-2 and non-H-2 genes in control of bacterial clearance from the spleen in Salmonella typhimurium-infected mice. Infect Immun 56: 2407–2411

Neauport-Sautes C, Morello D, Lemonnier F, Demant P (1977) Relationships between private and public specificities controlled by the H-2D region. Transplant Proc 9: 653–655

Neauport-Sautes C, Morello D, Freed JH, Nathenson SG, Demant P (1977) The private specificity H-2.4 and the public specificity H-2.28 of the D region are expressed on two independent polypeptide chains. Eur J Immunol 8: 511–515

Neauport-Sautes C, Joskowitz M, Demant P (1978) Molecular relationship between private and public H-2 specificities. Further evidence for two separate loci (H-2D and H-2L) in the D region of the H-2 complex. Immunogenetics 6: 513–527

Neefjes JJ, Breur-Vriesendorp BS, van Seventer GA, Iványi P, Ploegh HL (1986) An improved method for the analysis of HLA class-I antigens. Definition of new HLA class-I subtypes. Hum Immunol 16: 169–181

Nelson-Rees WA, Klement V, Peterson WD Jr, Weaver JV (1973) Comparative study of two RD-114 virus-indicator cell lines. KC and KB. JNCI 50: 1129–1135

Nesbitt MN, Skamene E (1984) Recombinant inbred mouse strains derived from A/J and C57BL/6J: A tool for the study of genetic mechanisms in host resistance to infection and malignancy. J Leukocyte Biol 36: 357–364

Nethanel T, Kinsky R, Moav N, Brown R, Ran M, Witz IP (1981) Separation of tumor-seeking small lymphocytes and tumor cells using percoll velocity gradients. J Immunol Methods 41: 43–56

Newbold CI, Schryer M, Boyle DB, McBride JS, McLean A, Wilson RJM, Brown KN (1984) A possible molecular basis for strain specific immunity to malaria. Mol Biochem Parasitol 11: 337–347

Newell AL, Malkovský M, Orr D, Taylor-Robinson D, Dalgleish AG (1987) Antigen test versus reverse transcriptase assay for detecting HIV. Lancet 2: 1146–1147

Neu N, Hála K, Wick G (1984) "Natural" chicken antibodies to red blood cells are mainly directed against the B-G antigen, and their occurence is independent of spontaneous autoimmune thyroiditis. Immunogenetics 19: 269–277

Neu N, Hála K, Dietrich H, Wick G (1985) Spontaneous autoimmune thyroiditis in obese strain chickens: A genetic analysis of target organ abnormalities. Clin Immunol Immunopathol 37: 397–405

Neu N, Hála K, Dietrich H, Wick G (1986) The genetic background of spontaneous autoimmune thyroiditis in the obese strain (OS) of chicken studied in hybrids with an inbred line. Int Arch Allergy Appl Immunol 80: 168-173

Neufeld E, Ritte U, Figueroa F, Klein J (1986) Low H-2 polymorphism in some Israeli wild mouse populations. Immunogenetics 24: 374-380

Nizetić D, Figueroa F, Klein J (1984) Evolutionary relationships between the *t* and *H-2* haplotypes in the house mouse. Immunogenetics 19: 311-320

Nizetić D, Figueroa F, Müller HJ, Arden B, Nevo E, Klein J (1984) Major histocompatibility complex of the mole-rat. I. Serological and biochemical analysis. Immunogenetics 20: 443-451

Nizetić D, Figueroa F, Nevo E, Klein J (1985) Major histocompatibility complex of the mole-rat. II. Restriction fragment polymorphism. Immunogenetics 22: 55-67

Nizetić D, Figueroa F, Dembić Z, Nevo E, Klein J (1987) Major histocompatibility complex gene organization in the mole rat *Spalax ehrenbergi:* Evidence for transfer of function between class II genes. Proc Natl Acad Sci USA 84: 5828-5832

Noumoff JS, Simon D, Heyner S, Farber M, Haydock SW, Pritchard ML (1988) Cytogenetics of an endometrial adenocarcinoma cell line and its implications. Gynecol Oncol (in press)

Oliver RTD, Pillai A, Klouda PT, Lawler SD (1977) HLA linked resistance factors and survival in acute myelogenous leukaemia. Cancer 39: 2337-2341

Ollier W, Doyle P, Alonso A, Awad J, Williams E, Gill D, Welch S, et al. (1985) HLA polymorphism in Saudi Arabs. Tissue Antigens 25: 87-95

Oomen LCJM, Demant P, Hart AAM, Emmelot P (1983) Multiple genes in the H-2 complex affect differently the number and growth rate of transplacentally induced lung tumours in mice. Int J Cancer 31: 447-454

Oomen LCJM, van der Valk MA, Hart AAM, Demant P, Emmelot P (1988) Influence of mouse major histocompatibility complex (H-2) on N-ethyl-N-nitrosourea-induced tumor formation in various organs. Cancer Res 48: 6634-6641

Opolski A, Kievits F, Iványi P (1986) Polymorphic and autoreactive monoclonal H-2-specific antibody isolated after injections of syngeneic virus-coated lymphocytes. Immunogenetics 24: 402-408

Opolski A, Degos L, Pla M (1988) Spendai virus infection of tumor cells increases the induction of autoreactive H-2-specific antibodies in syngeneic recipients. In: Iványi P (ed) MHC specific antibodies induced by foreign antigens. Springer, Berlin Heidelberg New York, pp 66-71

Oppenheim S, Kinsky RG, Voisin GA (1977) Immune status of mice tolerant of living cells. III. Presence and evolution of cells cytotoxic to the tolerated strain. Transplantation 24: 274-281

O'Toole C, Stejskal V, Perlmann P, Karlsson M (1974) Lymphoid cells mediating tumor specific cytotoxicity to carcinoma of the urinary bladder. Separation of the effector population using a surface marker. J Exp Med 139: 457

Ottenhoff THM, Klatser PR, Iványi J, Elferink DG, de Wit MYL, de Vries RRP (1986) *Mycobacterium leprae*-specific protein antigens defined by cloned human helper T cells. Nature 319: 66-68

Oudshoorn-Snoék M, Demant P (1983) Altered expression of MHC products on AKR lymphoma cells. Transplant Proc 15: 2104-2106

Oudshoorn-Snoék M, Demant P (1986) Correlation between quantitative expression of H-2K, H-2D and MuLV antigens on spontaneous AKR lymphomas. Int J Cancer 37: 303-310

Oudshoorn-Snoék M, Demant P (1987) Antigens of the Qa-2 family exhibit differential cellular expression. Transplant Proc 19: 864-865

Oudshoorn-Snoék M, Demant P (1988) Interaction of Qa-region with the beta-2-microglobulin and with non-Qa genes in determination of Qa phenotype. In: Iványi P (ed) MHC + X: Complex formation and antibody induction. Springer, Berlin Heidelberg New York, pp 134-137

Oudshoorn-Snoék M, Iványi D, Demant P (1981) Qualitative and quantitative aspects of anti-H-2Ld sera. Transplantation 32: 128-136

Oudshoorn-Snoék M, Demant P, Mellor AL, Flavell RA (1983) Antigenic characterization of products of cloned H-2b genes. Transplant Proc 15: 2027-2032

Oudshoorn-Snoék M, Mellor AL, Flavell RA, Demant P (1984) A new determinant Qa-m208, detected on T lymphocytes and transfected L cells by a Kb specific monoclonal antibody. Immunogenetics 19: 461-474

Paschall VL, Brown LA, Lawrence EC, Karol RA, Lotzová E, Brown BS, Shearer WT (1984) Immunoregulation in an isolated 12-year-old boy with congenital severe combined immunodeficiency. Pediat Res 18: 723-728

Passmore HC, Kubo JK, Singh SK, Klein J (1980) The histocompatibility-2 system in mice. XI. Ss and Slp properties of wild-derived *H-2* haplotypes. Immunogenetics 11: 397-405

Patchen M, Lotzová E (1982) Depression of B cell colony-formation by immunomodulating agent glucan. Biomed Pharmacother 36: 316-319

Patchen M, Lotzová E (1980) Modulation of murine hemopoiesis by glucan. Exp Hematol 8: 409-422

Patchen M, Lotzová E (1981) The role of macrophages and T-lymphocytes in glucan-mediated alteration of murine hemopoiesis. Biomedicine 34: 71-77

Paty D, Mervart H, Campling B, Rand C, Stiller C (1974) HLA frequencies in patients with multiple sclerosis. J Can Sci Neurol 1: 211-213

Paul P, Lepage V, Sayagh B, Metzger JJ, Pla M, Boumsell L, Douay C, et al. (1985) Serological expression after sequential double transfection with purified HLA-11 gene of mouse fibroblasts carrying human beta-2 microglobulin. Immunogenetics 22: 1-8

Pazderka F, Longenecker BM, Law GRJ, Ruth RF (1975) The major histocompatibility complex of the chicken. Immunogenetics 2: 101

Pazderka F, Longenecker BM, Law GRJ, Stone HA, Ruth RF (1975) Histocompatibility of chicken populations selected for resistance to Marek's disease. Immunogenetics 2: 93

Pazderka F, Dossetor JB, Falk J, Mervart H, Reeve CE, Sargent A, Singal DP, Stiller CR (1977) Canadian regional report. In: Bodmer WF, Batchelor JR, Bodmer JG, Festenstein H, Morris PJ (eds) Histocompatibility testing 1977. Munksgaard, Copenhagen, pp 413-422

Pazderka F, Dossetor JB, Falk JM, Mervart M, Reeve CE, Sargent A, Singal DP, Stiller C (1978) Joint report of the Canadian region to the 7th International Histocompatibility Workshop. In: Bodmer WF, Batchelor JR, Bodmer JC, Festenstein H, Morris PJ (eds) Histocompatibility testing 1977. Munksgaard, Copenhagen, p 413

Pazderka F, Dossetor JB (1980) "BW45". In: Terasaki PI (ed) Histocompatibility testing 1980. UCLA Tissue Typing Laboratory, Los Angeles, p 402

Pazderka F, Saidman S, Schlaut JW, Dossetor JB (1980) Heterogeneity of DRW antigens. In: Terasaki PI (ed) Histocompatibility testing 1980. UCLA Tissue Typing Laboratory, Los Angeles, p 914

Pazderka F, Angeles A, Kovithavongs T, Dossetor JB (1983) Induction of suppressor cells in autologous mixed lymphocyte culture (AMLC) in humans. Cell Immunol 75: 122

Pazderka F, Pazderka V, Kovithavongs T, Dossetor JB (1985) T lymphocyte subsets in renal allograft recipients. In: Chatterjee SN (ed) Monoclonal antibodies: diagnostic and therapeutic use in tumor and transplantation. PSG, Littleton, p 1

Pazderka F, Olson L, Dossetor JB (1988) Alloreactive T4 cell clone recognizing HLA class II antigen in linkage disequilibrium with HLA-A1. In: Dupont B, Barletta M, Flomenberg N (eds) Histocompatibility testing 1987. Springer, Berlin Heidelberg New York

Peck AB, Klein J, Wigzell H (1981) The mouse primed lymphocyte typing (mPLT) test. II. Detection of variant H-2K and D molecules in the typing analysis of the class I-associated lymphocyte-stimulating (LS) determinants, using the B10.W lines. Scand J Immunol 13: 453-460

Peck AB, Klein J, Wigzell H (1980) The mouse primed lymphocyte typing (mPLT) test. III. Dissociation of T lymphocyte-stimulating (LS) determinants and antibody-defined specificities of the I region-associated Ia antigens. J Immunol 125: 1078-1086

Pelletier M, Forget A, Bourassa D, Gros P, Skamene E (1982) Immunopathology of BCG infection in genetically-resistant and susceptible mouse strains. J Immunol 129: 2179-2185

Pelletier M, Forget A, Bourassa D, Skamene E (1984) Histological and immunopathological studies of delayed hypersensitivity reaction to tuberculin in mice. Infect Immun 46: 873-875

Pelton BK, North M, Palmer RG, Hylton W, Smith-Burchnell C, Sinclair AL, Malkovský M, et al. (1988) A search for retrovirus infection in systemic lupis and rheumatoid arthritis. Ann Rheum Dis 47: 206-209

Pentycross CR, Klouda PT, Lawler SD (1972) The HL-A system and the mixed lymphocyte reaction. Lancet 1: 95

Pentycross CR, Klouda PT, Lawler SD (1972) HL-A non-identical individuals with mutually negative mixed lymphocyte reaction. Transplantation 14: 657-658

Perlman P, Perlman H, Biberfeld P, Stejskal V (1970) Cytotoxicity of activated lymphocytes, mechanism of activation and target cell lysis. In: Miescher PA (ed) 6th International symposium on immunopathology. Schwabe, Basel, p 259

Perlmann P, Holm G, Stejskal V (1973) Cell-mediated cytotoxicity in vitro. Target cell recognition and effector cell requirements. Transplant Proc 4: 1625

Peterson AR, Klement V (1985) Oncogenic transformation of C3H/10T1/2 cells: Methods and mechanisms. Carcinogenesis 9: 337–354

Phillips JT, Duncan WR, Klein J, Streilein JW (1979) Immunochemical detection of hamster class II Mhc homologues by murine anti-Ia^k sera. Immunogenetics 9: 477–486

Phillips NC, Skamene E, Chedid L (1988) Correction of defective tumoricidal activity of macrophages from A/J mice by liposomal immunomodulators. Immunopharmacology 15: 1–10

Pietrangeli CE, Edelson PJ, Skamene E, Kongshavn PAL (1981) Measurement of 5' nucleotidase as index of macrophage stimulation in Listeriosis. Infect Immun 32: 1206

Pietrangeli C, Pang KC, Skamene E, Kongshavn PAL (1983) Characteristics of mononuclear phagocytes mediating antilisterial resistance in splenectomized mice. Infect Immun 39: 742–749

Pink JRL, Iványi J (1975) Close linkage between genes coding for allotypic markers on chicken IgG and IgM. Eur J Immunol 5: 506–507

Pippard MJ, Dalgleish A, Gibson P, Malkovský M, Webster ADB (1986) Acquired immunodeficiency with disseminated cryptococcosis. Arch Dis Child 61: 289–291

Pla M (1985) Le modèle murin: H-2. In: Dausset J, Pla M (eds) HLA, complexe majeur d'histocompatibilité de l'homme. Flammarion, Paris

Pla M (1989) Le modèle murin: H-2. In: Dausset J, Pla M (eds) HLA, complexe majeur d'histocompatibilité de l'homme. Flammarion, Paris

Pla M, Colombani JM (1979) Etudes des déterminants responsables de la stimulation lors de la réaction lymphocytaire mixte secondaire (MLR-II). C R Acad Sci Paris 289: 477–480

Pla M, Colombani JM (1980) Réactions lymphocytaires mictes primaire et secondaire chez la souris. Ann Inst Pasteur Immunol 131: 3–29

Pla M, Condamine H (1984) Recombination between two mouse t haplotype (t^{w12} tf and t^{Lub-1}): Mapping of the H-2 complex relative to centromere and tufted (tf) locus. Immunogenetics 20: 277–285

Pla M, Iványi P (1986) Cross-reactions of class-II histocompatibility antigens of different species. In: Solheim BG, Moller E, Ferrone S (eds) HLA class-II antigens. Springer, Berlin Heidelberg New York, pp 128–153

Pla M, Zakany J, Fachet J (1976) H-2 influence on corticosteroid effects on thymus cells. Folia Biol Praha 22: 49–50

Pla M, Birnbaum D, Guimezanes A, Colombani M, Colombani J (1981) Correlation between serologic and cellular methods for the definition of Ia specificities. Transplant Proc 13: 1051–1054

Pla M, Colombani M, Colombani J (1981) Inhibition of secondary mouse mixed lymphocyte reaction by anti-Ia sera. Immunogenetics 12: 285–295

Pla M, Rocca A, Guilbert G, Reboul M, Dastot H, Colombani J, Avrameas S (1986) Anti-H-2 monoclonal antibody recognizes self cytoskeletal structures. Immunogenetics 24: 122–124

Pla M, Rocca A, Gillet D, Villette J-M, Fiet J, Degos L (1988) Involvement of the H-2 complex in steroid metabolism. In: David SC (ed) H-2 antigens. Genes, molecules, function. Plenum, New York

Pla M, Opolski A, Rocca A, Degos L (1988) Immunization with the fibroblasts transfected with a cloned retroviral DNA induces H-2-specific antibodies in syngeneic recipients. In: Iványi P (ed) MHC specific antibodies induced by foreign antigen. Springer, Berlin Heidelberg New York, pp 61–65

Pollock RE, Lotzová E (1987) Surgical stress related suppression of NK activity: A possible role in tumor metastasis. Nat Immun Cell Growth Regul 6: 269–275

Pollock RE, Lotzová E, Stanford SD, Romsdahl MM (1987) Effect of surgical stress on murine natural killer cell cytotoxicity. J Immunol 138: 171–178

Potter M, O'Brien A, Skamene E, Gros P, Forget A, Kongshavn PAL, Wax JS (1983) A BALB/c congenic strain of mice that carries a genetic locus (Ity^r) controlling resistance to intracellular parasites. Infect Immun 40: 1234–1235

Powell PC, Hála K, Böck G, Dietrich H, Wick G (1987) Immune mechanisms in Rous sarcoma regression. In: Avian immunology. Liss, New York, pp 207–218

Powell PC, Hála K, Wick G (1987) Aberrant expression of Ia-like antigens on tumor cells of regressing but not of progressing Rous sarcomas. Eur J Immunol 17: 723–726

Praputpittaya K, Iványi J (1985) Detection of an antigen (MY4) common to *M. tuberculosis* and *M. leprae* by 'tandem' immunoassay. J Immunol Methods 79: 149-157

Praputpittaya K, Iványi J (1987) Stimulation by anti-idiotype antibody of murine T cell responses to the 38kD antigen of *M. tuberculosis*. Clin Exp Immunol 70: 307-315

Praputpittaya K, Iványi J (1987) Study of idiotypes expressed by monoclonal antibodies to the 38kD and 12kD antigens of *M. leprae*. Clin Exp Immunol 70: 298-306

Prasad N, Lotzová E, Thornby JI, Taber K (1989) MR imaging does not inhibit human NK cell cytotoxicity or stimulation of NK cells with interleukin-2. American J Roentgenology (in press)

Prasad N, Lotzová E, Thorneby JE, Madewell JE, Ford J, Bushong SC (1987) Effects of magnetic resonance imaging on murine natural killer cell cytotoxicity. AJR 148: 415-417

Price DA, Klouda PT, Harris R (1978) HLA and congenital adrenal hyperplasia linkage confirmed. Lancet 1: 930-931

Pruss RM, Herschman HR, Klement V (1978) 3T3 variant lacking receptors for epidermal growth factor are susceptible to transformation by Kirsten sarcoma virus. Nature 274: 272-274

Rakusanova T, Ben Porat T, Himeno M, Kaplan AS (1971) Early functions of the genome of herpesvirus. I. Characterization of the RNA synthesized in cycloheximide treated, infected cells. Virology 46: 877-899

Rakusanova T, Ben Porat T, Kaplan AS (1972) Effect of herpesvirus infection on the synthesis of cell specific RNA. Virology 49: 537-548

Rakusanova T, Kaplan JC, Smales WP, Black PH (1976) Excision of viral DNA from host cell DNA after induction of SV40 transformed hamster cells. J Virol 19: 279-285

Rakusanova T, Smales WP, Kaplan JC, Black PH (1978) Replication of simian virus 40 in SV40-transformed hamster kidney cells induced by mitomycin C or Co60-irradiation. Virology 88: 300-313

Rakusanova T, Smales WP, Kaplan JC, Black PH (1979) Effect of mitomycin C and Co60-irradiation on the replication of SV40 in cell lines of varying permissivity for SV40 replication. J Gen Virol 43: 235-239

Rakusanova TA, Juneja HS, Fleischmann WR Jr (1989) Inhibition of hemopoietic colony formation by human cytomegalovirus in vitro. J Infect Dis (in press)

Rammensee H-G, Klein J (1983) Complexity of the histocompatibility-3 region in the mouse. J Immunol 130: 2926-2929

Rammensee H-G, Klein J (1983) Polymorphism of minor histocompatibility genes in wild mice. Immunogenetics 17: 637-647

Rammensee H-G, Nagy ZA, Klein J (1983) Characterization of "veto" cells that cause nonresponsiveness to minor histocompatibility antigens. In: Pierce CW, Cullen SE, Kapp JA (eds) *Ir* genes, past, present, and future. Humana, Clifton, pp 383-387

Rammensee H-G, Juretić A, Nagy ZA, Klein J (1984) Class I restricted interaction between suppressor and cytolytic cells in the response to minor histocompatibility antigens. J Immunol 132: 668-672

Rao PN, Wang Y, Lotzová E, Khan AA, Rao SP, Stephens LC (1985) Antitumor effects of gossypol in mouse mammary adenocarcinoma 755. Cancer Chemother Pharmacol 14: 20-25

Ratcliffe MJH, Iványi J (1979) Allotype suppression in the chicken. I. Generation of chronic suppression in heterozygous but not in homozygous chickens. Eur J Immunol 9: 847-852

Ratcliffe MJH, Iványi J (1979) Allelic exclusion of surface IgM allotypes on spleen and bursal B cells in the chicken. Immunogenetics 9: 149-156

Ratcliffe MJH, Iványi J (1981) Allotype suppression in the chicken. II. Suppression in homozygous chickens with anti-allotype antibody and allotype-disparate B cells. Eur J Immunol 11: 296-300

Ratcliffe MJH, Iványi J (1981) Allotype suppression in the chicken. III. Analysis of the recovery from suppression by neonatally injected or maternal antibodies. Eur J Immunol 11: 301-306

Ratcliffe MJH, Iványi J (1981) Allotype suppression in the chicken. IV. Deletion of B cells and lack of suppressor cells during chronic suppression. Eur J Immunol 11: 307-310

Rees ADM, Praputpittaya K, Scoging A, Dobson N, Iványi J, Young D, Lamb JR (1987) T cell activation by anti-idiotypic antibody: evidence for the internal image. Immunology 60: 389-393

Rees ADM, Scoging A, Dobson N, Praputpittaya K, Young D, Iványi J, Lamb JR (1987) T cell activation by anti-idiotypic antibody: mechanism of interaction with antigen reactive T cells. Eur J Immunol 17: 197-201

Reichert RA, Jerabék L, Butcher EC, Weissman IL (1986) Ontogeny of lymphocyte homing receptor expression in the mouse thymus. J Immunol 136: 3535

Reynolds CP, Tomayko MM, Donner L, Helson L, Seeger RC, Triche TJ, Brodeur GM (1988) Biological classification of cell lines derived from human extracranial neural tumors. Prog Clin Biol Res 271: 291–306

Rhodes J, Iványi J, Cozens P (1986) Antigen presentation by human monocytes: Effects of modifying monocyte MHC class II antigen expression by means of recombinant interferons and hydrocortisone. Eur J Immunol 16: 370–375

Rittner C, Giles CM, Roos MH, Demant P, Mollenhauer E (1984) Genetics of human C4 polymorphism: Detection and segregation of rare and duplicated haplotypes. Immunogenetics 19: 321–333

Rocca A, Degos L, Pla M (1988) Immunization with fibroblasts expressing human β2-microglobulin induces H-2-specific antibodies in syngeneic recipients. In: Iványi P (ed) MHC specific antibodies induced by foreign antigens. Springer, Berlin Heidelberg New York, pp 72–76

Roitt IM, Male DK, Guarnotta G, de Carvalho LP, Cooke A, Hay FC, Lydyard PM, et al. (1981) Idiotypic networks and their possible exploitation for manipulation of the immune response. Lancet 1: 1041–1045

Röpcke E, Sluyser M, Demant P (1987) H-2 and the hormonal factors in mammary tumorigenesis. In: Davis C (ed) H-2 antigens: Genes, molecules, and functions. Plenum, New York, pp 681–690

Roos MH, Demant P (1982) Murine complement factor B (BF): Sexual dimorphism and H-2-linked polymorphism. Immunogenetics 15: 23–30

Roos MH, Mollenhauer E, Demant P, Rittner C (1982) A molecular basis for the two locus model of human complement component C4. Nature 298: 854–856

Roos MH, Giles CM, Demant P, Mollenhauer E, Rittner C (1984) Rodgers (Rg) and Chido (Ch) determinants on human C4: Characterization of two C4B5 subtypes, one of which contains Rg and Ch determinants. J Immunol 133 (5): 2634–2540

Roy-Burman P, Klement V (1975) Derivation of mouse sarcoma virus (Kirsten) by acquisition of genes from heterologous host. J Gen Virol 28: 193–198

Roy-Burman P, Dougherty M, Pal BK, Charman HP, Klement V, Gardner MB (1976) Assay for type-C virus in mouse sera based on particulate reverse transcriptase activity. J Virol 19: 1107–1110

Sackstein R, Roos MH, Demant P, Colten HR (1984) Subdivision of the S region of the mouse major histocompatibility complex by identification of genomic polymorphism of the class III genes. Immunogenetics 20: 321–330

Sadarangani C, Kongshavn PAL, Skamene E (1980) Radiation effect on anti-listerial response in genetically resistant and sensitive mice. Infect Immun 28: 381–386

Samaan A, Gillet D, Chopin M, Degos L, Pla M (1989) Mouse cytotoxic cells can recognize HLA-B27 antigen without H-2 restriction. Immunogenetics (in press)

Sansom DM, Bidwell JL, Klouda PT, Maddison PJ (1986) Restriction fragment length polymorphism in Felty's syndrome. Dis Markers 4: 185–189

Sansom DM, Bidwell JL, Maddison PJ, Campion E, Klouda PT, Bradley BA (1987) HLA DQα and DQβ restriction fragment length polymorphisms associated with Felty's syndrome and Dr4 positive rheumatoid arthritis. Hum Immunol 19: 267–278

Sansom DM, Bidwell JL, Klouda PT, Amin SN, Bradley BA, Maddison PJ (1988) HLA DQ polymorphism in rheumatoid arthritis. Lancet 1: 58–59

Sajid MA, Cerny J, McAlack RF, Friedman H (1971) "High dose" immunologic tolerance to *E. coli* lipopolysaccharide assessed by bacteriolytic and hemolytic plaque assay. Experientia 27: 454

Sajid MA, McAlack RF, Cerny J, Friedman H (1971) Antibody plaque response of mice injected as neonates with high and low doses of bacterial antigen with distinct determinants. J Immunol 106. 1301

Sarmay G, Sanderson A, Iványi J (1979) Modulation of Fc receptors on human peripheral blood lymphocytes by antisera against β^2 microglobulin, Ia or immunoglobulin. Immunology 36: 339–345

Sarmay G, Iványi J, Gergely J (1980) The involvement of a preformed cytoplasmic receptor pool in the reexpression of Fc receptors following their interaction with various antibodies. Cell Immunol 56: 452–464

Savary CA, Lotzová E (1986) Phylogeny and ontogeny of NK cells. In: Lotzová E, Herberman RB (eds) Immunobiology of natural killer cells, vol 1. CRC, Boca Raton, pp 45–61

Savary CA, Lotzová E (1978) Suppression of natural killer cell cytotoxicity by splenocytes from Corynebacterium parvum-injected, bone marrow-tolerant and infant mice. J Immunol 120: 239-243

Savary CA, Lotzová E (1987) Mechanism of decline of NK cell activity in *Corynebacterium parvum* treated mice: Inhibition by erythroblasts and Thyl.2 lymphocytes. JNCI 79: 533-541

Savary CA, Lotzová E (1988) Natural killer cell-mediated inhibition of growth of myeloid and lymphoid clonogenic leukemias. Exp Hematol (in press)

Savary CA, Lotzová E (1988) Down-regulation of human bone marrow cells and their progenitors by IL-2 activated lymphocytes. In: Lotzová E (ed) Role interleukin-2 activated killer cells in cancer. CRC, Boca Raton (in press)

Savary CA, Lotzová E, Gray KN, Jardine J (1985) Natural killer cell-mediated antitumor reactivity of Rhesus monkeys. Nat Immun Cell Growth Regul 4: 328-339

Savary CA, Lotzová E, Klostergaard J (1989) Interleukin-2-activated large granular lymphocytes: tumoricidal efficiency and mechanism. Immunol Letters (in press)

Savary CA, Phillips JH, Lotzová E (1979) Inhibition of murine natural killer cell-mediated cytotoxicity by pretreatment with ammonium chloride. J Immunol Methods 25: 1389-1392

Schauenstein K, Krömer G, Böck G, Rossi K, Hála K, Wick G (1987) T cell hyperreactivity in obese strain (OS) chickens. Different mechanisms operative in spleen and peripheral blood lymphocyte activation. Immunobiologic 175: 226-235

Schöpfer R, Figueroa F, Nizetic D, Nevo E, Klein J (1987) Evolutionary diversification of class II P loci in the Mhc of the mole-rat, *Spalax ehrenbergi*. Mol Biol Evol 4: 287-299

Schurr E, Skamene E, Nesbitt M, Hynes R, Gros P (1988) Identification of a linkage group including the Bcg gene by restriction fragment length polymorphism analysis. In: Mock B, Potter M (eds) Immunoregulatory genes workshop. Springer, Berlin Heidelberg New York, pp 310-315

Schuster JD, Rakusan TA, Chonmaitree T, Box QT (1984) Tuberculous osteitis of the skull mimicking histiocytosis X. J Pediatr 105: 269-271

Scollay R, Jacobs S, Jerabék L, Butcher E, Weissman I (1980) T cell maturation: thymocyte and thymus migrant subpopulations defined with monoclonal antibodies to MHC region antigens. J Immunol 124: 2845

Sconc R, Hála K, Wick G (1987) Relationship between the expression of class I antigen and reactivity of chicken thymocytes. Immunogenetics 26: 150-154

Sengar DPS, Mervart H, Hudson RW (1982) Histocompatibility antigens in varicocele. Tissue Antigens 19: 230-232

Sengar DPS, Mervart H, Hudson RW (1983) Histocompatibility antigens in varicocele. Tissue Antigens 21: 345-347

Sengupta U, Sinha S, Ramu G, Lamb J, Ivanyi J (1987) Suppression of delayed hypersensitivity skin reactions to tuberculin by *M.leprae* antigens in patients with lepromatous and tuberculoid leprosy. Clin Exp Immunol 68: 58-64

Servis C, Seckler R, Nagy ZA, Klein J (1986) Two adjacent epitopes on a synthetic dodecapeptide induce lactate dehydrogenase B-specific helper and suppressor T cells. Proc R Soc Lond [Biol] 228: 461-470

Shalev A, Pla M, Ginsburger-Vogel T, Echalier G, Logdberg L, Bjorck L, Colombani J, Segal S (1983) Evidence for β2-microglobulin-like and H-2-like antigenic determinants in drosophila. J Immunol 130: 297-302

Shand FL, Ivanyi J (1973) Developed γM haemolytic plaque-forming cells in chickens. Immunology 24: 759-770

Shand FL, Ivanyi J (1977) Inhibition of B cell function by Concanaval in-A-induced suppressor cells. Scand J Immunol 6: 1329-1332

Shand FL, Orme LM, Ivanyi J (1980) The induction of suppressor T cells by Concanavalin A is independent of cellular proliferation and protein synthesis. Scand J Immunol 12: 223-231

Sherr CJ, Fedele LA, Donner L, Turek L (1979) Restriction endonuclease mapping of unintergrated proviral DNA of Snyder-Thielen feline sarcoma virus: Localization of sarcoma-specific sequences. J Virol 32: 860

Shin DM, Gupta BV, Donner L, Chawla RB, Gutterman J, Blick M (1987) Aberrant oncogene expression in uncultured human sarcoma and melanoma. Anticancer Res 7: 1117-1124

Shin DM, Ince C, Shtalrid M, Lee JS, Ro JS, Gupta V, Donner L, Ferrell RE, Blick M (1988) Reduction to homozygosity of SIS/PDFG-2 locus in human mesenchymal tumors. Biochem Biophys Res Commun 155: 692-699

Short CD, Klouda PT, Smith L (1982) Campylobacter Jejuni enteritis and reactive arthritis. Ann Rheum Dis 41: 287-288

Shreffler DC, Klein J (1970) Genetic organization and gene action of the mouse H-2 region. Transplant Proc 2: 5-14

Shreffler DC, David CS, Passmore HC, Klein J (1971) Genetic organization and evolution of the mouse H-2 region: a duplication model. Transplant Proc 3: 175-179

Shreffler DC, David C, Götze D, Klein J, McDevitt H, Sachs D (1974) Genetic nomenclature for new lymphocyte antigens controlled by the *I* region of the *H-2* complex. Immunogenetics 1: 189-190

Silver LM, Hammer M, Fox H, Garrels J, Bucan M, Herrmann B, Frischauf A-M, et al. (1987) Molecular evidence for the rapid propagation of mouse t haplotypes form a single ancestral chromosome. Mol Biol Evol 4: 473-482

Simon D, Knowles BB (1986) Peripheral blood lymphocytes and a hepatocellular carcinoma cell line derived from the same patient contain common chromosome instabilities. Lab Invest 55: 657-665

Simon D, Aden DP, Knowles BB (1982) Chromosomes in human hepatoma cell lines. Int J Cancer 30: 27-33

Simon D, Searls D, Cao Y, Sun KL, Knowles BB (1985) Chromosomal site of HBV integration in a human hepatocellular carcinoma-derived cell line. Cell Genet Cytogenet 39: 116-120

Simon D, Valentine S, Heber-Katz E, Knowles BB (1988) A simple technique to distinguish rat from mouse chromosomes in T cell hybridomas. Hybridoma 7: 301-307

Simons K, Helenius A, Morein B, Balcarová J, Sharp M (1980) Development of effective subunit vaccines against enveloped viruses. In: Mizrah A (ed) New developments with human and veterinary vaccines. Liss, New York, p 217

Simonsen M, Crone M, Koch C, Hála K (1982) The MHC haplotypes of the chicken. Immunogenetics 16: 513-532

Signal DP, Blajchman MA, Joseph S, Frame B, Ludwin D, Mervart H (1988) In vitro production of antiidiotypic antibodies by EBV-transformed B-cell lines from renal transplant recipients. Hum Immunol 23: 147-148

Singer PA, Lauer W, Dembić Z, Mayer WE, Lipp J, Koch N, Hämmerling G, Dobberstein B (1984) Structure of the murine Ia-associated invariant (Ii) chain as deduced from a cDNA clone. EMBO J 3: 873-877

Singh PP, Gervais F, Skamene E, Mortensen RF (1986) Serum amyloid P-component induced enhancement of macrophage listericidal activity. Infect Immun 52: 688-694

Singh SK, Wakeland EW, Vucak I, Nagy ZA, Klein J (1981) An *H-2* haplotype possibly derived by crossingover between the $(A_\alpha A_\beta)$ duplex and the $E\beta$ locus. Immunogenetics 14: 273-281

Singh SK, Wakeland EW, Klein J (1982) Serological and biochemical characterization of class II antigens in B10.W lines. Tissue Antigens 19: 42-52

Sinha S, Sengupta U, Ramu G, Ivanyi J (1983) A serological test for leprosy based on competitive inhibition of monoclonal antibody binding to the MY2a determinant of *M.leprae*. Trans R Soc Trop Med Hyg 77: 869-871

Sinha S, Sengupta U, Ramu G, Ivanyi J (1984) Serological survey of leprosy and control subjects by a monoclonal antibody-based immunoassay. Int J Lepr 53: 33-38

Skamene E (1980) Genetic control of resistance to bacterial infections. In: Skamene E, Kongshavn PAL, Landy M (eds) Genetic control of natural resistance to infection and malignancy. Academic, New York, pp 209-214

Skamene E (1983) Genetic regulation of host resistance to bacterial infection. Rev Infect Dis 5: S823-S831

Skamene E (1985) Susceptibility of BALB/c sublines to infection with *Listeria monocytogenes*. Curr Top Microbiol Immunol 122: 128-133

Skamene E (1986) Genetic control of resistance to mycobacterial infection. Curr Top Microbiol Immunol 124: 49-66

Skamene E (1988) Genetic control of susceptibility to mycobacterial infections. Rev Infect Dis (in press)

Skamene E, Chayasirisobhon W (1977) Enhanced resistance to Listeria monocytogenes in splenectomized mice. Immunology 33: 851-858

Skamene E, Forget A (1988) Genetic basis of host resistance and susceptibility to intracellular pathogens. In: Eisenstein TK, Hanna N, Bullock W (eds) Host defenses and immunomodulation to intracellular pathogens. Plenum, New York, pp 23-37

Skamene E, Gold P (1976) Organ transplantation. In: Freedman SO, Gold P (eds) Clinical immunology. Harper and Row, London

Skamene E, Gros P (1983) Role of macrophages in resistance against infectious diseases. In: Herberman RB (ed) Clinics in immunology and allergy, vol 3. Saunders, Philadelphia, pp 539-560

Skamene E, Kongshavn PAL (1979) Phenotypic expression of genetically controlled host response to *Listeria monocytogenes*. Infect Immun 25: 345-351

Skamene E, Kongshavn PAL (1983) Cellular mechanisms of resistance to Listeria monocytogenes. Adv Exp Med Biol 162: 217-225

Skamene E, Russell PS (1971) A quantitative study of the binding of ALS to various cell types. Clin Exp Immunol 2: 195

Skamene E, Stevenson MM (1985) Genetic control of macrophage response to infection. In: Van Furth R (ed) Mononuclear phagocytes. Characteristics, physiology, and function. Nijhoff, Dordrecht, pp 647-653

Skamene E, Hawkins D, Shuster J, Gold P, Freedman SO (1972) Studies on nephrotoxic antibody in antilymphocyte globulin. Transplantation 13: 9

Skamene E, Chayasirisobhon W, Kongshavn PAL (1978) Increased phagocytic activity of splenectomized mice infected with Listeria monocytogenes. Immunology 34: 901

Skamene E, Kongshavn PAL, Sachs DH (1979) Resistance to Listeria monocytogenes in mice is genetically controlled by genes which are not linked to the H-2 complex. J Infect Dis 139: 228

Skamene E, Forget A, Gros P, Kongshavn PAL (1982) Chromosome 1 locus: A major regulator of natural resistance to intracellular pathogens. In: Herberman RB (ed) NK cells and other natural effector cells. Academic, New York, pp 313-318

Skamene E, Gros P, Forget A, Kongshavn PAL, St Charles C, Taylor BA (1982) Genetic regulation of resistance to intracellular pathogens. Nature 297: 506-510

Skamene E, Stevenson MM, Kongshavn PAL (1982) Natural cell-mediated immunity against bacteria. In: Herberman RB (ed) NK cells and other natural effector cells. Academic, New York, pp 1513-1520

Skamene E, Stevenson E, Lemieux S (1983) Murine malaria: Dissociation of natural killer (NK) cell activity and resistance to *Plasmodium chabaudi*. Parasite Immunol 5: 557-565

Skamene E, Gros P, Forget A, Patel PJ, Nesbitt MN (1984) Regulation of resistance to leprosy by chromosome 1 locus in the mouse. Immunogenetics 19: 117-124

Skamene E, James SL, Meltzer MS, Nesbitt MN (1984) Genetic control of macrophage activation for killing of extracellular targets. J Leukocyte Biol 35: 65-69

Smith RE, Ivanyi J (1980) Pathogenesis of virus-induced osteopetrosis in the chicken. J Immunol 125: 523-530

Snoek M, Demant P (1979) Analysis of the expression of H-2 and H-2-linked antigens on mammary tumor cells. Int J Cancer 24: 165-167

Snoek M, Ivanyi D, Nusse R, Demant P (1979) A new H-2.1-positive D region allele, Ddx, controlling two molecules, H-2Ddx and H-2Ldx. Immunogenetics 8: 109-125

Snoek M, Ivanyi D, Nusse R, Demant P (1979) H-2D and H-2L molecules in the products of H-2.21 positive allele Ddx. Immunogenetics 9: 310

Snyder G, Kinsky R, Voisin GA (1964) Evaluation of homograft prolongation methods. Plast Reconstr Surg 33: 110-119

Somerfield SD, Skamene E (1988) Modulation of the respiratory burst by naturally occurring substances. In: Sbarra AJ, Strauss RR (eds) The respiratory burst and its physiological significance. Plenum, New York, pp 191-201

Somerfield SD, Gervais F, Skamene E (1985) Bee venom melittin blocks neutrophil O_2-production. Inflammation 10: 175-182

Somerfield SD, Stach J-L, Mraz C, Gervais F, Skamene E (1984) Bee venom inhibits superoxide production by human neutrophils. Inflammation 8: 385-391

Spits H, Breuning MH, Iványi P, Russo C, de Vries JE (1982) In vitro isolated human cytotoxic T-lymphocyte clones detect variations in serologically defined HLA antigens. Immunogenetics 16: 503–512

Sprangrude GJ, Aihara Y, Weissman IL, Klein J (1988) The stem-cell antigens Sca-1 and Sca-2 subdivide thymic and peripheral T lymphocytes into unique subsets. J Immunol (in press)

Sprangrude GJ, Klein J, Heimfeld S, Aihara Y, Weissman IL (1988) Two monoclonal antibodies identify thymicrepopulating cells in mouse bone marrow. J Immunol (in press)

Stach J-L, Gros P, Forget A, Skamene E (1984) Phenotypic expression of genetically-controlled natural resistance to *Mycobacterium bovis* (BCG). J Immunol 132: 888–892

Stejskal V (1976) Species-specific lymphocyte target cell interaction in vitro. In: Eijsvoogel VP, Roos D, Zeijlemaker WP (eds) Proceedings of the 10th leucocyte culture conference. Academic, New York, p 659

Stejskal V (1975) Species specificity of of lymphocyte-target cell interaction in vitro. Scand J Immunol 4: 765

Stejskal V (1976) Differential cytotoxicity of activated lymphocytes on allogeneic and xenogeneic target cells. IV. Competitive inhibition of target cell lysis by addition of unlabeled cells. Scand J Immunol 5: 479

Stejskal V, Perlmann P (1976) Differential cytotoxicity of activated lymphocytes on allogeneic and xenogeneic target cells. III. Species-specificity of lymphocyte-target cell recognition in vitro. Eur J Immunol 6: 347

Stejskal V, Perlmann H, Perlmann P (1972) Cytotoxicity in vitro of lymphocytes precultivated with antibody-treated target cells. Acta Pathol Microbiol Scand [B] 80: 174

Stejskal V, Holm G, Perlmann P (1973) Differential cytotoxicity of activated lymphocytes on allogeneic and xenogeneic target cells. I. Activation by tuberculin and by staphylococcus filtrate. Cell Immunol 8: 71

Stejskal V, Lindberg S, Holm G, Perlmann P (1973) Differential cytotoxicity of activated lymphocytes on allogeneic and xenogeneic target cells. II. Activation by phytohemagglutinin. Cell Immunol 8: 82

Stejskal V, Härfast B, Holm G, Perlmann P (1974) Cytotoxicity of human lymphocytes induced by pokeweed mitogen or in mixed lymphocyte culture. Specificity and nature of effector cells. Eur J Immunol 4: 126

Stejskal V, Härfast B, Holm G, Perlmann P (1974) Cytotoxicity of human lymphocytes induced by PWM or by PHA. Differences in cytotoxic efficiency and cellular requirements. In: Lindahl-Kiessling K, Osoba D (eds) Proceedings of the 8th leucocyte culture conference. Academic, New York, p 371

Stejskal V, Havu N, Malmfors T (1982) Necrotizing vasculitis as an immunological complication in toxicity study. Arch Toxicol [Suppl] 5: 283–286

Stejskal V, Olin R, Forsbeck M (1983) Diagnosis of drug-induced occupational allergy by lymphocyte transformation test. In: Hayes AW, Schnell RC, Miya TS (eds) Developments in the science and practice of toxicology. Elsevier, Amsterdam, pp 559–562

Stejskal V, Olin R, Forsbeck M (1986) The use of lymphocyte transformation test for diagnosis of drug-induced occupational allergy. J Allergy Clin Immunol 77: 420–426

Stejskal V, Forsbeck M, Olin R (1987) Side chain-specific lymphocyte responses in workers with occupational allergy induced by penicillins. Int Arch Allergy Appl Immunol 82: 461–464

Stevenson MM, Skamene E (1985) Murine malaria: Resistance of AXB/BXA recombinant inbred mice to *Plasmodium chabaudi*. Infect Immun 47: 452–456

Stevenson MM, Skamene E (1986) Modulation of primary antibody responses to sheep erythrocytes in *Plasmodium chabaudi*-infected resistant and susceptible mouse strains. Infect Immun 54: 600–602

Stevenson MM, Kongshavn PAL, Skamene E (1980) Macrophage inflammatory responses in Listeria-resistant and Listeria-sensitive mice. In: Skamene E, Kongshavn PAL, Landy M (eds) Genetic control of natural resistance to infection and malignancy. Academic, New York, pp 565–574

Stevenson MM, Kongshavn PAL, Skamene E (1981) Genetic linkage of resistance to Listeria monocytogenes with macrophage inflammatory responses. J Immunol 127: 402–407

Stevenson MM, Lyanga JJ, Skamene E (1982) Murine malaria: Genetic control of resistance to plasmodium chabaudi. Infect Immun 38: 80–88

Stevenson MM, Kongshavn PAL, Skamene E (1983) Natural resistance to *Listeria monocytogenes* as a function of macrophage inflammatory response. Adv Exp Med Biol 162: 235-244

Stevenson MM, Gervais F, Skamene E (1984) Natural resistance to listeriosis: Role of host inflammatory responsiveness. Clin Invest Med 7: 297-301

Stevenson MM, Lemieux S, Skamene E (1984) Genetic control of resistance to murine malaria. J Cell Biochem 24: 91-102

Stevenson MM, Shenouda G, Thomson DMP, Skamene E (1985) Genetically-determined defect in chemotactic responsiveness of inflammatory macrophages from A/J mice. Prog Leukocyte Biol 3: 577-584

Stevenson MM, Skamene E, McCall RD (1986) Macrophage chemotactic response in mice is controlled by two genetic loci. Immunogenetics 23: 11-17

Stevenson MM, Skamene E (1988) Genetic control of macrophage antitumor responses. In: Heppner GH, Fulton A (eds) Macrophages and cancer. CRC, Boca Raton (in press)

Stewart CC, Skamene E, Kongshavn PAL (1980) The genetic basis of macrophage colony formation. In: Skamene E, Kongshavn PAL, Landy M (eds) Genetic control of natural resistance to infection and malignancy. Academic, New York, pp 499-509

Stewart-Phillips JC, Lough J, Skamene E (1988) Genetically determined susceptibility and resistance to diet-induced atherosclerosis in inbred strains of mice. J Lab Clin Med 112: 36-42

Stewart-Phillips JL, Lough J, Skamene E (1989) Ath-3, a new gene for artherosclerosis in the mouse. Clin Invest Med (in press)

Stiller RA, Cerny J (1976) Immunosuppression by spleen cells from Moloney leukemia. II. Studies on the mechanism of suppression and failure to detect an extracellular suppressive product. J Immunol 117: 889

Stout TS, Strickland F, Cerny J (1985) Regulation of idiotope expression. I. The effect of antigen dose on expression of certain T15 idiotopes during primary IgM response to *S.pneumoniae* R36a. J Immunol 134: 1926

Strambachova-McBride J, Micklem HS (1978) Immunosuppression in murine malaria. III. Induction of tolerance and immunological memory by soluble bovine serum albumin. Immunology 36: 607-614

Strambachova-McBride J, Micklem HS (1979) Immunosuppression in murine malaria. IV. The secondary response to bovine serum albumin. Parasite Immunol 1: 141-157

Strambachova-McBride J, McBride WH, Weir DM (1980) Are 'new' antigenic determinants exposed on aggregated bovine serum albumin? Clin Exp Immunol 39: 233-239

Streilein JW, Klein J (1977) Neonatal tolerance induction across regions of the *H-2* complex. J Immunol 119: 2147-2150

Streilein JW, Klein J (1979) Neonatal tolerance to *K* and *D* region alloantigens of the *H-2* complex: *I-J* region requirements. Transplant Proc 11: 732-735

Streilein JW, Klein J (1980) Neonatal tolerance induction across H-2 mutational disparity: Induction and specificity of tolerance. Immunogenetics 10: 113-123

Streilein JW, Klein J (1980) Neonatal tolerance of H-2 alloantigens. I. *I* region modulation of tolerogenic potential of K and D antigens. Proc R Soc Lond [Biol] 207: 461-474

Strickland F, Hamilton SL, Blalock E, Cerny J (1985) Shared idiotypy betwen phosphorylcholine-specific antibody and acetylcholinesterase detectable by a monoclonal antibody. J Immunol 134: 1053

Strickland F, Gleason J, Cerny J (1987) Re-expression of T15 idiotope on mutant immunoglobulins following the binding of another anti-idiotopic antibody. J Immunol 138: 3868

Strickland F, Gleason J, Cerny J (1987) Serologic and molecular characterization of the T15 idiotype. I. Topologic mapping of idiotopes on TEPC15. Mol Immunol 24: 631

Strickland F, Gleason J, Cerny J (1987) Serologic and molecular characterization of the T15 idiotype. II. Structural basis of independent idiotype expression on phosphorylcholine specific monoclonal antibodies. Mol Immunol 24: 637

Strickland FM, Cerny J, Currier P, Infante AJ (1988) Restricted idiotypic profile of anti-phosphorylcholine antibodies induced by helper T cell clones. Eur J Immunol (submitted)

Strickland F, Cronkhite R, Cerny J (1989) Regulation of idiotope expression. II. Effect of multiple immunizations with *S.pneumoniae* R36a or phosphocholine-keyhole limpet hemocyamin on T15 idiotopic diversity. Immunology (submitted)

Strong PN, Wood JN, Ivanyi J (1984) Characterization of monoclonal antibodies against β-Bungarotoxin and their use as structural probes for related phospholipase A_2 Enzymes and presynaptic phospholipase neurotoxins. Eur J Biochem 142: 145–151

Sturm S, Figueroa F, Klein J (1982) The relationship between *t* and *H-2* complexes in wild mice. I. The *H-2* haplotypes of 20 *t*-bearing strains. Genet Res 40: 73–88

Styrna J, Klein J (1981) Evidence for two regions in the mouse *t* complex controlling transmission ratios. Genet Res 38: 315–325

Sullivan FP, Ricardi C, Hauptfeld V, Lacy PE (1987) Effect of low temperature culture and site of transplantation on hamster islet xenograft survival (hamster to mice). Transplantation 44: 465–468

Szarfman A, Walliker D, McBride JS, Lyon JA, Quakyi IA, Carter R (1988) Allelic forms of gp195, a major blood-stage antigen of *Plasmodium falciparum*, are expressed in liver stages. J Exp Med 167: 231–236

Szymura JM, Klein J (1982) Mapping of the mouse *Upg-1* locus. Immunogenetics 16: 89–90

Szymura JM, Klein J (1981) Linkage of a gene controlling urinary pepsinogen with the major histocompatibility complex of the mouse. Immunogenetics 13: 267–271

Szymura JM, Wabl MR, Klein J (1981) Mouse mitochondrial superoxide dismutase locus is on chromosome 17. Immunogenetics 14: 231–240

Szymura JM, Taylor BA, Klein J (1982) *Upg-2:* A urinary pepsinogen variant located on chromosome 1 of the mouse. Biochem Genet 20: 1211–1219

Teele DW, Dashefsky B, Rakusan T, Klein JO (1981) Meningitis after lumbar puncture in children with bacteremia. N Engl J Med 305: 1079–1081

Tempelis CH, Hála K, Krömer G, Schauenstein K, Wick G (1988) Failure to alter neonatal transplantation tolerance by the injection of interleukin-2. Transplantation 45: 449–451

Terasaka R, Lacy PE, Hauptfeld V, Bucy RP, Davie JM (1986) The effect of cyclosporine A, low-temperature culture and Ia antibodies on prevention of rejection of rat islet allografts. Diabetes 35: 83–88

Tewarson S, Figueroa F, Klein J (1982) Identification of *D*-locus alleles in mouse B10.W lines. Immunogenetics 16: 273–278

Tewarson S, Figueroa F, Klein J (1982) Monoclonal antibodies specific for class I and class II molecules controlled by the mouse *H-2* complex. Immunogenetics 16: 373–379

Tewarson S, Zaleska-Rutczynska Z. Figueroa F, Klein J (1983) Polymorphism of Qa and Tla loci of the mouse. Tissue Antigens 22: 204–212

Thaithong S, Beale GH, Fenton B, McBride J, Rosario V, Walker A, Walliker D (1984) Clonal diversity in a single isolate of the malaria parasite *Plasmodium falciparum*. Trans R Soc Trop Med Hyg 78: 242–245

Thomson DMP, Stevenson MM, Skamene E (1985) Correlation between chemoattractant-induced leukocyte adherence inhibition, macrophage chemotaxis and macrophage inflammatory responses in vivo. Cell Immunol 94: 547–557

Torano A, Houssaint E, Ivanyi J (1984) Post-natal ontogenesis of graft-versus-host reactivity of peanut agglutinin lectin-negative thymocytes in the chicken. Cell Immunol 88: 540–544

Tosi R, Tanigaki N, Sorrentino R, van Mourik P, Iványi P (1982) Human Ia molecules carrying DC1 or BRx7 determinants are not homologous to murine I-E molecules. Immunogenetics 16: 187–199

Trentin JJ, Gallagher MT, Lotzová E (1976) Xenogeneic and genetic resistance to leukemia surveillance. In: Dupont B, Good RA (eds) Immunobiology of bone marrow transplantation. Grune and Stratton, New York, pp 137–142

Trentin JJ, Gallagher MT, Lotzová E (1976) Xenogeneic and genetic resistance to bone marrow transplantation: Relationship to leukemia surveillance. Transplant Proc 8: 463–468

Uhr JW, Vitetta E, Klein J, Poulik M, Klapper D, Capra J (1977) Structural studies of H-2 and TL alloantigens. Cold Spring Harbor Symp Quant Biol 41: 363–368

VandeBerg JL, Klein J (1978) Localization of mouse *Pgk-2* gene at the *D* end of the *H-2* complex. J Exp Zool 203: 319–324

Van de Meugheuvel W, van Seventer G, Demant P (1985) A new Tla region antigen Qa-11, similar to Qa-2 and associated with B-type beta2-microglobulin. J Immunol 134: 2507–2512

Van Mourik P, Petranyi G, Gyodi E, Lindblom B, Holmlund G, Kastelan A, van der Reijden HJ, Iványi P (1983) Alloimmune anti-Ia^k sera of individual mice detect HLA-DR-associated polymorphism on human B cells. Tissue Antigens 22: 134–141

Van Nie R, Ivanyi D, Demant P (1978) A new H-2 linked mutation, rds, causing retinal degeneration in the mouse. Tissue Antigens 12: 106–108

Van Rood JJ, van Leeuwen A, Iványi P, Cats A, Breur-Vriesendorp BS, Dekker-Saeys AJ, Kijlstra A, van Kregten E (1985) A blind trans-ocean workshop confirms Geczy's data on Dutch AS patients. Lancet 2: 943–944

Van Seventer G, Ijssel H, Breuning M, Spits H, Breur B, van Poelgeest A, Huis B, et al. (1984) Heterogeneity of HLA-B7 as detected by cytotoxic T-cell clones. In: Albert ED, Baur MP, Mayr WR (eds) Histocompatibility testing 1984. Springer, Berlin Heidelberg New York, pp 479–480

Van Seventer GA, Huis B, Melief CJM, Ivanyi P (1986) Fine specificity of human HLA-B7-specific cytotoxic T-lymphocyte clones. I. Identification of HLA-B7 subtypes and histotopes of the HLA-B7 CREG. Hum Immunol 16: 375–389

Van Seventer GA, van Lier RAW, Spits H, Ivanyi P, Melief CJM (1986) Evidence for a regulatory role of the T8 (CD8) antigen in antigenspecific and anti-T3-(CD3)-induced lytic activity of allospecific cytotoxic T-lymphocyte clones. Eur J Immunol 16: 1363–1371

Van Seventer GA, Spits H, Ijssel H, Melief CJM, Ivanyi P (1988) Differential recognition by human cytotoxic T-cell clone of human M1 fibroblasts transfected with an HLA-B7 gene (JY150) provides evidence for the existence of two different HLA-B7 genes in the cell line JY (HLA-A2,2; B7,7; Cw-,-; DR4,w6). J Immunol 141: 417–422

Van Seventer GA, van der Horst AR, Semeijn J, Lardy NM, Krom FEJM, Breur-Vriesendorp BS, de Waal LP, Ivanyi P (1988) Six subtypes of HLA-B7 defined by histotypes, epitopes and 1D-IEF. In: Histocompatibility testing 1987. Munksgaard, Copenhagen

Van Seventer GA, van der Horst AR, de Waal LP, Reekers P, Ivanyi P (1988) Public determinants of the HLA-B7 CREG defined by antibodies and T-cell clones. In: Histocompatibility testing 1987. Munksgaard, Copenhagen

Valentova V, Cerny J, Ivanyi J (1971) Immunological memory of IgM and IgG type of antibodies. I. Requirements of antigen dose of induction and time interval for development of memory. Folia Biol (Praha) 13: 100

Vega MA, Bragado R, Ivanyi P, Pelaez JI, López de Castro JA (1986) Molecular analysis of a functional subtype of HLA-B27. A possible evolutionary pathway for HLA-B27 polymorphism. J Immunol 137: 3557–3565

Vidović D, Juretić A, Nagy ZA, Klein J (1981) Lyt phenotypes of primary cytotoxic T cells generated across the A and E region of the H-2 complex. Eur J Immunol 11: 499–504

Vidović D, Simon MM, Nagy ZA, Klein J (1983) Lyt-phenotype conversion of cytotoxic T lymphocytes specific for the A and E class II major histocompatibility complex molecules. Scand J Immunol 17: 583–586

Vidović D, Klein J, Nagy ZA (1984) The role of T cell subsets in the generation of secondary cytolytic responses in vitro against class I and class II major histocompatibility complex antigens. J Immunol 132: 1113–1117

Vidović D, Klein J, Nagy ZA (1985) Recessive T cell response to poly (Glu^{50}Tyr^{50}) possibly caused by self tolerance. J Immunol 134: 3563–3568

Vinček V, Nižetić D, Golubić M, Figueroa F, Nevo E, Klein J (1987) Evolutionary expansion of Mhc class I loci in the mole-rat, *Spalax ehrenbergi*. Mol Biol Evol 4: 483–491

Vitetta ES, Klein J, Uhr JW (1974) Partial characterization of Ia antigens from lymphoid cells. Immunogenetics 1: 82–90

Vitetta ES, Capra JD, Klapper DB, Klein J, Uhr JW (1976) The partial amino acid sequence of an H-2K molecule. Proc Natl Acad Sci USA 73: 905–909

Vitetta ES, Poulik MD, Klein J, Uhr JW (1976) Beta 2-microglobulin is selectively associated with H-2 and TL alloantigens on murine lymphoid cells. J Exp Med 144: 179–192

Vitetta ES, Uhr JW, Klein J, Pazderka F, Moticka EJ, Ruth RF, Capra JE (1977) Homology of (murine) H-2 and (human) HLA with a chicken histocompatibility antigen. Nature 270: 535–536

Vlahov K, Kinsky RG, Voisin GA (1983) Modification of immune responsiveness to tumor grafts (enhancement or inhibition) induced in mouse foster mothers by allogeneic embryos. Folia Biol (Praha) 29: 419–423

Volf D, Dolejskova-Hauptfeld V, Kastelan A (1975) A thymus role in T-lymphoytopoiesis in prethymic hemopoietic tissue. Transplant Proc 7: 869–872

Volf D, Kastelan A, Dolejskova-Hauptfeld V (1976) The effect of thymectomy on the competitive potential of C57BL/6 bone marrow graft. Exp Hematol 4: 201–208

Voisin GA, Kinsky RG (1962) Protection against runting by specific treatment of newborn mice, followed by increased tolerance. In: Wolstenholme GW, Cameron MP (eds) Ciba Foundation symposium on transplantation. Churchill, London, pp 286–326

Voisin GA, Kinsky RG, Jansen FK (1966) Tranplantation immunity: localization in mouse serum of antibodies responsible for hemagglutination, cytotoxicity and enhancement. Nature 210: 138–139

Voisin GA, Kinsky RG, Maillard J (1967) Protection contre la maladie homologue par facilitation immunologique (enhancement phenomenon) induite passivement et activement. Ann Inst Pasteur 113: 521–547

Voisin GA, Kinsky RG, Maillard J (1968) Protection against homologous disease in hybrid mice by passive and active immunological enhancement-facilitation. Transplantation 6: 187–202

Voisin GA, Kinsky RG, Maillard J (1968) Réactivité immunitaire et anticorps facilitants chez des animaux tolérants aux homogreffes. Ann Inst Pasteur 115: 855–880

Voisin GA, Kinsky R, Bernard C, Chouroulinkov I (1969) Recherches d'immuno-pathologie expérimentale sur la silicose. IV. Influence des réactions d'hypersensibilité envers des antigènes exogènes et endogènes sur la fibrose silicogène. Rev Fr Etudes Clin Biol 14: 486–499

Voisin GA, Kinsky RG, Jansen F, Bernard C (1969) Biological properties of antibody classes in transplantation immune sera. Transplantation 8: 618–632

Voisin GA, Kinsky RG, Jansen F, Bernard C (1970) Biological properties of antibody classes in transplantation immune sera. Transplantation 9: 428

Voisin GA, Kinsky RG, Duc HT (1972) Immune status of mice tolerant of living cells. II. Continuous presence of facilitating (enhancing) antibodies in tolerant animals. J Exp Med 135: 1185–1203

Voisin JE, Kinsky RG, Voisin GA (1971) Protection contre le syndrome secondaire des souris irradiées au moyen de sérums immuns facilitants. CR Acad Sci [D] 273: 2180–2182

Voisin JE, Kinsky RG, Voisin GA (1972) Choc immuno-allogenique provoqué chez des souris par des sérums immuns de transplantation. CR Acad Sci [D] 275: 293–296

Voisin JE, Kinsky RG, Voisin GA (1973) Immunoallogenic shock in adult mice treated with allotransplantation immune sera. Transplantation 15: 206–210

Voisin JE, Kinsky RG, Voisin GA (1973) Protection against secondary syndrom by facilitating immune sera. Ann Immunol (Paris) 124: 75–85

Voisin JE, Kinsky RG, Voisin GA (1986) Maternal alloimmune reactions towards the conceptus and GVHR. II. Inhibition of priming by placental extracts. J Reprod Immunol 9: 85–94

Vucak I, Juretić A, Nagy ZA, Klein J (1982) Cytolytic T cells activated by H-2-controlled E molecules cross-react with A molecules. Immunogenetics 15: 519–527

Vucak I, Raska K, Nagy ZA, Klein J (1983) Frequency of responsiveness to the H-Y antigen among the B10.W lines. J Immunol 131: 325–328

Vucak I, Juretić J, Vidović D, Nagy ZA, Klein J (1984) Qa-like gened defined by CTL analysis of B10.W lines. J Immunol 132: 2232–2236

Vujanović N, Duc HT, Kinsky RG, Voisin GA (1973) Distinction morphologique des lymphocytes thymo-dépendants et thymo-indépendants de la souris. Expériences différentielles analytiques et préparatives in vitro. CR Acad Sci [D] 277: 377–380

Vujanović N, Kinsky RG, Voisin GA (1973) Persistance des différences morphologiques entre lymphocytes thymo-dépendants et thymo-indépendants de la souris après sollicitation antigénique sélective de l'une ou de l'autre population. CR Acad Sci [D] 277: 901–904

Vujanović N, Kinsky RG, Duc HT, Voisin JE, Voisin GA (1974) Morphological differences between thymus - and bone marrow - derived lymphocytes. I. A light microscopic and experimental study in unstimulated mice. Differentiation 2: 107–117

Wakeland EK, Klein J (1979) Structural comparisons of serologically identical IA- and IE encoded antigens from inbred and wild mice. Immunogenetics 9: 535–550

Wakeland EK, Klein J (1979) The histocompatibility-2 system in wild mice. VII. Serological analysis of 29 wildderived *H-2* haplotypes using antisera to inbred I-region antigens. Immunogenetics 8: 27–39

Wakeland EK, Klein J (1980) The polymorphism of I region encoded antigens among wild mice. In: Reisfeld R, Ferrone S (eds) Current trends in histocompatibility, vol 1. Plenum, New York, pp 289–305

Wakeland EK, Klein J (1983) Evidence for minor structural variations of class II genes in wild and inbred mice. J Immunol 130: 1280–1287

Walden P, Klein J (1986) Unfragmented proteins can be recognized by T lymphocytes. Ann Inst Pasteur Immunol 137 D: 297–349

Walden P, Klein J (1987) Antigen presentation without antigen processing. In: Sercarz EE, Berzofsky JA (eds) Immunogenicity of protein antigens: repertoire and regulation, vol 1. CRC, Boca Raton, pp 147–152

Walden P, Nagy ZA, Klein J (1985) Introduction of regulatory T-lymphocyte responses by liposomes carrying major histocompatibility complex molecules and foreign antigen. Nature 315: 327–329

Walden P, Nagy ZA, Klein J (1985) Antigen presentation by liposomes. In: Neth R, Gallo RC, Greaves MF, Janka G (eds) Modern trends in human leukemia VI. Springer, Berlin Heidelberg New York, pp 481–485

Walden P, Nagy ZA, Klein J (1986) Major histocompatibility complex – restricted and unrestricted activation of helper T cell lines by liposome-bound antigens. J Mol Cell Immunol 2: 191–197

Wallis M, Ivanyi J, Surowy TK (1982) Binding specificity of monoclonal antibodies towards the size variants of human growth hormone. Mol Cell Endocrinol 28: 363–372

Webster ADB, Dalgleish AG, Malkovský M, Beattie R, Patterson S, Asherson GL, North M, Weiss RA (1986) Isolation of retroviruses from two patients with "common variable" hypogammaglobulinaemia. Lancet 1: 581–583

Webster ADB, Dalgleish AG, Malkovský M, Beattie R, North M, Millrain M, Thorpe R, Mellor A (1986) Isolation of retroviruses from patients with acquired 'common variable' hypogammaglobulinaemia. In: Vossen J, Griscelli C (eds) Progress in immunodeficiency research and therapy, vol 2. Elsevier, Amsterdam, pp 467–472

Wedell J, Meier zu Eissen P, van Kalker H, Blanco A, Fiedler R, Koldovsky P, Schlipköter HW (1980) Das Anastomosenrezidiv nach anterior Resektion wegen Rektumkarzinom – ein Beitrag zur Problematik der diagnostischen CEA-Bestimmung. Zentralbl Chir 105: 833

Weissman IL, Gutman GA, Friedberg SH, Jerabek L (1976) Lymphoid tissue architecture. III. Germinal centers, T cells, and thymus dependent vs. thymus-independent antigens. In: Feldman, Globerson (eds) Immune reactivity of lymphocytes. Plenum, New York, p 229

Weissman I, Lannin D, Jerabek L, Barclay T (1973) Cellular immunity to heterologous erythrocytes in vitro. I. The role of surface adherent cells and specific mediators in an effector mechanism. Cell Immunol 7: 222

Weissman IL, McGrath MS, Pillemer E, Hollander N, Rouse RV, Jerabek L, Stevens SK, et al. (1981) Normal and neoplastic lymphocyte maturation. J Supramol Struct Cell Biol 15 (3): 303

Weissman I, Pillemer E, Kooistra D, Tsukamoto A, Jerabek L, Humphrey D, Coffman R, et al. (1982) Tumor antigen antibody interactions in murine lymphomas: possible implications for human lymphomas. In: Rosenberg SA, Kaplan HS (eds) Advances in malignant lymphomas: Etiology, immunology, pathology, treatment. Academic, New York, pp 131–153 (Third annual Bristol-Myers Symposium on cancer research, Stanford University, Nov 20–21, 1980, vol 3)

Weissman IL, Jerabek L, Greenspan S (1984) Tolerance and the H-Y antigen: male T cells, and not B cells are required to induce tolerance. Transplantation 37: 3

Werner C, Eugster M, Klouda PT, Jeannet M (1976) Some methodological studies on effector cells in the lymphocyte-dependent cytotoxic antibody assay. J Immunol Methods 10: 279–288

Werner C, Klouda PT, Correa MC, Vassalli P, Jeannet M (1977) Isolation of B and T lymphocytes by nylon fiber columns. Tissue Antigens 9: 227–229

Wernet D, Klein J (1979) Unrestricted cell-mediated lympholysis to antigens linked to the *Tla* locus in the mouse. Immunogenetics 8: 361–365

Wernet D, Klein J (1981) Cell-mediated lympholysis in H-2K/D identical congenic strain combinations. In: Cunningham D, Goldwasser E, Watson J (eds) Control of cellular division and developments, part A. Liss, New York, pp 573–577

Wettstein PJ, Bailey DW, Mobraaten LE, Klein J, Frelinger JA (1978) T lymphocyte response to H-2 mutants. I. Proliferation is dependent on Ly-1^+2^+ cells. J Exp Med 147: 1395–1404

Wettstein PJ, Bailey DW, Mobraaten LE, Klein J, Frelinger JA (1979) T lymphocyte response to H-2 mutants: Cytotoxicity effectors are Ly-1^+2^+. Proc Natl Acad Sci USA 76: 3455–3459

Wick G, Hála K (1981) Xenogeneic and allogeneic surface determinants of chicken mononuclear cells. In: The immune system, vol 2. Karger, Basel, pp 265-272

Wick G, Boyd RL, Hála K, de Carvalho L, Kofler R, Müller PU, Cole RK (1981) The obese strain (OS) of chickens with spontaneous autoimmune thyroiditis. Curr Top Microbiol Immunol 91: 109-128

Wick G, Boyd RL, Hála K, Thunhold S, Kofler H (1982) Pathogenesis of spontaneous autoimmune thyroiditis in obese strain (OS) chickens. Clin Exp Immunol 47: 1-18

Wick G, Oberhuber G, Boyd RL, Hála K (1984) Obese strain (OS) chickens with spontaneous autoimmune thyroiditis have a deficiency in thymic nurse cells. Top Aging Res Eur 3: 39-46

Wick G, Hála K, Wolf H, Boyd RL, Schauenstein K (1984) Distribution and functional analysis of B-L/Ia positive cells in the chicken: expression of B-L/Ia antigens on thyroid epithelial cells in spontaneous autoimmune thyroiditis. Mol Immunol 21: 1259-1265

Wick G, Möst J, Schauenstein K, Krömer G, Dietrich H, Ziemiecki A, Fässler R, et al. (1985) Spontaneous autoimmune thyroiditis - a birds eye view. Immunol Today 6: 359-364

Wick G, Hála K, Wolf H, Ziemiecki A, Sundick RS, Stöffler-Meilicke M, deBaets M (1986) The role of genetically-determined primary alterations of the target organ in the development of spontaneous autoimmune thyroiditis in obese strain (OS) chickens. Immunol Rev 94: 113-136

Wick G, Krömer G, Neu N, Fässler R, Ziemiecki A, Müller RG, Ginzel M, et al. (1987) The multi-factorial pathogenesis of autoimmune disease. Immunol Lett 16: 249-258

Wick G, Krömer G, Dietrich H, Schauenstein K, Hála K (1987) Genetic basis of spontaneous autoimmune thyroiditis. In: Pinchera A, Ingbar SH, McKenzie JM, Fenzi GF (eds) Thyroid autoimmunity. Plenum, New York, pp 199-206

Widmer MB, Omedei-Zorini C, Bach ML, Bach FH, Klein J (1973) Importance of different regions of H-2 for MLC stimulation. Tissue Antigens 3: 309-315

Wille GW, Koldovsky P, Schlipköter HW (1981) Einfluß von chronischer Bleibelastung auf die Entwicklung von Lungenmetastasen in einem syngenischen System. Zentralbl Bakteriol Hyg 173: 319

Wilson CF, Anand R, Clark JT, McBride JS (1987) Topography of epitopes on a polymorphic schizont antigen of *Plasmodium falciparum* determined by the binding of monoclonal antibodies in a two-site radioimmunoassay. Parasite Immunol 9: 737-746

Wolf H, Hála K, Boyd RL, Wick G (1984) MHC- and non-MHC-encoded surface antigens of chicken lymphoid cells and erythrocytes recognized by polyclonal xeno-, allo- and monoclonal antibodies. Eur J Immunol 14: 831-839

Wong SY, Pazderka F, Longenecker BM, Law GRJ, Ruth RF (1973) Immobilization of lymphocytes at surfaces by alloantibodies. Immunol Commun 1: 597

Wong SY, Longenecker BM, Pazderka F, Ruth RF (1975) Immobilization of lymphocytes at surfaces by lectins. Exp Cell Res 92: 428

Wood Jr WJ, Lotzová E (1989) Adriamycin induced resistance to NK mediated cytotoxicity. Cancer (in press)

Wright JR Jr, Lacy PE, Unanue ER, Muszynski C, Hauptfeld V (1986) — Interferon-mediated induction of Ia antigen expression on isolated murine whole islets and dispersed islet cells. Diabetes 35: 1174-1177

Wright JR Jr, Lacy PE, Unanue ER, Hauptfeld V (1987) Induction of class II MHC antigens on human and rodent islet parenchymal cells in vitro. Diabetologia 30: 441

Wright JR, Epstein HR, Hauptfeld V, Lacy PE (1988) Tumor necrosis factor enhances interferon-induced Ia antigen expression on murine islet parenchymal cells. Am J Pathol 130: 427-430

Yang E, Wong KH, Ferrone S, Mervart H (1986) Recognition of a variant of HLA-A2 with a human monospecific alloatiserum. Hum Immunol 17: 145-146

Yang YHJ, Rhim JS, Rasheed S, Klement V, Roy-Burman P (1979) Reversion of Kirsten sarcoma virus transformed human cells: Elimination of the sarcoma virus nucleotide sequences. J Gen Virol 43: 447-451

Yorston D, Whicker T, Chambers R, Klouda P, Easty D (1985) The acute phase response in acute anterior uveitis. Trans Ophthalmol Soc UK 104: 166-170

Young DB, Ivanyi J, Cox JH, Lamb JR (1987) The 65kD antigen of mycobacteria - a common bacterial protein? Immunol Today 8: 215-219

Young DB, Kent L, Rees A, Lamb JR, Ivanyi J (1986) Immunological activity of a 38 kilodalton protein purified from *Mycobacterium tuberculosis*. Infect Immun 54: 177-183

Young RA, Bloom BR, Grosskinsky CM, Ivanyi J, Thomas D, Davis RW (1985) Dissection of *Mycobacterium tuberculosis* antigens using recombinant DNA. Proc Natl Acad Ski USA 82: 2583–2587

Zaleska-Rutczynska Z, Klein J (1977) Histocompatibility-2 system in wild mice. V. Serological analysis of sixteen B10.W congenic lines. J Immunol 119: 1903–1911

Zaleska-Rutczynska Z, Figueroa F, Klein J (1983) Sixteen nes *H-2* haplotypes derived from wild mice. Immunogenetics 18: 189–203

Zaleski M, Klein J (1974) Immune response of mice to Thy-1.1 antigens: Genetic control by alleles at the *Ir-5* locus, loosely linked to the *H-2* complex. J Immunol 113: 1170–1177

Zaleski M, Klein J (1975) A new loxus *(Ir-5)* controlling immune response to Thy-1.1 (OAKR) antigen. Transplant Proc 7: 101–107

Zaleski M, Klein J (1976) Immune response of mice to Thy-1.1 antigen: Intra-*H-2* mapping of the complementary *Ir-Thy-1* loci. J Immunol 117: 814–817

Zaleski M, Klein J (1977) *H-2* mutation affecting immune response to Thy-1.1 antigen. J Exp Med 145: 1602–1606

Zaleski MB, Klein J (1978) Mapping the *Ir-Thy-1* locus to the *K* region of the *H-2* complex. In: McDevitt HO (ed) Ir genes and Ia antigens. Academic, New York, pp 44–54

Zaleski MB, Klein J (1978) Genetic control of the immune response to Thy-1 antigens. Immunol Rev 38: 120–162

Zaleski MB, Gorzynski T, Klein J (1978) Effect of H-2 incompatibility between recipient and donor on the magnitude of response to Thy-1.1 antigen. Immunogenetics 6: 553–560

Zaleski MB, Gorczynski T, Klein J (1979) The H-2 and Thy-1 alloantigens: Effect of H-2 antigens on the primary anti-Thy-1 response. Transplant Proc 11: 1359–1362

Zeromski J, Thorén-Tolling K, Bergqvist R, Stejskal V (1984) DNA binding proteins in canine sera. A method for removal of nonspecific DNA binding in the Farr assay. Vet Immunol Immunopathol 7: 169–183

Ziemiecki A, Krömer G, Müller RG, Hála K, Wick G (1988) Ev 22, a new endogenous avian leukosis virus locus found in chickens with spontaneous autoimmune thyroiditis. Arch Virol 100: 267–271

Zinkernagel R, Klein J (1977) H-2-associated specificity of virus-immune cytotoxic T cells from *H-2* mutant and wild-type mice: M523 *(H-2^{ka})* and M505 *(H-2K^{bd})* do, M504 *(H-2D^{da})* and M506 *(H-2K^{ba})* do not cross-react with wildtype H-2K or H-2D. Immunogenetics 4: 581–590

Zinkernagel R, Callahan G, Streilein J, Klein J (1977) Neonatally tolerant mice fail to react against virusinfected tolerated cells. Nature 266: 837–839

Zinkernagel RM, Althage A, Cooper S, Kreeb G, Klein PA, Sefton B, Flaherty L, et al. (1978) *Ir* genes in *H-2* regulate generation of anti-viral cytotoxic T cells. Mapping to *K* or *D* and dominance of unresponsiveness. J Exp Med 148: 592–606

Zinkernagel RM, Klein PA, Klein J (1978) Host-determined fine specificity for self-H-2 in radiation bone-marrow chimeras of standard C57BL/6 *(H-2^b)*, mutant Hz1 *H-2^{ba})*, and F$_1$ mice. Immunogenetics 7: 73–77

Zinkernagel RM, Callahan GN, Althage A, Cooper S, Streilein JW, Klein J (1978) The lymphoreticular system in triggering virus plus self-specific cytotoxic T cells: Evidence for T help. J Exp Med 147: 897–911

Zinkernagel RM, Callahan GN, Klein J, Dennert G (1978) Cytotoxic T cells learn specificity for self H-2 during differentiation in the thymus. Nature 271: 251–253

Zinkernagel RM, Callahan GN, Althage A, Cooper S, Klein P, Klein J (1978) On the thymus in the differentiation of "H-2 self-recognition" by T cells: Evidence for dual recognition? J Exp Med 147: 882–896

Zinkernagel RM, Althage A, Waterfield E, Pincetl P, Calahan G, Klein J (1979) Two stages of H-2 dependent T cell maturation. In: Le Douarin N (ed) Cell lineage, stem cells and cell determination. Elsevier, Amsterdam, pp 251–260

Appendix A: FONDATION DE FRANCE

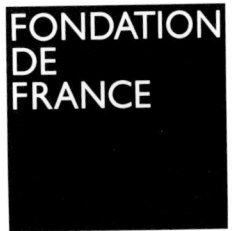

Organisme privé, reconnu d'utilité publique, sans but lucratif, la FONDATION DE FRANCE a été créée en 1969 à l'initiative du Général De Gaulle et d'André Malraux.

Au point de rencontre de la générosité des Français, des besoins et des aspirations de nos contemporains, la FONDATION DE FRANCE catalyse les solidarités en remplissant une double mission: elle collecte des fonds auprès des particuliers et des entreprises en faveur d'actions sociales, culturelles, scientifiques et offre parallèlement à toute personne ou entreprise désirant poursuivre, à titre personnel, une action d'intérêt général, la possibilité de la mener à bien sous son égide.

Elle agit selon des programmes prioritaires qu'elle définit, face à la diversité des projets qu'elle reçoit. Un effort exemplaire a été engagé en faveur de la recherche scientifique et médicale, particulièrement dans le domaine de la Leucémie.

En 1982, la FONDATION DE FRANCE et un groupe de médecins spécialistes des maladies du sang, placé sous la présidence du Professeur Jean Bernard, ont, par une volonté commune, décidé de créer un Fondation contre la Leucémie dans le but de soutenir des recherches vers des directions neuves, d'aider à l'amélioration des conditions de cure et de post-cure des malades, de favoriser de nouvelles voies de traitement des leucémies ainsi que d'encourager et susciter des échanges internationaux.

C'est dans cette perspective que le symposium "Realm of Tolerance", organisé en octobre 1988 à Ommen/Amsterdam, a retenu l'attention de la Fondation contre la Leucémie. Tout en rappelant la mémoire du Professeur Milan Hašek, cette rencontre internationale a permis de confronter les travaux actuels des chercheurs issus de cette école, dans divers domaines de l'immunologie, de la génétique et de la cancérologie.

La FONDATION DE FRANCE est heureuse de s'associer à cette action de concertation scientifique précieuse pour le développement de la Recherche.

Appendix B: Memoranda

Jean Dausset:

Il était une fois un géant, géant à tout point de vue, stature impressionnante, force de la nature, coeur d'une générosité sans limite, esprit d'une grande hauteur et largeur de vue, d'un humanisme courageux et d'un dynamisme et d'un entrain irrésistibles, en un mot plein de talent, voire de génie. Tel fut celui que nous avons connu et aimé: Milan Hašek. On n'abat pas les chênes et pourtant il fut hélas abattu.

C'est à lui que l'on doit l'extraordinaire école biologique tchèque, née de rien sinon de lui-même dans une ville dévastée par la guerre mais dont l'âme était indestructible et où brûlait toujours la flamme de la vieille et profonde culture tchèque.

J'ai eu l'insigne privilège de connaître Milan Hašek alors déjà au sommet de sa gloire, alors qu'il aurait dû, au moins, partager le Prix Nobel avec F. Macfarlane Burnet et Peter Medawar pour la grande découverte de la tolérance immunitaire. Le matériel dont il disposait pour y parvenir nous paraît aujourd'hui rudimentaire: quelques animaux, beaucoup d'imagination, d'habileté expérimentale et surtout d'intelligente interprétation.

Mais ce n'est pas tout.

Ce fut un grand chef d'école, comme trente ans après cette découverte mémorable le prouve l'hommage que tiennent à lui rendre ses multiples élèves dispersés de par le monde, mais réunis de coeur et de langue pour célébrer sa mémoire par ce colloque d'Amsterdam/Ommen et la publication de ce volume.

En effet, Milan Hašek avait su rassembler autour de lui de brillants élèves et insuffler son optimisme, sa culture intellectuelle et avait ainsi formé une pépinière d'immunogénéticiens de premier plan. Il était tout naturel que cette école s'attaquât à l'étude du complexe majeur d'histocompatibilité des différentes espèces: la poule, la souris et bien sûr l'homme.

J'ai eu la chance d'accueillir dans mon laboratoire, en 1965, au tout début de la grande aventure de l'histocompatibilité humaine Pavol et Dagmar Iványi. Mettant à profit les techniques patientes et systématiques apprises à Prague nous avons ensemble décrit le système Hu-1, devenu plus tard HL-A puis HLA.

Ainsi s'est créée la "Paris-connection" avec Prague. Il n'est, sans doute, pas déplacé de conter ici l'histoire de l'appartement de l'avenue Rapp. Dans un immeuble voué à une démolition prochaine nous avions pu loger dans des conditions très économiques mais aussi très précaires, nos amis Iványi. La démolition tarda plusieurs années au cours desquelles sont venus à tour de rôle et parfois entassés ensemble bien des scientifiques tchèques. Malgré l'exiguïté et le manque de confort ce petit appartement devint un véritable phalanstère, un foyer de liberté tchèque.

Il m'a donc été donné par ce moyen assez inattendu de connaître et d'apprécier l'amitié qui unissait dans la joie et l'enthousiasme tous ces jeunes gens. Il faut le souligner, ils n'avaient aucun contact sur le plan international et pourtant étaient tous animés d'une belle ambition qui, on le voit aujourd'hui, était pleinement justifiée.

Ces liens m'ont valu plusieurs voyages mémorables à Prague et dans les environs. J'ai pu visiter l'Institut de Génétique Expérimentale alors dirigé par Milan Hašek, constater que les laboratoires, quoique pauvrement équipés, étaient bourrés d'idées.

Quant à la ville elle-même, malgré la tristesse du décor, la pesanteur ambiante de toutes ces pierres noires, de toutes ces ruelles mal éclairées jaillissaient un humour, un dynamisme, une vitalité sans égale qui criaient le refus d'un peuple fier, aux racines intellectuelles millénaires forgées par des centaines d'années d'oppression.

Sans doute après l'humour du pauvre soldat Švejk, après le 6/4 griffonné sur tous les murs le soir du match de football contre l'équipe russe vaincue 6 à 4, après les talents artistiques dont par exemple celui du théâtre des ombres si original, après les peintures surréalistes plus ou moins clandestines, et la musique de Dvořák ou d'autres compositeurs, le travail était-il la meilleure des réponses.

L'effort le plus considérable s'est porté sur l'étude du complexe majeur d'histocompatibilité et avec Bar Harbor, Prague devint le deuxième centre mondial spécialisé dans le système H-2.

Faut-il encore ici évoquer la réunion mémorable au Château de Liblice situé près de Prague où Georges Snell présenta l'immense tableau des multiples loci et allèles supposés exister dans le complexe murin. Le tableau mesurait plusieurs mètres de haut et de large.

C'est à Peter Démant que l'on doit d'avoir établi le lien entre l'homme et la souris. Allant quelques mois plus tard en année sabbatique à Bar Harbor il y apporta la conception du complexe humain composé seulement (à l'époque) de 2 loci (HL-A et B) présentant plusieurs allèles. Grâce à l'application de ce concept à la souris, l'immense tableau de Snell se simplifia, s'ordonna lui aussi en deux séries alléliques K et D. Ce fut là, peut-être, la contribution la plus importante que le complexe HLA a offerte au complexe H-2 en témoignage de reconnaissance pour tout ce qu'il lui devait.

Par ailleurs, Pavol Iványi et son équipe ont ouvert une nouvelle vision des diverses fonctions, en particulier endocriniennes, que le complexe H-2 pouvait exercer, préfigurant ainsi la découverte ultérieure des gènes "squatters" de classes III et IV.

C'est dans ce contexte studieux et particulièrement efficace qu'éclata le coup de Prague. Nous étions au Japon, Milan Hašek, Pavol Iványi, Jan Klein et moi-même ce jour-là et je me souviens de leur émotion et surtout du douloureux débat de conscience qui fut le leur. Chacun a pris sa décision selon ses critères personnels, tous respectables.

La conséquence, chacun la connaît, ce fut l'éclatement de l'école d'immunogénétique qui fut petit à petit vidée de sa sève. Milan Hašek perdit son outil de travail et la plupart de ses élèves s'égaillèrent à travers le monde.

En nombre considérable, plus d'une vingtaine, ils sont partis et ont fondé en dehors de Tchécoslovaquie de nombreux foyers d'immunogénétique pour la plupart de la souris mais aussi de la poule, du chimpanzé, etc. ...

A ce propos la contribution de Jan Klein mérite une mention spéciale. Autre géant qui est à la base de la découverte des autres gènes du complexe H-2, ceux de classe II dont on sait toute l'importance en immunologie. A son tour il a créé une belle école dont l'éclat et l'originalité n'ont rien à envier à celle de Milan Hašek.

Marquant d'un drapeau sur une mappemonde les villes où se trouvent les élèves de Hašek on serait étonné de constater leur dispersion à Amsterdam, Paris, Miami, etc. ...

Mais cette dispersion géographique n'a pas empêché que des liens étroits persistent entre ces laboratoires, malgré les distances qui les séparent – d'ailleurs en science la distance n'existe plus. La famille Hašek est restée une famille unie. Cette réunion d'Amsterdam/Ommen et ce volume en sont la preuve.

Ses élèves demeurent unis non seulement par le souvenir mais aussi par la culture tchèque, la langue et la formation scientifique coulées dans un même moule.

J'ai eu le privilège d'être le témoin de cette aventure que certains peuvent qualifier, sans doute avec juste raison, de drame mais qui dans la difficulté, voire le malheur s'est révélée en définitive bénéfique pour la science en général, sinon pour la science tchèque.

J'ai pu admirer l'abnégation, le stoïcisme de beaucoup, l'absence de découragement, la volonté de surmonter les difficultés. En fin de compte la réussite de cette diaspora immunogénétique aura peut-être rendu plus de service à la science que si elle n'avait pas eu lieu.

Ce volume est à mon sens un hommage à la fois au grand savant, au grand chef d'école que fut Milan Hašek et aussi à l'extraordinaire rôle catalyseur de tous ses élèves dans le monde.

La dernière image que j'ai de lui, à la Gare de l'Est, quelques mois avant sa mort est celle d'un visage heureux, d'un homme satisfait d'être venu au Collège de France donner une série de leçons.

Octobre 1988　　　　　　　　Jean Dausset
　　　　　　　　　　　　　　Professeur au Collège de France
　　　　　　　　　　　　　　Président du
　　　　　　　　　　　　　　Centre d'Etude du Polymorphisme Humain
　　　　　　　　　　　　　　Lauréat du Prix Nobel

Francois Jacob:

Une stature imposante. Un visage large et ouvert sous une chevelure abondante. Un regard direct et plein d'enthousiasme. Une voix très grave. Bref une "présence" d'acteur ou de tribun. Quand on avait une fois, une seule fois, vu Milan Hašek, on ne l'oubliait plus. Je l'ai rencontré en août 1965 à Brno, lors du Symposium organisé par l'Académie des Sciences de Tchécoslovaquie pour commémorer le centième anniversaire du premier mémoire de Mendel. C'était le "printemps" là-bas. On avait restauré le jardin où Mendel cultivait ses pois et remis sur pied sa statue. Deux cents biologistes américains et deux cents biologistes soviétiques avaient, dans l'église attenant au monastère où avait jadis vécu Mendel, assisté, côte à côte, à une messe dite par un évêque qui ressemblait à Max Delbrück.

La veille au soir, une grande réception était donnée par l'Académie tchèque. La génétique mondiale discutait, mangeait, buvait avec entrain à la mémoire du Fondateur. Soudain, je m'aperçus que Lise, ma femme, avait disparu. Je la cherchai dans tous les groupes. Pas de Lise. Inquiet, je courus jusqu'à l'hôtel. Pas de Lise. Je revins à la réception pour la chercher dans tous les salons. Toujours pas de Lise. Je finis par la découvrir. Elle était tranquillement installée dans une petite pièce réservée aux Académiciens et organisateurs du Symposium. Là, au lieu de pâté et de bière, on dégustait caviar et vodka. Lise était engagée dans une longue discussion philosophique avec Milan Hašek!

Je n'ai revu Milan Hašek que vingt ans plus tard. Quelques mois avant sa mort. Il était venu à Paris faire des conférences à l'invitation de Jean Dausset. Il avait changé. Mais il avait toujours ce port imposant et cette voix très grave. Toujours la même présence.

Milan Hašek a eu de nombreux disciples. Beaucoup d'entre eux sont devenus des chercheurs et professeurs renommés dans les pays les plus variés. Il faut les remercier d'avoir organisé un Colloque et publié ce livre à la mémoire de celui qui fut un des plus grands biologistes de ce siècle.

Octobre 1988

François Jacob
Professeur au Collège de France
et à l'Institut Pasteur
Lauréat du Prix Nobel

Name and Subject Index

abl prot-oncogene 226
acquired tolerance 14, 38
adenocarcinoma, endometrium 226
-, intestinal 83
-, liver 83
adoptive transfer experiments 139
Adriatic coast 76
allergen-specific IgE synthesis 213
alloantigenic function of HLA-B27 on transgenic cells 120
allogenic anaphylactic mast cell degranulation 5
Alprenolol 218, 222
- epoxide 222
Amilakvari, Thamar 13
amino acid sequences from the N-terminal part, GP43-53K antigen 158
2-aminoethylisothio-uronium bromide hydrobromide (AET) 60
AMLC-induced suppression 66
AMLC-stimulated T cells, phenotypes 64
AMLR (Autologous Mixed Lymphocyte Reaction) 60
anaphylactic shock 223
antibody Plaque-Forming Cells (PFC) 21
antigen, B-F, class I 43
-, B-G 44
-, B-L, class II 44
-, F-, L- and G 43
- receptors, variable domains 18
antigenic modulation 170
antiviral and immunological effects of interferons 31
autoactivated blasts 68
autocrine regulation 199

B cell lymphoma line, transfection (BCL1) 21
B cell receptors 129
B cell repertoire 125
B locus, chicken 154
B regions 43
B-F antigen, class I 43

B-G antigen 44
B-L antigen, class II 44
Bacampicillin 216
background strain 86
BALBccSTS, colon tumors 87
-, genetics of susceptibility 87
-, hormonally induced mammary tumors 87
-, intestinal tumors 87
-, liver tumors 87
-, lung tumors 87
-, virally tumors 87
Barbacid, Mariano 190
BCG (Bacille Calmette-Guerin) 139, 147, 170
-, vaccine 139
Beg congenic mice 149
- gene, linkage group 148
- -, mapping 148
- -, molecular genetics 148
- -, phenotypic expression 149
- -, population genetics 147
- macrophages 150
beneficially matches 91
Berns, Ton 131
beta-2-microglobulin 94, 119
Billingham 169
biological response modifiers 170
Biozzi mice 146
Black, Paul H. 160
blastogenesis 62
blasts, autoactivated 68
blot analysis, southern 96
Bobe, Pierre 16
Brachyury (T) 109
breast cancer cells, human 181
Brent 169
Burkitt's lymphoma 226
Burnet, F. Macfarlane 3, 10, 58

C57BL/10Sn, colon tumors 87
-, genetics of susceptibility 87
-, hormonally induced mammary tumors 87
-, intestinal tumors 87

C57BL/10Sn, liver tumors 87
-, lung tumors 87
-, virally tumors 87
cancer cytogenetics 226, 236
- therapy 181
carcinogenesis, virus induced 160
carcinogens, chemical 82
-, mutagen N-ethyl-N-nitrosourea 82
CD2 31
CD3 31
CD4 31
CD4 molecule 31
CD8 31
CD11a 31
CD18 31
cell clones 96
- line T4-EF 25
-, suppressor 53
- surface markers, T cell lines 22
-, T veto 55
-, T8 60
cell-mediated lympholysis 40
cell-to-cell interaction 19
CFS-1, macrophage growth factor, receptor 191
Chaouat, Gerard 15
chemotherapy 138
chicken, B locus 154
-, histocompatibility 123
-, inbred lines 43
- MCH 43, 44
- -, structure 43
- -, haplotypes, nomenclature 44
-, Obese Strain (OS) 45
chimpanzee 77
ChLA antigen 77
choriocarcinoma 170
chromosome 10 abnormalities 236
- marker, T6T6 15
chronic myelogenous leukemia 226
Cibotti, Ricardo 16
class I antigen, B-F 43
- - and class II molecules, interactions 40
- -, H-2 molecules 110
- -, HLA molecules 94
- -, MHC products 81
class II antigens 60
- - -, B-L 44
- - -, RSV-induced tumors 48
- - molecules 94
class III, MHC products 81
classification of leprosy 140
Clomethiazole 218, 219
clonal abortion 51
Cloxacillin 216
CMV (Congenital Cytomegalovirus), infants with congenital, neutropenia 162

- infection 161, 164
- -, effect, GM colony formation 164
- -, inhibition of hemopoetic colony formation 165
c-*myc* expression in tumors 193
Colombani, J. 117
colon cancer 227
colonic formation, hemopoetic 162
competitive radioimmunoassay 23
complement components 2, 4 and factor B 111
Costa, Jose 191
c-sis, giant cell tumors of bone 193
Cyclosporin 90
cytofluorometric analysis 119
cytogenetic abnormalities, endometrial adenocarcinoma 228
cytokeratins 229
cytokines, NK cells 199
cytoskeleton marker for epithelial cells 229
cytotoxic activity, suppression 61
- and proliferative response 61
- T cell lympholysis 16

D, class I 36
Daudi cells 120
Dausset, Jean 5, 6, 14, 90, 101, 117, 123
David, Chella 114
Demant, Peter 4, 93, 114, 124
DNA technology, recombinant 118
Doric, Miljenko 16
Douvas, Georg 15
DR matching 91
drug allergy 213
DTH (Delayed-Type Hypersensitivity) skin reactions 139
Dubbs 189
duct carcinomas of breast, neu oncogene 192
Dux, A. 81

Eijsvoogel, Vincent 131
electrophoresis, gel 96
ELISA (Enzyme-Linked Immuno-adsorbent Assay) studies 16
embryonal parabiosis 169
endometrial andenocarcinoma 226
- -, cytogenetic abnormalities 228
Engelfriet, Paul 131
enhancements 14
-, passive 15
enzyme 21-hydroxylase 111
epidermal growth factor receptor 181
- - - - gene 192
epithelial cells, cytoskeleton marker 229
Erickson 189
Escher, M.C. 30
expression of H-2 molecules 110

Name and Subject Index

F-antigen 43
FACS (Fluorescence-Activated Cell Sorter) 16
factor B 111
feline sarcoma virus 189, 190
– – – mutans 190
fenoterol 221
fertile crescent 75
fes oncogene 190
flow cytometry 191
Flucloxacillin 216
fms oncogene 191
formaldehyde 220
–, lymphocyte proliferation 223

G-antigen 43
gamma Interferon (IFN) 139
Gardner, Murray 187
gel electrophoresis 96
gene conversion 125
– mapping 85
–, non-MHC-linked 81
– pool 75
–, tumor suspectibility 81
genealogical tree of the t chromosome 115
genetic of generation of suppressor cells 62
genomic DNA, hybridisation analysis, parasites 157
Gillam, Ian 138
Glucocorticoid (GC)-induced teratogenesis 83
Glycoprotein, GP43-53K 155
GM (Granulocytic/Macrophage) colonies 163
– colony formation, effect of CMV infection 164
GP43-53K antigen, amino acid sequences from the N-terminal part 158
GP43-53K gene 157
–, glycoprotein 155
–, serological variants 156
graft rejection 37, 51
– survival 90, 91
– – and HLA matching in first cadaver graft recipients 91
– – rate 91
Graph, Ralph 80
growth factor receptor, epidermal 181
Grozdanovic, Jan 168
Gupta, Gopal 16
GVH (Graft-Versus-Host) disease 13
– Reaction (GVHR) 8, 13, 16, 44
– –, local, role of histamine in modulation 16

H-2 complex 74
– – mapping 109
– congenic strains 111

– genotype 82
– haplotypes 82
– heterozygous tumors 73
– molecules, class I 110
– –, expression 110
– –, tryptic peptide mapping 76
– polymorphism 75, 115
– serology 124
– –, non-conventional 130
– specific antibodies, naturally occurring 128
– system 4, 15, 36
– tumor variants 74
H-Y antigen work 51
–, immune deficiency 51
Hala, Karel 154
Halas, Frantisek 109
Harper, Peter 138
Hartley, Janet 187
Hašek, Milan 3, 4, 6, 9, 13, 15, 17, 29, 42, 43, 50, 58, 73, 80, 90, 94, 117, 137, 154, 168, 180, 189, 195, 213
Hashimoto thyroiditis 45
Haskova, Vera 8, 168, 169
heat shock proteins 140
HeLa cell line 189
hemopoetic colony formation 162
HER-2/neu oncogene 181
Hermann, Günther 16
Hilgert, Ivan 14, 15
histamine in the modulation of local GVH reactions 16
histocompatibility antigens, tolerance to minor 55
– complex, major 4
–, chicken 123
–, rabbit 123
HIV (Human Immunodeficiency Virus) infection 31, 139
– receptor 31
HLA 3, 90–95, 101, 120, 142
– class I subtypes 101
– class II association 142
– gene expression 120
– matching 90
– – and graft survival in first cadaver graft recipients 91
– molecules, class I 94
– subtypes 94
– system 90, 94
– –, nomenclature 94
– typing 96
HLA-A (A locus) specificities 95
– matching 91
HLA-ABC, neuroblastomas 191
–, neuroepitheliomas 191
HLA-B (B locus) specificities 96
– matching 91

309

HLA-B27 molecules in transgenic mice, expression 119
- on transgenic cells, allogenic function 120
HLA-C (C locus) specificities 98
HLA-DQ (DQ locus) specificities 100
HLA-DR (DR locus) specificities 98
HLA-transgenic mice 118
Hort, Jan 168
Howard, James 14
Hraba, Tomas 42, 168
Hrubesova, Mirka 7
HSV-2 (Herpes Simplex Virus, Type 2) 189
HT-29 tumor, growth 172
Hu-1 system 3, 90
Huebner, Robert 187
human breast cancer cells 181
- retroviruses 29
Humphrey, John 7, 9
hybrid zone 76
hybridisation analysis of genomic DNA parasites 157
hypersensitivity, immediate 214
hypophysis, estrogen receptors 83

I-A, class II 36
I-E Mls antigens 56
I-E, class II 36
Idh-1 (Isocitrate dehydrogenase) 148
idiotype binding studies on long-term T cell lines 24
-, network hypothesis 18
-, T15 19
IFN's 200
Ig isotypes 14
IgE synthesis, allergen-specific 213
IL-2 (Interleukin-2) 29–31, 33, 60, 213, 236
- exhaustion 65
- induced DNA synthesis in lymphocytes, effects of IFNs 33
- receptor (IL-2R) 30, 31, 141, 236
IL-2-activated lymphocytes, characterization 204
- - in the treatment of leukemia 202
immediate early viral messenger RNA 160
immune complexes 15, 21
- deficiency to H-Y 51
- paralysis 14
- repertoire 141
- response (Ir) 18, 36, 74, 114
- response-associated (Ia) antigens 36
- responsiveness 51
immunity, protective 139
immunoglobulins, monoclonal antibodies 25
immunological and antiviral effects of Interferons 31
- tolerance 10, 17, 18, 27, 29, 42, 123, 169
-, transplantation 14

immunomodulating effects of placental glycoproteins 16
immunoparasitology 154
immunoregulation and human retroviruses 29
immunosuppressive drugs 36
incidence of neutropenia 162
induction of unresponsiveness 31
infectious mononucleosis 161
integrins 149
interactions between class I and class II molecules 40
Interferon (IFN) 163
-, immunological and antiviral effects 31
interleukin receptors 31
intestinal adenocarcinomas 83
- tumors, mouse 82
intra-H2 recombinants 36
Ir gene 30
Iranian plateau 75
isoelectric focusing 96, 105
Isoprenaline 221
Ivan, K. 154
Ivanyi, Dagmar 3
-, *Pavol* 3, 4, 50, 80, 90, 93, 117
Ivaskova, Eva 93

Jacob, Francois 6
Jakoubkova 170
Janecek, Ota 109
Janeway 18
Jenkins 31
Jerne 18, 58
Jutland peninsula 76

K and D, class I 36
Kafka 48
Kaplan, Albert S. 160
kidney transplant 91
killer cells, nonspecific 31
Kinsky, Radslav 169
KIT 189
Klein Eva 73
-, *George* 73
-, *Jan* 4, 36, 50
Knödel 48
Köhler 115
Kokoschka 48
Koldovsky, Pavel 13, 16
Kourilsky, Raoul 13

L3T4 22
L-antigen 43
L-myc, oncogene 192
LAK (Lymphokine Activated Killer) cells 171, 200
- -, therapy 171

Langerhans, β cells 37
laryngeal carcinoma, growth 172
LcA (lentil lectin) 15
Ld molecule 126
LDH-C4 (sperm Lactate Dehydrogenase) 16
Lebouteiller, Philippe 16
Leghorns, white 46
leishmania donovani, response 149
Len-1, gamma crystallin gene 148
Lengerova, Alena 15, 42
leprosy, classification 140
-, mortality 139
Leu2 (T8) cells 62
Leu3 (T4) cells 62
Leu3/Leu2 ratios 62
leukemia by Gross-MuLV, mouse 82
linkage disequilibrium 92
- group IX 109, 111
Linkova, Eva 168
lipoarabinomannan 140
liver adenocarcinomas 83
Lord, John 138
LTT (Lymphocyte Transformation Test) 213
lung tumors, mouse 82
lymphocyte proliferation, formaldehyde 223
- -, penicillins 217
- passenger 37
- Reaction, Autologous Mixed (AMLR) 60
- -, mixed 16
lymphocytotoxicity test 123
Lymphokine-(IL-2)-Activated Killer (LAK) activity 31
lymphokines 36
-, secretion 141
lymphoma 191
-, Burkitt's 226
Lyt2+ (CD8) T cells 53

M511 22
Mac 101
macrophage activation 150
-, Beg 150
- dysfunction 151
- growth factor CSF-2, receptor 191
malaria antigens, polymophisms 154
-, incidence 154
-, vaccines 154
malignant fibrous histiocytoma 193
Martinek, Ludek 168
mast cell degranulation, allogenic anaphylactic 15
McAllister, Robert 187
McDonough, Susan 190
MCH, chicken 43, 44
McLaren 9
Medawar, Peter 3, 9, 10, 58, 169
Mekori, Thamar 16

melanoma 193
Melief, Kees 131
memory cells 213
Mendel 6, 48
Merchant, Donald J. 110
metoprolol 218, 219
- epoxide 222
MHC antigens, ontogenesis 44
- chicken, genetic organization 44
- function 45
- interspecies cross-reactions 125
- polymorphism 77
- products, class I 81
- -, class III 81
- restricition of T cells 125
MHC-linked tumor susceptibility 82
MHC-restricted antibodies 129
MHC+X 128
mice, sources 76
Michie, Donald 9
Michurinism 8
Mickey 90
Mickova, Milada 124
microglobulin, β-2 119
microlymphocytotoxic test 119
microlymphocytotoxicity 96
Milstein 115
Mitchell, Peter 7
Mitchison, Aviron 8, 14, 169
Mitomycin C 61
MLR (Mixed Lymphocyte Reaction) 40
Mls antigens, I-E 56
molecules class I and class II, interactions 40
Moloney virus specific response 125
monoclonal antibodies 115
- -, immunoglobulins 25
mononucleosis, infections 161
Moreno 140
mouse leukemia by gross-MuLV 82
- populations 75
muramyldipeptide 140
Mus domesticus 76
- *musculus* 76
myc proto-oncogene 226
mycobacterial disease 138
- infections, animal models 146
- -, susceptibility 145

N-*myc*, oncogene 192
-, retinoblastomas 192
neodeterminants 129
neolithic agricultural revolution 75
neuraminidase-1 (Neu-1) locus 111
neuroblastomas 191
neurofibrosarcoma 193
neutropenia, incidence 162

neutropenia, in infants with congenital CMV 162
-, virus-induced 161
Nie, van, R. 81
NK (Natural Killer) cells 170, 171, 195–201, 208
- -, cell-augmenting activity 200
- -, cell-related suppressor cells 200
- -, cytokines 199
- -, cytotoxicity, correlation to tumor resistance 197
- -, -, suppression 201
- -, cytotoxic mechanism 208
- - in defense against human cancer 198
- - - - infectious disease 199
- -, definition 196, 197
- - resistance cells 33
non-MHC-linked genes 81
Nonpenicillin drugs 218

Obese Strain (OS) chicken 45
occupational allergy 213
- hypersensitivity 218
oncogene expressions in tumors 192
-, fes 190
-, fms 191
-, L-myc 192
-, N-myc 192
-, neu, duct carcinomas of breast 192
oncogenesis 126
-, MHC antigens 44
Oomen, Lauran 81
Orciprenaline 221
Oudshoorn-Snoek, Margriet 81
ovarian cancer 198
Owen 58

pancreatic islet transplants 37
parabiosis 15
passenger lymphocytes 37
Patrick, W.J. 154
PCA (Passive Cutaneous Anaphylaxis) 15
PCR (Polymerase Chain Reaction) 157
PcV (Phenoxymethylpenicillin) 216
penicillin 216
- hapten 223
-, lymphocyte proliferation 217
-, nonpenicillin drugs 218
-, treatment 223
Pep-3 (dipeptidase 3) 148
Perlmann, Peter 213
PFC (Plaque-Forming Cells) 16, 21
-, antibody 21
Phenoxymethylpenicillin 216
pituitary isografts 83
placental glycoproteins, immunomodulating effects 16

plasmodium falciparum 154
Ploegh, Hidde 131
polymorphism, malaria antigens 154
- of P. falciparum antigens 155
Porat, Tamar Ben 160
proliferative responses 25, 26
- responses, T cell lines 26
proto-oncogenes 181
pulmonary tuberculosis association 142

quinidine 218

rabbit histocompatibility 123
racism 138
radiation enhanced oncogenic expression 181
- on immunological tolerance 80
radioimmunoassay, competitive 23
radiotherapy 170
Ramazeilles, Claude 16
RAST (Radio-Allergosorbent Test) 223
rb-1 locus 227
RCS (Recombinant Congenic Strains), colon tumors 87
-, colon tumors 87
-, genetics of susceptibility 87
-, hormonally induced mammary tumors 87
-, intestinal tumors 87
-, liver tumors 87
-, lung tumors 87
-, production 85
-, virally tumors 87
realm of tolerance 143
Recombinant Congenic Strains (RCS) 85, 86
- DNA technology 118
- interleukins 170
red blood cells, tolerance 43
renal carcinoma 227
response, cytotoxic and proliverative 61
- of macrophages to lymphokines 141
-, proliferative 25, 26
Ressl 48
restriction fragment 148
retinoblastoma 227
-, N-myc 192
retroviruses, human 29
RFLP (Restriction Fragment Length Polymorphism) 96
- analysis 148
rIL-1 (recombinant interleukin-1) 166
RIS (Recombinant Imbret Strains), production 85
RNA, immediate early viral messenger 160
Rous Sarcoma Virus (RSV)-induced tumours 45
Rowe, Wallace P. 187
RSV-induced tumours, expression of class II antigens 48

Name and Subject Index

– –, regression 46
Russel, Bertrand 138
Rychlikova, Milena 93

S-region genus, C4 87
– –, Slp 87
salbutamol 221
salmonella typhimurium, response 149
SAT (Spontaneous Autoimmuno Thyroiditis) 45
–, major genes 46
–, minor genes 46
Sawyer, Tom 36
Schwartz 35
secretion of lymphokines 141
self-tolerance 58
Sherr, Charles 190
shock, anaphylactic 223
Shreffler, Donald, C. 114
Silverberg, Steve 191
Simonsen, Morton 8, 10
SK-BR-3, human breast cancer cell line 181
skin allograft rejection 39
 – Delayed-Type Hypersensitivity (DTH) reactions 139
Snell, George D. 4, 80
sources of mice 76
southern blot analysis 96
speciation 75
sperm Lactate Dehydrogenase (LDH)-C4 16
SRCA (Subrenal Capsule Assay) 172
Sterzl, Jaroslav 7, 9, 10
Stimpfling, Jack 114
strains, background 86
–, H-2 congenic 111
–, Recombinant Congenic (RCS), production 85
–, – inbred (RIS), production 85
Streptococcus Pneumoniae R36a (Pn) 19
Streptozotocin 37
suppression 21
 – of cytotoxic activity 61
suppressor cell activity 64
 – cells 53, 60, 62, 68
 – –, genetic of generation 62
suppressor-effectors 68
suppressor-inducer cells 68
Surrogate mothers 16
susceptibility to mycobacterial infections 145
SV 40 (simian papova virus, small DNA virus) 160
Svoboda, Jan 180
Swann, Michael 7

T4-EF cell line 25
T6T6 chromosome marker 15
T8 cells 60

T15 idiotype-bearing immunoglobulins, binding 25
T15 idiotypes 19
T cell activation 20, 31
– –, AMLC-stimulated, phenotypes 64
– – anergy 141
– – lines, cell surface markers 22
– – –, long-term, idiotype binding studies 24
– – –, proliferative responses 26
– – lympholysis, cytotoxix 16
– –, Lyt2+ (CD8) 53
– – receptor 26, 31, 56, 58, 126, 129
– – – repertoire 58
– – repertoire 126
– – restriction 129
– – unresponsiveness 30, 31
t chromosome, genealogical tree 115
t complex 115
T veto cells 55
TAA (Tumor-Associated Antigen) 170
Tadaro, George 189
TEPC15 22
Terasaki 90, 91
terbutaline 218, 221
therapy with LAK cells 171
Thy-1,2/FITC 22
thyroiditis, HASHIMOTO 45
–, Spontaneous Autoimmune (SAT) 45
TIL (Tumor-Infiltrating Lymphocytes) 205
–, characterization 205
TNP (Trinitropheny) coupled to Brucella Abortus (BA)-(TNP-BA) 21
tolerance, acquired 14, 38
–, active 14
–, immunological 17, 18
 – induction 14
 – to minor histocompatibility antigens 55
 – to red blood cells 43
–, self- 58
trans-species hypothesis 77
transfection of a B Cell Lymphoma line, BCL1 21
transfer of tolerance 51
transgenes 118
transgenic mice 86, 87, 118
– –, unigenic analytic system 87
translocation 230
 – break T138Ca 109
transplant immunology 90
–, kidney 91
transplantation anaphylaxis 15
 – immunity 36, 169
 – immunology 9, 14
 – tolerance 51
 – – to H-Y 54
transregulatory factors 87
Triche, Timothy 191

Trnka, Zdenek 7
tryptic peptide mapping, H-2 molecules 76
tubercle bacilli, growth rate 139
Tuberculin (PPD) 141
tuberculosis in inbred strains of mice 146
–, mortality 139
tufted 101
tumor biology 81
– immunity 169
–, intestinal, mouse 82
–, lung, mouse 82
– necrosis factor 111
– resistance 81, 197
– suppressor genes 181
– susceptibility 81
– – genes 81, 86
– virology 190
tumorigenesis 82

unresponsiveness, induction 31
–, T cell 30, 31
urticaria 223

Valk, van der, Martin 81
variable domains of the antigen receptors 18
veto cells 55
Violacea 73
viral P85 glycoprotein 190
virulence of mycobacteria 140
virus induced carcinogenesis 160
– neutropenia 161
Vlachov, Kolja 16
Vojtiskova, Marta 13, 15, 168

Weissman, Irving 50, 58
Wilm's tumor 227
Witz, Isaac 16
Woude, van de, George 190

Young, R.A. 140
Yujanovic, Nikola 16

Zimelidine 219, 222